Alzheimer's Disease: Activity-Focused Care

Alzheimer's Disease: Activity-Focused Care

Second Edition

Carly R. Hellen, O.T.R./L.
Director of Alzheimer's Care,
The Wealshire, Lincolnshire, Illinois

With a foreword by
Jacob H. Fox, M.D.
Chairman, Department of Neurology,
Rush-Presbyterian-St. Luke's Medical Center
and Co-Director, Rush Alzheimer's Disease
Center, Chicago

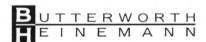

Boston   Oxford   Johannesburg   Melbourne   New Delhi   Singapore

Butterworth–Heinemann supports the efforts of American Forests and the Global ReLeaf program in its campaign for the betterment of trees, forests, and our environment.

Library of Congress Cataloging-in-Publication Data
Hellen, Carly R.
    Alzheimer's disease : activity-focused care / Carly R. Hellen ;
with a foreword by Jacob H. Fox. -- 2nd ed.
      p. cm.
    Includes bibliographical references and index.
    ISBN 0-7506-9908-6
    1. Alzheimer's disease -- Patients -- Care. I. Title
    [DNLM: 1. Alzheimer's Disease -- rehabilitation. 2. Activities of
Daily Living. 3. Occupational Therapy.   WT 155 H477a 1998]
RC523.H45 1998
362. 1'96831 -- dc21
DNLM/DLC
for Library of Congress   98-20819
                                                              CIP

British Library Cataloguing-in-Publication Data
A catalogue record for this book is available from the British Library.

The publisher offers special discounts on bulk orders of this book.
For information, please contact:

Manager of Special Sales
Butterworth–Heinemann
225 Wildwood Avenue
Woburn, MA 01801-2041
Tel: 718-904-2500
Fax: 718-904-2620

For information on all Butterworth–Heinemann publications available,
contact our World Wide Web home page at: http://www.bh.com

10 9 8 7 6 5 4 3 2

Printed in the United States of America

With love and appreciation to all residents with Alzheimer's disease, their families, and my colleagues for their support and wisdom sharing throughout the years

Contents

Foreword   *xv*
Preface   *xvii*
Acknowledgments   *xix*

1. Activity-Focused Alzheimer's Care   **1**
Activity-Focused Care: Defined   1
The "Activity" of Life: Search for Meaning   2
Ability Centering: Upholding and Maintaining Competence   3
Cognitive and Physical Ability Centering and Challenges   3
Ability-Centered Plan of Care   7
Caregiving: Defined as Purposeful Activity   7
The 10 Commandments of Alzheimer's Care   8
Health Care Provider and Staff Issues   9
Summary   11
Suggested Reading   11
Appendixes
    1-1 Alzheimer's Disease: Symptoms and Challenges   **13**
        Persons with Dementia: Mild Impairment   13
        Persons with Dementia: Moderate Impairment   14
        Persons with Dementia: Severe Impairment   14
    1-2 Ability-Centered Plan of Care   **15**

2. Maintaining Personhood: Psychosocial Aspects of Support   **19**
Promoting Life's Meaning and Personhood   19
Psychosocial Ability Centering and Challenges   20
Being Valued, Not "Discounted"   21
An Alzheimer's Disease Patient's Bill of Rights   22
Residents with an Integrated Self-Image   23
Residents with a Compromised Self-Image   24
Depression: Overwhelming Sadness   25
Interventions and Support of Psychosocial Needs   26
Being Included: Respected Connectedness   30
Couples with Dementia: Finding Balance   31
Development of a Psychosocial Support Group for Residents with
    Moderate Impairment   35
Staff Personhood: A Staff Statement of Respect   40
Health Care Provider and Staff Issues   41
Summary   41
References   42
Suggested Reading   42
Appendixes
    2-1 Dementia Support Group Theme Facilitation Plan Example **43**
        Theme Title: Identification of Self   43

2-2 Support Group Game   45
2-3 Staff Empowerment Considerations   47
2-4 Administrators Walk in Assistants' Shoes   49
2-5 Form for Resident Case Study   51

3. LifeStory Book: LifePreserver for LifeAffirmation   55
   LifeStory Book Indicators: LifeAffirmation   55
   LifeStory Book: Contraindications for Use   56
   Book Format Suggestions   57
   LifeAffirmation: Book Content Recommendations   58
   Family Suggestions and Quality Involvement   58
   Guidelines for Staff Use of Books   59
   Health Care Provider and Staff Issues   60
   Summary   61
   Suggested Reading   61
   Appendix
      3-1 LifeStory Book Letter to Families   63

4. Communication: Understanding and Being Understood   67
   Words: Bloomers or Witherers?   67
   Communication: Guidelines for Connecting   68
   Vocal and Spoken Communications   71
   Nonverbal and Implied Communication   76
   Language of Touch   78
   Assessing Communication in Late-Stage Dementia   78
   Assessing the Environment for Promotion of Communication   78
   Health Care Provider and Staff Issues   79
   Summary   79
   Suggested Reading   80
   Appendixes
      4-1 Communication and Environmental Assessment Form   81
      4-2 Communication Assessment Profile Form for Residents
           with Late-Stage Dementia   83

5. Daily Living Care Activities   87
   Dementia Factors Affecting Daily Care Activities   87
   Using a Sensory Profile   89
   Activities of Daily Living Guidelines   90
   Hands-On Care Strategies   92
   Bathing, Hygiene, and Oral Care   93
   Dressing and Disrobing   97
   Finding and Using the Toilet Appropriately and Incontinence   100
   Health Care Provider and Staff Issues   103
   Summary   104
   Suggested Reading   105
   Appendixes
      5-1 Daily Life Tasks: Resident Abilities, Challenges,
           and Assistance Needed   107

5-2 Sensory Profile 111
5-3 Nursing Assistants' Care Conference Activities
    of Daily Living Report Form 115
5-4 Resident Basic Care Information Form 119
5-5 Sample Dressing Policy and Procedures: Supporting the
    Symbolism of Clothing 121
5-6 Sample Staff Support Policy and Procedures: "Do What You
    Have to Do" 125

6. Eating and Mealtimes: An Activity of Consequence   **127**
Eating: How Do You Promote Success? 128
Eating and Mealtime Interventions and Facilitation ... 129
Eating Behaviors Exhibited and Problems Encountered ... 131
Possible Causes or Antecedents of Eating Problems: Cognitive
    Challenges 132
Possible Causes or Antecedents of Eating Problems: Physical
    Challenges 133
Possible Causes or Antecedents of Eating Problems: Psychosocial
    Challenges 134
Possible Causes or Antecedents of Eating Problems: Environmental
    Challenges 136
The Humiliation of Being a "Feeder" 136
Increasing Food Consumed and Nutrition: Approaches and Interventions 138
Dietary Department: Food Modifications and Mealtime Support 141
Dining Environment and Equipment Support 142
Mealtime Assistance: Activities Involvement and Other Staffpersons 143
Family Involvement at Mealtime 145
Late or Terminal Care Nutritional Assessment and Challenges 146
Health Care Provider and Staff Issues 148
Summary 149
Suggested Reading 150
Appendixes
  6-1 Sample Policy and Procedures: Supporting Optimal Nutrition
     for Residents with Dementia 151
  6-2 Finger Food Suggestions 153
    Finger Food Ideas for Breakfast 153
    Finger Food Ideas for Lunch and Snacks 153
    Finger Food Ideas for Desserts 154
    Finger Food Ideas for Dinner 154
  6-3 Nutrient-Dense Recipes 155

7. Physical Wellness: Mobility and Exercise   **159**
Dementia Factors Affecting Mobility 160
Promoting Mobility and Independent Ambulation 162
Assisting Mobility 165
Caregiving for Immobile Residents 166
Assessing for Falls 167
Functional Maintenance and Rehabilitation Programs 169

Physical Restraints: Definition, Issues, and Efficacy   171
Dementia Factors Affecting the Use of Restraints   172
Negative Effects of Restraints   173
Alternatives to Restraints   174
Restraint Use Considerations: Can There Be Positive Outcomes?   176
Health Care Provider and Staff Issues   179
Summary   180
References   180
Suggested Reading   180
Appendixes
   7-1 Exercises, Balance, and Strengthening   **183**
   7-2 Fitness Trail   **187**
      Examples of Exercises for Fitness Trail   187
   7-3 Activity-Focused Mobility Task Example: Getting into a Car **189**
   7-4 Sample Fall Assessment Form   **191**

8. Behaviors: Understanding, Creative Interventions, and Refocusing   **195**
Behaviors as Expressions of Abilities and Inabilities   196
Risk Factors Precipitating Behavioral Manifestations   198
Guidelines for Understanding and Refocusing Behaviors   198
Implementing a Behavior Profile   200
Tracking Behavioral Patterns: A Behavior Observation Form   205
Problem Solving: A Behavior Analysis Form   205
Safety in the Community: Elopement and a Police Dispatch Form   206
Behavior Analysis Examples   207
Safety Issues: Physically Aggressive, Combative, or Violent Situations   211
Resident Behavioral Responses   216
  Anxiety and Agitation   216
  Catastrophic Reactions   217
  Combativeness and Aggression   218
  Sundowning   218
  Inappropriate Sexual Responses: Hypersexuality and Stripping 220
  Picking or Repetitious Movements   220
  Hyperorality   220
  Wandering and Pacing   220
  "Redistribution of Stuff"—Rummaging   221
  Sleep Disturbances and Nocturnal Wandering   221
  Demonstration of Hallucinations, Aberrations, and Delusions   221
  Demonstration of Accusing, Demanding, and Paranoia   223
  Screaming, Yelling, Calling, and Asking Repetitious Questions 224
  Demonstration of Withdrawal, Apathy, and Inability
    to Initiate Activity   225
Health Care Provider and Staff Issues   225
Summary   226
Suggested Reading   226
Appendixes
   8-1 Behavior Profile Form   **227**

8-2   **Behavior Observation Form**   229

8-3   **Behavior Analysis Form**   231

8-4   **Community and Civic Professionals Training Outline**   235

8-5   **Lincolnshire Police Department Resident Checklist for
      The Wealshire (Lincolnshire, Illinois)**   237

8-6   **Catastrophic Reaction Analysis**   239

9. Meaningful Activities: Daily Life Stuff   **243**

Daily Life Stuff: How Do You Spell Success?   244

Objectives of an Activity   244

Criteria for a Successful Activity   245

Qualities of an Activity: Cognitive, Physical, Psychosocial, and Spiritual   245

Activity Analysis: Can "Anything" Be a Meaningful Activity?   247

Identifying the Therapeutic Value of an Activity   249

Activity Assessment and Grouping Residents for Effective Activities   250

Who Does Daily Life Stuff? Connecting Multifaceted
    Creative Therapies   251

Making It Happen   253

Basic Stuff Needed   253

Thinking Activities: Encouraging Cognitive Participation   255

Movement Activities: Encouraging Physical Participation   258

Psychosocial Activities: Encouraging Participation   260

Spiritual Activities: Compassionate Connectedness   261

Life Work and Normalization Activities   262

Community Partnership and Service for Others Activities   263

Intergenerational Activities: Fun for All   264

Activities for Engaging Male Participation, Enjoyment, and Satisfaction   265

Shoestring and Wearable Activities for Residents with Short
    Attention Spans   266

One-to-One Activities: Personalized Activities   267

Sensory Stimulation and Activities for Late-Stage Dementia Care   268

Activities for Behavioral Refocusing and Effective Intervention   269

Activities for Therapeutically Reducing the Prevalence, Onset,
    or Intensity of Aggressive or Combative Behaviors   270

Activities for Residents Who Pace and Wander   273

Activities for Refocusing "Searching and Discovering"   274

Activities for Loneliness, Sadness, and Depression   274

Health Care Provider and Staff Issues   275

Summary   276

Suggested Reading   276

Appendixes

9-1   **Activity Analysis Example: Using a Beach Ball**   277

9-2   **Reminiscing Kits**   281

9-3   **Sample Policy and Procedures: What Is an Age-Appropriate
    Activity?**   285

    Discussion   285

    Procedures   286

9-4 **Sample Policy and Procedures: What Is a Life Work or Normalization Activity?** 287
    Discussion 287
    Procedures 288
9-5 **Life Work Activity Examples** 289
    Each One Teach One: Pride in Activities of Sharing Wisdom and Skills 289
    Hands for Others: Pride in Activities of Service 290
    Neighborly Celebrations: Pride in Activities of Hospitality 291
    Ordinary and Orderly: Pride in Activities of Homemaking 292
    On the Job: Pride in Activities of Life's Work 293
9-6 **Community Partnership Example Letter: Creating Meaningful Activity Opportunities for Nursing Home Residents** 295
    Meaningful Activities for Nursing Home Residents 296
9-7 **Community Partnership and Collaborating Forces to Enhance Quality of Life: Much More Than Just Entertainment** 299
9-8 **Activity Therapist Job Description Example** 303
9-9 **Activity Therapy Care Conference Report Form** 305
9-10 **Activity Therapy Care Conference Report Form Information: Therapeutic Value** 307

10. **Expressions of Intimacy: Giving and Receiving Affection** 311
Inclusiveness of Intimacy 312
Intimacy-Related Responses: Enabling Strengths and Diminishing Challenges 313
Using an Intimacy Profile 314
Masturbation: Self-Directed Intimacy and Caregiving Interventions 315
Overt or Hypersexuality: Issues and Caregiving Interventions 316
Guidelines for Intimacy Expressions in Care Facilities 320
Health Care Provider and Staff Issues 322
Summary 324
Reference 324
Suggested Reading 324
Appendixes
  10-1 **The Changing Face of Intimacy** 325
  10-2 **The Joy of Life: Compassionate Relationships** 327
  10-3 **Expressions of Intimacy Guidelines for Persons with Dementia Residing in Care Facilities** 329
    Reference 331
  10-4 **Expressions of Intimacy: Analysis** 333
  10-5 **Intimacy Profile** 337

11. **Spirituality: Compassionate Connectedness and Well-Being** 339
Appraising Spiritual Well-Being and Needs 339
The Clergy, Caring Congregation, and Confused Worshipper 340
Clergy Support for Persons with Dementia and Their Families 340
The Congregation's Shared Communion of Love and Support 341
The Confused Worshipper 343

Creative Ministry: Uniting an Alzheimer's Care Center and a Local
   Congregation   343
Creating a Praise, Thanksgiving, and Worship Center   345
Activity-Focused Adapted Worship Service Guidelines   346
Activity-Focused Worship Example: Holy Hands   347
Activity-Focused Worship Example: To Be Called By Name   348
Service of Remembrance: Celebrating Our Friend   349
Health Care Provider and Staff Issues   350
Summary   351
Suggested Reading   352
Appendix
  **11-1 Religious, Spiritual, and Sacred Center Assessment of
    Compassionate Connectedness**   **353**

12. Terminal Care: Final Storm Weathered   **355**
A Cherished Sentinel   355
Family Grief: Sadness without End   356
Pain: Recognizing and Responding to the Message   357
Hospice: Final Days with a Caring Team   358
Terminal Care Considerations   358
Medical Issues and Impending Death   359
Psychosocial Issues: Emotional Support and Preservation of Personhood   361
Communication: "Talking Touch"   362
Activities of Daily Care: Enabling Dignity   363
Nutrition and Eating: Demonstration of Caring   364
Mobility: Assisted and Passive Movement   365
Behavior: Challenging Demonstrations   367
Activities: Honoring Simplicity   368
Spiritual Support: Compassionate Connectedness   369
Death: Creation of a "Cherished Sentinel"   369
Autopsy: The Opportunity of Gifting Others   371
Health Care Provider and Staff Issues   371
Summary   372
Suggested Reading   372
Appendixes
  12-1 Alzheimer's Patient Hospital Transfer Information   **373**
  **12-2 Alzheimer's Patient Hospital Transfer Information Explanation
    and Worksheet**   **375**
    Awareness and Orientation   375
    Communication, Approaches, Language   375
    Physical Movement and Mobility   376
    Eating: Needs and Behaviors   376
    Bowel and Bladder: Needs and Behaviors   376
    Dressing and Hygiene: Approaches and Assistance   376
    Psychosocial Support   377
    Behaviors: Responses and Assistance   377
    Safety Concerns   377
    Activity Support   377

13. Family Caregivers: Needs, Partnership, and Support   **379**
   Grief and Loss   380
   Making Nursing Home Placement Decisions   380
   Nursing Home's Response: Building the Bridge   382
   Admission Day: Suggestions on Getting the Resident to the Home   384
   Admission Day: Family Mourning   386
   Caregiving Partnership: Staff and Family   387
   New Family Orientation Program   389
   Developing a Family Mentor Program   389
   Partnership in Action: Family Council   390
   Facilitating Change: A Family Survival Handbook   391
   Involvement: "Coulds" Versus "Shoulds"   392
   Visiting: An Opportunity for Connectedness and Volunteering   393
   Special Opportunities: Holidays, Family Weddings, and Special Events   394
   Partnership in Action: Plan-of-Care Conference   396
   Family Support: One to One or Groups   396
   Family Support: When Both Parents Have Dementia   397
   Partnership: Educational Opportunities and Families as Teachers   397
   Partnership: Research Opportunities   399
   Family and the Dying Resident   399
   Health Care Provider and Staff Issues   400
   Summary   400
   Suggested Reading   400
  Appendixes
    13-1 Twelve Steps for Caregivers   **403**
    13-2 Care for Caregivers: Grappling with Guilt   **405**
    13-3 Preadmission Information Form   **407**
    13-4 Activity-Focused Nursing Home Visits   **409**
      Objectives and Criteria for an Activity   409
      Normalization Activities   410
    13-5 Coping with the Holidays and Gift Suggestions   **413**
    13-6 Family Care Conference Form   **417**

**Ability-Centered Plan-of-Care Glossary of Terms for Residents
  with Dementia**   **419**

Index   **423**

Foreword

Alzheimer's disease has gone from obscurity to being a national and even international preoccupation. From the time that Dr. Alois Alzheimer described the illness that bears his name in 1907 until the later 1960s, Alzheimer's disease was thought to be an uncommon dementing illness occurring in young people. When it was realized that, in fact, Alzheimer's disease becomes progressively more common as people age, and that most people previously thought to be "senile" or have "hardening of the arteries" in fact have Alzheimer's disease, its importance became obvious. We now think that at least 10% of Americans age 65 years or older may have Alzheimer's disease, and almost half of those age 85 years and older may be affected. Because the aged population in the United States is expected to double by 2028, the number of Alzheimer's victims will increase dramatically.

No clear cause of Alzheimer's disease has been discovered. Genetic and environmental influences have been suggested and studied, but no definite conclusions have been drawn. Alzheimer's disease is a progressive illness that starts mainly with memory disorder, progresses to more general confusion, and ends with an inability to care for one's self and to communicate. Physical decline does not occur until the very end of the illness in an otherwise healthy person. No effective treatments are currently available. We are dealing, therefore, with an illness that impairs the mind but spares the body and for which there is currently no effective treatment.

Alzheimer's disease is associated with behavioral disorders in a significant number of patients with advanced dementia. The tendency has been to treat these patients with medications or physical restraint. These measures have led to excessive disability for patients and emotional turmoil for families.

Carly Hellen has been my colleague and friend for many years. She has studied and developed ways to care for Alzheimer's patients by stressing their abilities and avoiding excessive use of medication and restraints. Part of this effort has been to teach professional and family caregivers how to deal with their patients and loved ones in a way that maximizes the quality of their lives. This book represents a distillation of Carly's wisdom and experience and should serve as an extraordinarily useful guide for care-givers in dealing with patients with dementia. It can be used as both a practical guide and as a source of comfort and inspiration for all of us committed to the care of patients with Alzheimer's disease.

Jacob H. Fox, M.D.

Preface

This edition of *Alzheimer's Disease: Activity-Focused Care* wrote itself . . . therefore, I accept the role as facilitator and scribe. Residents with dementia, family members, and caregivers have been my teachers. Nursing assistants have shared with me their valuable insights, care information, and recipes for using and maintaining patience. But above all, the residents themselves, traveling the journey of dementia, have been my mentors. As their student, I have learned from the residents' ongoing internal wisdom and verbal and nonverbal communications, and have been blessed by their great capacity to accept my attempts to connect with them.

Activity-focused care involves practical, often simple, innovative care approaches that do not demean, humiliate, or infantalize persons with dementia. If all of life is an activity of being and doing, then all of life requires a commitment to provide or be provided with purposeful and meaningful opportunities. Activity-focused care revolves around encouraging the resident to participate, to be connected, to benefit from care that *includes* them, not care that is done *to* them. Caregivers are challenged to think, to integrate this book's suggestions and insights, and offer residents assistance based on compassion, sensitivity, and understanding.

What have I learned since the first edition of this book was published? Obviously, a lot; this edition is much longer and much better! I have deepened my commitment to supporting the wholistic wellness of persons with dementia. I have improved greatly in speaking and understanding the "language of dementia" (see Chapter 4). My residents have taught me well.

I am embarrassed by what I left out of the first edition because my awareness was limited. For example, the new chapter on expressions of intimacy, the beauty of sexuality, and the giving and receiving of affection as it enhances the resident's sense of self describes this integral part of life (see Chapter 10). The expansion of meaningful activities as the essence of daily life "stuff" offers insight and suggestions for encouraging in residents a positive sense of personhood and well-being (see Chapter 9). Identifying the therapeutic values of an activity ensures that the residents' abilities are supported. The uniqueness of caring for spouses with dementia requires finding the balance between each individual's well-being and abilities while respecting their unity as a couple. Creative interventions can refocus behaviors if all caregivers are "speaking the same language" of dementia care that does not allow the behavior to define expectations or the resident. Daily life care can become a ministry in the hands of compassionate caregivers. Whether it is offering cookies during shower time to refocus the resident's anxiety, using bridging as a sensory facilitation technique, or reducing the humiliation of being fed, the residents' inner sense of self is honored as they are offered opportunities to feel in control.

The gift of a LifeStory Book (see Chapter 3) affirms and supports the emphasis on valuing, not discounting, the resident. The answer is in the continued compassionate connectedness with the resident. This linkage may be made through activity-focused worship that calls forth the resident's spiritual center (see Chapter 11). Certainly, persons with dementia who feel safe, accepted, and loved discover companionship for their journey.

The uniqueness of *Alzheimer's Disease: Activity-Focused Care* is the emphasis on the resident with dementia's tireless search for a life of meaning, connectedness, and respect. Identifying the residents' abilities, not focusing on their inabilities, enables "shoulds" and "can'ts" to become "coulds" and "cans." Caregivers are offered problem-solving techniques so they can make informed decisions at the time needed for the resident seeking assistance. One size does not fit all, never has, and certainly never will when it comes to dementia care. The suggestions in this book have been tried and found successful in everyday caregiving. They come from caregivers who know the most, the ones who truly dedicate themselves to activity-focused Alzheimer's care, day after day. I admire and give them thanks.

Carly R. Hellen

Acknowledgments

With heartfelt thanks, I am grateful for my parents of the Quaker faith who actively live with their faith, offering respect and kindness for all persons. Throughout my life, I have honored respect and kindness as essential life qualities. Family, friends, and colleagues, especially from Bethany Methodist Terrace (Morton Grove, Illinois), Rush Alzheimer's Disease Center (Chicago, Illinois), and The Wealshire (Lincolnshire, Illinois), have filled my daily living with these qualities, and for them, I am thankful.

I am truly grateful for Karen Oberheim, Medical Editor, Butterworth–Heinemann, who has been my encourager and faithful helper before and throughout this second edition. I also appreciate the insight and suggestions from Jane Bangley McQueen, Production Editor, Silverchair Science + Communications, Inc.

Thanks also to my family, even though they only allowed, "Just one Alzheimer's story, Mom," at dinner each evening. Above all, I could never say a big enough "Thank you" to Jim, my husband and friend, who gives the words *respect* and *kindness* the ultimate meaning in my life.

Alzheimer's Disease: Activity-Focused Care

1

Activity-Focused Alzheimer's Care

"Life" exists in the activities of being and doing. Often, "life" becomes segmented into endeavors such as working, playing, sleeping, eating, and exercising. Each area, then, of life's involvement becomes viewed and endowed with its own meaning and significance. Realistically and practically, the tasks of life cannot stand alone but are interconnected parts of the whole. The activities of giving a response or being a participant connect and bring together all of life's components. Working, playing, sleeping, and other aspects of everyday living therefore require an inclusive, redefined frame of reference; these elements should not be evaluated as only separate tasks or taken-for-granted performances. A person's response to life's stimuli, within or outside of himself or herself, becomes his or her current or momentary activity. The "frame of activity," therefore, encompasses all of life.

ACTIVITY-FOCUSED CARE: DEFINED

Activity-focused care is the nurturing and supportive care that surrounds and honors the ongoing living of life as a person's activity. All of life is an activity of being and doing. The tasks of life are interconnected parts of the whole. Persons with Alzheimer's disease or related dementia do not lose this basic activity component that gives support and meaning to their lives, but they are confronted with many changes. Commonly held views of illness as signifying dysfunction often make it become all too easy to position the person with dementia into a medically focused concept of caregiving. This medical model centers on illness and equates symptoms and inappropriate responses as problems. Just using the word "problems" can color or predetermine the reactions of the person with Alzheimer's or the caregiver into a negative context or one that perceives the person and his or her daily activity as being unacceptable.

Similarly, the word "patient" emphasizes a medical or disease-related frame surrounding the person with dementia, which leads to preconceived judgments based on concepts of ill health or inabilities. Retirement and nursing care facilities prefer to call their community members "residents." Because all persons are engaged in the activity of being residents in one place or another, this more positive term will be used in this book to refer to persons with Alzheimer's disease or related dementia disorders.

Considering and defining a reaction or response as an activity, rather than a problem, appear to give both the resident and the caregiver permission to be creative and flexible. The focus then can change from one of illness or problems to one of wellness or possibilities and abilities rather than inabilities. Residents with dementia are often more capable than either they or their caregivers realize or expect. When daily living involvement is simplified, broken down into steps, or adapted to meet specific needs, residents can be more involved and better able to respond. An activity-supported ability may extend from the ultra-simple to the complex. For example, a resident may be able to bathe and dress independently and completely or may only be able to respond by holding a washcloth while receiving care. One resident may be able to handle a knife and fork while eating, while another may be unable to eat without being spoon-fed but may still maintain the ability to respond to cues for swallowing when pureed food is placed in his or her mouth.

If residents live in an environment that does not encourage participation or one that surmises that they cannot do for themselves, they easily fall prey to feelings of inadequacy and a role of passive involvement. Caregivers can become caught up in doing "to" or "for" the resident, rather than "with" the resident. Activity-focused care requires caregivers to be willing to change and be adaptive. Caregivers must enter the resident's world, not manipulate or force the resident with dementia into the caregivers' world. Awareness of the resident's abilities and identification of these abilities within the framework of supportive, activity-focused care and participation enable a positive affirmation of both the caregiver and the resident.

THE "ACTIVITY" OF LIFE: SEARCH FOR MEANING

The "activity" of life is a search for meaning and purpose. Dignity and the inner sense of worth arise from "work" or integrated occupations, including daily living activities and recreation. Activity involvement and encouraged responses can draw residents into a reality commensurate with their level of understanding. Involvement in meaningful relationships is shared through purposeful communication expressed as verbal and nonverbal messages, gestures, and rituals. Communication continues even when effective words are not accessible. Experiences void of meaning or without purpose can lead to fears, paranoia, catastrophic reactions, and depression. Throughout progressive dementia, adult feelings and needs continue, and when they are nurtured and answered appropriately, residents find value in living and themselves. Meaning and purpose become part of the framework of activity-focused caregiving, endowing the residents' responses and participation with value and acceptance.

Depicting "life" within this framework of activity that includes both caregivers and residents contributes to the significant centering that becomes wholistic support. Activity-focused caregiving identifies the total person cognitively, physically, emotionally, and spiritually. Residents with dementia are, first of all, persons: Persons, worthy of respect, with a treasured life story, who *also happen to* have a dementing condition. All of their responses, all of their losses, and all of their abilities or inabilities become integral considerations in supporting a positive quality of life. Caregivers cannot separate a resident's actions, behaviors, or inabilities from the whole person. A resident is not just a "troublemaker" because he or she rummages through other people's bureau drawers or deserving of being labeled as "combative" because of striking out during bathing. Upholding the resident as a person of worth who is dementia challenged facilitates integrated rather than segregated approaches to care. Residents often have increased sensitivity to their own inade-quacies and to the responses of others. Caring, supportive approaches and inter-ventions strive to avoid or minimize these inabilities.

ABILITY CENTERING: UPHOLDING AND MAINTAINING COMPETENCE

> Elizabeth, age 51 years, noticed the staff training outline on Carly's desk. She asked, "What are ADLs?" Carly explained that ADLs [activities of daily living] include information on bathing, dressing, hygiene, toileting, and eating and how they affect the resident with Alzheimer's disease. "Can I come?" Elizabeth asked. "I have Alzheimer's disease." Carly replied that she would very much like her to come. Realizing that Elizabeth appeared to have something more to say, Carly asked her if she would like to share how Alzheimer's disease had affected her life. Elizabeth firmly stated, "I want to tell them to stop doing for me what I can do for myself."

Honoring each resident's abilities offers persons with dementia a life of quality that moves away from letting the disease define the person. Certainly, the resi-dent's abilities will decline as the dementia progresses, but within ability-centered care the resident's strengths can still be identified and supported.

The reality is that the medical community places disease continuums into stages (see Appendix 1-1). Although stages assist in providing a common definition for study and research and perhaps knowledge for predicting the future, they have the tendency to depersonalize the person with the disease. Caregivers who say, "Edward is mid-stage" automatically make assumptions about Edward's abilities and challenges. These often imperfect indicators or labels of where the resident is in the disease process sometimes find that the person "does not quite fit" the description of symptoms or manifestations of the disease. Another difficulty with fitting residents into stages is that the person with dementia can vary day to day and, in fact, abilities and inabilities can fluctuate within a day.

Each person with dementia progresses through the disease process at a different rate. This unpredictable course challenges caregivers to enable the resident's abili-ties within all aspects of daily life. Searching for, identifying, and centering on abil-ities and competencies, not limitations, provides caregivers with the mind-set that the resident *is* capable, especially when caregiving is adapted and modified for suc-cessful resident support.

COGNITIVE AND PHYSICAL ABILITY CENTERING AND CHALLENGES

Identifying the person with dementia's cognitive and physical strengths enables caregivers to incorporate these abilities within all aspects of daily life activity. Abilities that are not called forth or integrated into actuality may risk the possibility of becoming lost or forgotten. Challenges are inevitable, but by centering the emphasis on cognitive and physical abilities, challenges can be refocused or adapted in ways that reduce their negative impact. See Chapter 2 for a discussion of psychosocial ability centering and challenges.

Cognitive and Physical Ability Centering and Challenges: Mild Dementia Impairment

The awareness of cognitive and physical difficulties affects residents with mild dementia impairments. Meaningful connection with the resident can be maintained when strengths and abilities are validated and facilitated. Challenges experienced during mild dementia can be depressing to the resident, possibly leading to withdrawal from past enjoyed activities or personal relationships. Such challenges may be redirected or diminished when daily living is adapted to promote the resident's success.

Cognitive Centering

- Can respond to an emergency stimuli or situation
- Follows simple directions of two or three steps
- Responds to reminders, can mirror a daily life task resulting in success
- Is able to benefit from reality-based orientation
- Personal opinions are expected and respected by resident's peer groups
- Understands verbal and visual cueing and memory triggers
- Responds safely to the environment with monitoring
- Is able to sometimes initiate participation in activity and will respond successfully to active involvement initiated by another person sharing the activity or being present
- Responds to volunteer and service activities
- Enjoys and benefits from validation and use of a LifeStory Book (see Chapter 3)
- Is timely with ADLs and responds to reminders for accomplishing details such as teeth brushing and hair combing
- Uses instruments of daily living appropriately or responds to cueing (silverware, glasses, etc.)
- Can usually self-report needs (e.g., hunger and illness) and can benefit from monitoring

Physical Centering

- Responds safely to physical limitations
- Is able to participate in ADLs if not impeded by other physical problems such as arthritis, Parkinson's disease, and so on
- Wandering is usually safe and will respond to redirection when needed
- Can usually use adapted equipment appropriately and safely (e.g., walkers, canes)
- Accepts light or standby assistance for physical movement
- Usually responds favorably to wellness and fitness programs

Cognitive and Physical Ability Centering and Challenges: Moderate Dementia Impairment

Centering on abilities during residents' experience of moderate dementia calls for increased adapting and daily life simplification by the caregiver. Meaningful connections between resident and caregiver becomes paramount as cognitive and physical challenges increase and impact overall resident responses and wellness. Caregiving needs to continue to support the resident's remaining abilities, using them within daily life tasks. Ability centering requires doing "with," not "to" or "for," the resident. Only then can the resident's positive sense of self be upheld.

Cognitive Centering

- Accepts and needs assistance for emergency stimuli or situation response
- Follows directions when visual and verbal cueing systems are included
- Benefits from task sequencing and breakdown (simplification) for success
- Tolerates reminding and benefits from one-step directions
- Accepts ongoing monitoring to assure environmental safety and way-finding assistance
- Demonstrates interest in activities and accepts assistance due to limited initiation of activities, therefore benefiting from the presence of a caregiver to assure focus and ability to continue participation
- May not use instruments of daily living appropriately but usually is able to respond to simplification and redirection for assuring success
- Is able to communicate using some words or phrases and nonverbal reflections of desired information to be shared
- Commonly unable to self-report needs but often can demonstrate needs via nonverbal cues
- Usually responds to and benefits from therapeutic orientation rather than reality orientation
- Often participates fully in normalization activities with assistance (e.g., folding clothing, wiping tables, sweeping the floor, raking leaves)
- Usually accepted by peer group members but can handle being on the perimeter of gathered residents or on the edges of an activity; therefore, benefits from involvement of "being there," although not as an active participant

Physical Centering

- May need or benefit from total assistance to respond to an emergency that requires moving from a harmful stimulus or situation
- Benefits from monitoring due to physical limitations impacting dementia care and triggering risks for falls, and so on
- Participation in ADLs allows partnership and active assistance from the caregiver
- Wandering can be encouraged with continual monitoring to uphold resident safety
- Uses multisensory cues successfully for ADLs, physical involvement, and participation

- Accepts hand-over-hand assistance and chaining (i.e., assistance at the introduction of a task, after which the resident can take over)
- Benefits from and requires direct caregiver contact for enabling abilities

Cognitive and Physical Ability Centering and Challenges: Severe Dementia Impairment

The symptoms of severe dementia may greatly diminish residents' cognitive and physical wellness as well as the continued ability to respond to daily life tasks. Strengths are facilitated when one-to-one care allows for meaningful connections between the resident and the caregiver. Challenges are experienced, especially as they affect communications and overall cognitive and physical awareness. The wellness of the physical body systems become compromised. Caregivers able to connect with the resident as a person of great worth can continue a supportive and nurturing relationship despite encountered difficulties.

Cognitive Centering

- Benefits from and needs one-to-one support for cognitive needs and meaningful activity
- Responds to reassurance orientation
- Can increase nonverbal communications for displaying emotions and making needs known
- Has limited ability but may respond to cueing systems
- Benefits from total assistance for responding to environmental safety
- Can be successful with staff-initiated activities, especially when carried out on a one-to-one basis
- Benefits from staff assistance due to limited ability or inability to use instruments of daily living
- Staff and family are the basis of the resident's peer group
- Reflects cognitive wellness within personal ability level when receiving a high intensity of staff support

Physical Centering

- Benefits from increased health monitoring, as physical care issues usually supersede dementia needs
- Caregivers offer the resident nurturing and are responsible for implementing all ADLs with the resident involved as much as possible (e.g., providing hand-over-hand assistance)
- Benefits from ambulation assistance but is usually a high risk for falls
- Responds to positioning and monitoring when immobile
- May benefit from pain control and hospice care
- Responds to increased touch and light massage
- Often benefits from a passive range of motion
- Benefits from focus on skin care
- Reflects physical wellness when receiving appropriate staff support

Alzheimer's Disease: Activity-Focused Care

ABILITY-CENTERED PLAN OF CARE

Creating a plan of care, whether the resident is cared for at home or within a health care facility, helps caregivers identify the resident's strengths and difficulties. The plan of care is most effective when all aspects of daily life are considered as the resident's activity. This philosophy of activity-focused care allows and facilitates the planning of care to focus on the residents' abilities and strengths. However, a plan of care very often starts with naming all the problems the resident is experiencing, for example:

1. Resident urinates on the floor, cannot find the bathroom.
2. Resident takes personal items belonging to others.
3. Resident strikes out during bathing.

When the approach to care starts with accentuating the resident's remaining abilities and strengths, the perception of a difficult-to-care-for resident can often be shifted into a resident challenged because of dementia. An ability-centered plan of care might look at the care challenges in the previous list in the following way:

1. Resident can respond to multisensory cueing and benefit from the promotion of independence (e.g., place a picture of a toilet on the bathroom door).
2. Resident can find comfort, meaning, and a feeling of being in control when gathering items as though reenacting past life roles (e.g., housekeeping [place available items for resident to sort and carry on the kitchen table]).
3. Resident can be more cooperative and strikes out less when holding items and actively participating in the bathing process, which refocus the resident's fearfulness and hands (e.g., give resident a washcloth to hold and use hand-over-hand bathing).

Therefore, before care difficulties are addressed, the resident's abilities are listed in the plan of care. These abilities can then be incorporated in the care approaches or interventions (see Appendix 1-2).

Caregiving for residents with dementia requires adapted approaches and innovative interventions. The plan of care that starts by identifying the resident's abilities will reflect dementia-specific caregiving skills and their implementation. Each resident will have approaches to care that are personally unique, meaningful, and reflective of activity- and ability-centered care (see the Glossary at the end of the book). As each plan of care is discussed and developed, the question to ask is, does the plan of care demonstrate the resident's unique abilities, and are they incorporated into reducing challenges by the implementation of ability-centered caregiving?

CAREGIVING: DEFINED AS PURPOSEFUL ACTIVITY

Family caregivers search for meaning and purpose as they wrestle with their personal physical and emotional responses to their loved one's illness and decline. If caregivers can "frame" or acknowledge a resident's behavior, such as pacing, as the resident's activity rather than an annoying negative behavior, they are more capable of releasing former expectations and open to redefining parameters of acceptance. Caregivers seek to experience their own involvement with the resident as a purposeful, meaningful activity. The caregivers' abilities also must be recognized and promoted, and their inabilities minimized or compensated with support, assistance, and empathy. The caregivers' own lives crave an inner sense of meaning or ministry that will enable them to participate in the activity of giving care to themselves and others.

Family caregivers need holistic self-acceptance and support from significant others. They are more than caregivers, wives, husbands, children, or any of the other many roles they play. First and foremost, they are persons requiring love, understanding, and support of their cognitive, physical, emotional, and spiritual needs. Strength for the joys and sorrows of caregiving emanates from inner integrity.

Professional health care staff dedicated to supporting and nurturing the well-being of their residents, may also become emotionally involved in caregiving. Caregiving is often more than a skill or a job. Caregiving is meaningful, fulfilling, and often viewed as a ministry. Negative feelings, frustration, and sadness are also part of the continuum of emotions for health care workers. Acceptance, support, and respect are basic for enabling the staff to successfully manage the joys and sorrows of their chosen work.

Framing caregiving as an activity initiates the desired flexibility that goes hand in hand with caring. Flexibility calls for the ability to change and to reevaluate a situation, behavior, or response. Change is often difficult, but it is easier or more acceptable when supported by creativity and a sense of humor. For example, yesterday's aggressive behavior in the shower might be avoided today with a distraction technique, such as offering cookies or singing. The many losses, precipitated by the progressive dementia and experienced by both the resident and the caregiver, can be survived only if change is expected and accepted and if flexibility of attitudes and involvement is granted and tolerated.

THE 10 COMMANDMENTS OF ALZHEIMER'S CARE*

Health care staff, challenged with caring for a person with dementia, usually attend classes to expand their knowledge about caregiving. The truly effective staffpersons are aware and sensitive to their residents' dementia experience. This sensitivity calls for staff to be flexible, creative, and willing to enter the resident's world by providing safe and nurturing caregiving. The following 10 commandments of Alzheimer's care are indeed a tribute to the caring spirit of the nursing assistant.

1. Realize that *you* do the adapting and the modifying of your response to their behavior.
2. Realize that *you* enter their reality rather than pull them into yours.

---

*A special thank you to Cynthia Belle, A.C.C., Director of Training and Education, and the March 1994 Alzheimer's Nursing Assistant Class of The Methodist Home, Chicago, Illinois.

Alzheimer's Disease: Activity-Focused Care

3. Realize that one size does *not* fit all, when it comes to what will and will not work for each individual.
4. Realize that approaches and techniques are not 100% failure-free and that you must learn to be flexible.
5. Realize that *normalization* is important in giving residents a sense of participating in their own lives as they see fit.
6. Realize that *success* means adapting the task to whatever the individual's highest level happens to be.
7. Realize that the *process* is more important than the net result, and celebrate that process regardless of the outcome.
8. Realize that you need to "do what it takes" when the tried and true methods have not been effective.
9. Realize that the family is an equal partner in the caregiving process and that educating them is up to you.
10. Realize that through your caregiving, *you* hold the key to the success of the resident's journey through this disease and that because of this, you are a rare and special person.

HEALTH CARE PROVIDER AND STAFF ISSUES

Health care providers advertising specialized care for residents with Alzheimer's disease need to exhibit commitment to activity-focused care based on each resident's abilities. This commitment starts with the administration and must be supported by all staffpersons. The staff team can create a philosophy of care that identifies needs, goals, and a plan for facilitating an Alzheimer's program. Elements of the philosophy of dementia care include all aspects of care throughout the day, the creation of a therapeutic environment, trained staff that are sensitive to the experience of dementia, and a commitment to involve family members as part of the caregiving team. Accepting a resident into a dementia program should require evidence that a competent evaluation has been completed before admission. If the evaluation is questionable, the care center can insist that a reassessment be implemented.

At The Wealshire Alzheimer's care center in Lincolnshire, Illinois, the staff identified specifically the care goals they had for their residents, goals for families as partners in care, and goals for supporting staff. The following mission statement was created by uniting the common threads woven into each area of care: resident, family, and staff.

> The Mission of The Wealshire is to honor the ongoing living
> of life, enjoying dignity and well-being in a shared, caring
> relationship with residents, family, and staff.

Health care providers dedicated to activity-focused care may be in a position to model unique care approaches that differ from or modify current health care facility regulations. The differences are unique because they uphold the recognition and facilitation of the residents' remaining abilities. For example, a resident may be able to walk barefooted but not with shoes on. Developing a policy and procedure explaining the rationale for walking barefoot and including approaches and intervention on the resident's plan of care bring ability-centered care within acceptable boundaries.

From a caregiver's point of view, what is so different about activity- and ability-focused care for residents with dementia? Caregivers have identified the following specific areas:

1. *Caregiving is an activity.* The focus is on the resident, not the job. Upholding all of life as an activity expands possibilities, provides an opportunity to demystify the resident with dementia whose response to life is his or her activity at that time, and allows the caregiver and the resident to uphold responses and reactions as meaningful activity.
2. *A paradigm change is required.* Abilities and strengths are respected and facilitated; problems or challenges are refocused; care is personalized; the resident is first a person, not a disease; and staff recognize the fallacy of labeling problems, thereby making the resident "responsible" for the problem, not the staff.
3. *Being asked to do something "with" the resident, not "to" or "for" the resident.* Increased holistic involvement, commitment, and energy are required; the resident is valued; and the resident's abilities are respected and called forth into the activities of daily life.
4. *The resident sets the pace.* Caregivers enter the resident's world; expectations and outcomes are resident-centered, not staff-centered; and whatever the resident is involved with at the time is the resident's activity.
5. *"Work" is ongoing, and the job is never "done."* Some residents with dementia always want more; and residents can "un-do" about as fast as the staff can "do."
6. *Staffpersons may not be valued.* For example, during bathing or toileting the resident is not able to understand the significance of the caregiving being offered and may strike out at the staffperson; appreciation may not be verbalized due to communication dysfunctions or possible mask-like face; families may not value the staffperson when they are in denial of their loved ones' inabilities or are projecting anger from a difficult relationship; facility management does not understand or value the staffperson sharing a simple activity (e.g., a cup of tea) with the resident or asks why John's room isn't cleaned up, when John has been packing and unpacking as his activity for the past hour (see Staff Personhood: A Staff Statement of Respect in Chapter 2).
7. *Caregiving means accepting variability, change, inconsistency, and unexpectedness.* Resident moods are unpredictable; caregiving involvement is always changing; nothing is ever where the staffperson just left it; creativity is required to alter approaches and interventions; and staff must be problem solvers and able to think on their feet.

Staff, understanding the uniqueness of their position and the uniqueness of the residents they care for, are able to combine an activity-focused care approach with ability centering. Care plan meetings, family conferences, and formal and informal staff meetings that start with the identification of the resident's remaining strengths and abilities further strengthen the focus on "all of life" as an activity of great meaning. The listings earlier in this chapter of centering ability and challenges for residents at different levels of impairment can be used to assist in decisions when a resident is being considered for a move to more assistance and monitored care. This is especially helpful when a program for residents with

dementia has different levels of care that require the resident to move. The relocation of a resident is almost always an emotional and difficult process. An accurate
plan of care, therefore, is an important component of the decision-making process.

The "bottom line" for making activity-focused care a reality? Staff. Staff need to
have great patience, flexibility, humor, and genuine care for their residents.

SUMMARY

Activity, therefore, is a basic structure surrounding residents and their caregivers in
all daily life tasks. Activity-focused care understands and honors all that involves
the resident as his or her meaningful activity. Peer support, open communications,
plus respect for the resident are essential for caregivers, whose tasks include daily
care, encouraging eating, supporting mobility, understanding behaviors, promoting activities, and delivering terminal care. There cannot be a "cookbook"
approach to providing care because no two people are the same, nor does dementia
affect residents in totally similar ways. The challenge is for the caregiver to be flexible, creative, and able to change, because the resident usually cannot. The caregiver must enter the resident's world of just "the present moment" as the resident
attempts to cope and live his or her life with dignity. Persons with dementia grasp
at themselves and those around them as they search for a meaningful frame to surround and hold together their identity and perception of self-worth. An activity-
focused and ability-centered foundation or structure for calling forth residents'
wellness answers this search. Being "valued" becomes the cornerstone for finding
meaning and dignity within the "activity" of life.

SUGGESTED READING

Alzheimer's Association. Guidelines for Dignity. Chicago: Alzheimer's Disease and Related
    Disorders Association, 1992.
Alzheimer's Association. Key Elements of Dementia Care. Chicago: Alzheimer's Disease
    and Related Disorders Association, 1997.
Alzheimer's Association. Terms and Tips: An Alzheimer's Care Handbook. Chicago:
    Alzheimer's Disease and Related Disorders Association, 1995.
Bell V, Troxler D. The Best Friends Approach to Alzheimer's Care. Baltimore: Health Pro-
    fessions Press, 1997.
Davis R. My Journey into Alzheimer's Disease. Wheaton, IL: Tyndale House, 1989.
Floyd SP, Kuhn DR (eds). The Rush Manual for Caregivers (3rd ed). Chicago: Rush
    Alzheimer's Disease Center, 1996. (Call 312-942-4463 for information.)
Hoffman SB, Kaplan M (eds). Special Care Programs for People with Dementia. Baltimore:
    Health Care Professions Press, 1996.
Kitwood T, Bredin K. Towards a theory of dementia care: personhood and wellbeing. Ageing
    Soc 1992;12:269–287.
Mace NL, Rabins P. The 36-Hour Day (rev ed). Baltimore: Johns Hopkins University Press,
    1991.
Rader J. Individualized Dementia Care: Creative, Compassionate Approaches. New York:
    Springer, 1995.

A1-1
Alzheimer's Disease: Symptoms and Challenges

Dementia is not a normal part of aging. Aging is a time of change when forgetfulness does occur within the realm of "normalcy." Dementia, meaning a loss of intellectual functions, such as thinking and memory, is not a disease itself, but a collection of symptoms. These include memory loss; impaired judgment, orientation, and calculation skills; difficulties with learning new things or remembering recent events; and problems with abstract thinking.

Alzheimer's disease, affecting more than 4 million Americans, is the leading cause of dementia. Other causes include multi-infarct or vascular dementia, Parkinson's disease, Pick's disease, Lewy bodies, and Creutzfeldt-Jakob disease. Information on Alzheimer's and related dementias can be obtained by contacting a local chapter of the Alzheimer's Association. This information can include reversible dementias (e.g., those due to medication misuse, depression, metabolic dysfunctions, and normal-pressure hydrocephalus), risk factors for Alzheimer's disease, how the diagnosis is made, pathologic findings, medical treatment, current research, drug trial availability, medication information, autopsy information, educational opportunities, and support group information. The Alzheimer's Association can also provide information on area assessment centers as well as a listing of the federally recognized Alzheimer's centers.

Alzheimer's disease is diagnosed by careful assessment and mental status testing to determine the severity of the dementia. The clinical diagnosis is reached by looking at the person's medical history, neurologic examination findings, general physical results, blood work screening, brain scan, and any additional tests indicated by the person's history.

The following are generalized descriptions of the personal challenges for persons with Alzheimer's disease, based on level of impairment.

PERSONS WITH DEMENTIA: MILD IMPAIRMENT

- Memory loss, especially of recent events, misplacing things
- Mild word-finding difficulties
- Difficulty with calculations, decision making

- Decreased concentration, difficulty performing familiar tasks
- May experience depression or apathy, less spontaneity, less initiative
- Poor judgment (e.g., unsafe driving, being sold items not needed)
- Disorientation related to time, place
- Reminders needed at times (e.g., for activities of daily living [ADLs], involving personal care such as dressing, bathing, toileting, and daily life tasks, including using the telephone, preparing a meal, raking leaves)

PERSONS WITH DEMENTIA: MODERATE IMPAIRMENT

- Increase in memory loss, including names, places
- Word-finding difficulties leading to talking around the subject, making up words, or withdrawing from conversations
- Problems tracking conversations and television programs; reading stops
- May become lost easily, poses possible risk to self (e.g., by leaving the stove on, dressing inappropriately for the weather), cannot be alone
- May experience visual-spatial perceptual problems
- Possible mood disturbances and behavioral outbursts and agitation
- May exhibit paranoia, thinking that someone is stealing from him or her
- Possible hallucinations, auditory or visual, or both
- Motor activity includes pacing and wandering
- Increased risk for falling
- Reminders and often a standby assist for ADLs needed
- May experience urine incontinence
- Simplification of directions and tasks required to ensure success

PERSONS WITH DEMENTIA: SEVERE IMPAIRMENT

- Inability to perform daily care independently; may need assistance with feeding; becomes incontinent
- Immobility may be experienced; if walking, the resident is often at high risk for falls; trunk and extremities can become rigid
- Mute or limited communication abilities
- May experience weight loss, swallowing difficulties, stopping of eating or drinking
- Skin integrity often compromised
- Need for high-touch care

A1-2
Ability-Centered Plan of Care

Name: _____   Diagnosis: _____

Doctor: _____

Date	Abilities	Problems	Goals	Goal Date	Responsible Discipline	Interventions: Family and Staff
	Self-Care					
	Nutrition					
	Current weight: _____					
	Mobility					

Name: _____   Diagnosis: _____

Doctor: _____

Date	Abilities	Problems	Goals	Goal Date	Responsible Discipline	Interventions: Family and Staff
	Social Function					
	Sensory/Perception					
	Bowel and Bladder					
	Cognition					

Alzheimer's Disease: Activity-Focused Care

Name: _____   Diagnosis: _____
Doctor: _____

Date	Abilities	Problems	Goals	Goal Date	Responsible Discipline	Interventions: Family and Staff
		Safety				
		Other				

2

Maintaining Personhood: Psychosocial Aspects of Support

The psychosocial aspects of care and support are focused on residents' needs for acceptance and validation as persons of worth. Residents strive for a continuation of a purposeful life and sense of emotional, social, and spiritual well-being within their personal spheres of ability.

PROMOTING LIFE'S MEANING AND PERSONHOOD

Residents seek to hang onto and grasp meaning and full humanity within their lives. Meaning is not something happened on or stumbled across, like the missing puzzle piece or the answer to a trivia question. Meaning is something built into life, out of the past, talents, values, affections—out of the experience of being human. The components of meaning and personhood are still there, even if or when dementia is present. The components may change from the once brilliant colors of intense feelings and dedication to a more subtle hue, but the components of one's tapestry of meaning are still very much there, despite the dementia and along with the dementia. The person is not the dementia. "Personhood" refers to one's sense of self, the "I" within each resident. A person with dementia can experience relative well-being and can continue to know that he or she is a person. Kitwood and Bredin (1992) described the 12 indicators of personhood and well-being in persons with dementia as

1. The assertion of desire or will
2. The ability to experience and express a range of emotions
3. Initiation of social contact
4. Affectional warmth
5. Social sensitivity
6. Self-respect
7. Acceptance of other persons with dementia
8. Humor

9. Creativity and self-expression
10. Showing evident pleasure
11. Helpfulness
12. Relaxation

PSYCHOSOCIAL ABILITY CENTERING AND CHALLENGES

Centering or focusing on residents' psychosocial abilities and challenges allows caregivers to identify the changes they are responsible for making so that each resident's psychosocial well-being and personhood is enhanced. See Chapter 1 for a discussion of the cognitive and physical components of ability centering.

Psychosocial Ability Centering and Challenges: Mild Dementia Impairment

Persons with dementia experiencing the losses and changes associated with memory deficits may become depressed or respond by withdrawing from former daily living activities. Encouragement, support, and acceptance by family, friends, and caregivers are essential components for enabling the resident to continue to maintain a positive sense of self and well-being.

- Enjoys validation as a person of worth
- Responds appropriately in social situations
- Interacts with others with tolerance, and is not at risk to self or others
- Can self-direct mood changes
- Can accept mood refocusing from others (e.g., sadness, fearfulness, anxiety)
- Is able to receive praise and appreciation for participation in ability-based activities
- Reflects or displays infrequent episodes of anxiety
- Can be redirected during times of stress
- Benefits from opportunities to serve others, especially in the community
- Involvement with group-oriented "success" offers meaning and well-being
- Responds to resident-directed support groups
- Responds independently to identification with LifeStory Book

Psychosocial Ability Centering and Challenges: Moderate Dementia Impairment

Residents confronted with the psychosocial challenges related to moderate dementia require sensitivity and compassionate care. Remaining abilities can be enabled and continue to uphold personhood if all aspects of residents' daily living experiences are adapted for their successful involvement. It is in the meaningful connection of well-being and feelings of being loved, accepted, and safe that residents' psychosocial abilities are called forth and maintained.

- Is able to be redirected if experiencing outbursts or other inappropriate responses in social settings

- Is usually friendly but may demonstrate limited tolerance for others
- Accepts monitoring and redirection if at risk to self and others
- Responds to opportunities when persons and programs from the community are brought into the care center
- Accepts and usually needs assistance for successful involvement in psychosocial events
- Responds to staff-directed support groups
- Accepts and benefits from increased use of a LifeStory Book by staff as the basis of emotional support and needs by adapting and processing information for feelings of safety and assurance

Psychosocial Ability Centering and Challenges: Severe Dementia Impairment

Impairments due to severe dementia require caregiving centered on respect, nurturing, and compassion. Residents can continue to demonstrate their psychosocial abilities and needs if caregivers are willing to pause, focus, listen, and "see" the person before the dementia.

- Can display limited social responses when involved in one-to-one interactions
- Profits from one-to-one assistance to assure emotional well-being
- Responds to and benefits from a high-touch milieu and use of music
- Can demonstrate needs or emotions through verbal outbursts, sounds, or nonverbal body or facial responses
- May experience emotional responses that do or do not relate to the present experience

BEING VALUED, NOT "DISCOUNTED"

Promoting self-esteem starts with self-acceptance. The experience of dementia can be one of vulnerability. The ability to find respect for one's self, feelings of safety and acceptance, enjoyment, and the ability to participate in a socially supportive milieu can remain throughout almost the entire course of the dementing disease. Building on residents' social skills becomes the nucleus about which care revolves. With acceptance and positive affirmations of residents as "real people," feelings of security empower them to respond holistically (cognitively, physically, emotionally, and spiritually) to themselves, their caregivers, and their "world." Residents feel valued as persons of worth and great dignity.

Residents require caregivers who offer them the respect and dignity needed for feeling honored and valued. Residents' orientation and self-awareness gives caregivers a guide for interpreting and understanding residents' attitudes, behaviors, and responses. Appropriate approaches and interventions to support the psychosocial aspects of care are enhanced when the components of a therapeutic environment, caregiver training, and understanding of residents' physical and cognitive abilities, challenges, and needs come together to allow for maximum emotional and social well-being.

The opposite of wellness and personal validation is being "discounted." Being discounted, in other words, feeling like a nonperson, can occur when caregivers do not see the importance of their care approaches in upholding residents as persons of worth or are too exhausted to care. Caregivers can discount residents in many ways, including

- Walking by a resident who is calling or reaching out and not acknowledging his or her presence
- Not responding to a resident's look of anguish or pain
- Shoveling food into the resident's mouth at mealtime without regard for socialization
- Limiting eye contact or presence when a resident is trying to talk
- Not waiting for the resident to finish his or her conversation
- Looking hurried, harassed, too busy to be engaged
- Forgetting promises made to the resident
- Reminding the resident by using the *"just"* word (e.g., "You *just* ate breakfast, Harry," "I *just* took you to the toilet 5 minutes ago.")
- Talking about the resident in front of him or her
- Not including the resident in decision making
- Talking down to a resident in a non-adult manner
- Leaving a resident stranded in a wheelchair
- Seeing the dementia *before* seeing the person

Some forms of discounting as subtle ways of negating the resident are less obvious, but the message is the same.

> Joyce had enjoyed her cup of tea, and the empty cup sat before her on the dining room table. The nursing assistant noticed that the cup was empty and picked it up on her way to the kitchen.

This scene sounds like the nursing assistant is working effectively, attending his or her resident. But, the scene could be different.

> Joyce had enjoyed her cup of tea, and the empty cup sat before her on the dining room table. The nursing assistant noticed that the cup was empty and said to Joyce, "You have finished your cup of tea? Please pass me the cup and I'll take it to the kitchen for you." Or, "You have finished your cup of tea? Please help me out and take the cup to the kitchen."

Both of these endings to the scene help to engage the resident and ask for a response. Discounting is when the cup is taken away, without interfacing with the resident, just doing it. The resident becomes a nonperson, assumed to be incapable of being asked about the cup and discounted as though she were not even there.

AN ALZHEIMER'S DISEASE PATIENT'S BILL OF RIGHTS

An Alzheimer's disease patient's bill of rights surrounds and supports persons with dementia with a framework of respect. Bell and Troxel (1994) created a list of rights

Alzheimer's Disease: Activity-Focused Care

from their vast experience working with persons with dementia. Their bill of rights states that, "Every person diagnosed with Alzheimer's disease or a related disorder deserves:

To be informed of one's diagnosis

To have appropriate, ongoing medical care

To be productive in work and play as long as possible

To be treated like an adult, not a child

To have expressed feelings taken seriously

To be free from psychotropic medications if at all possible

To live in a safe, structured, and predictable environment

To enjoy meaningful activities to fill each day

To be out-of-doors on a regular basis

To have physical contact including hugging, caressing, and hand holding

To be with persons who know one's life story, including cultural and religious traditions

To be cared for by individuals well-trained in dementia care."

RESIDENTS WITH AN INTEGRATED SELF-IMAGE

Residents with a positive sense of self are able to participate in authentic living in a supportive environment. Life has meaning to these residents, and they desire and attempt to be helpful. They have a positive response to others and are able to be part of a "family" or peer community. There is a flexibility to accept change. Choices can be made with relative ease. Strangers and new situations are not perceived as threatening. General behavioral problems are diminished and responses to stress do not seem to escalate to combativeness. Although word-finding problems increase, attempts are made to continue using verbalization as the basis for communication.

> Frances welcomed each and every person who visited the nursing home Alzheimer's disease unit. She would greet them with a big smile and extended hand. Her conversation always included a compliment about the visitor's pretty dress or good-looking tie. Frances enjoyed social activities, especially parties. She often sat at the table with a contented smile. When the meal arrived, Frances became very concerned if people were standing and not sharing the food. Because the staff were available to show her to her room when she could not find it and all tasks were broken down into a single step at a time, Frances was able to obtain the support she needed to maintain her positive self-image and to continue to feel in control.

RESIDENTS WITH A COMPROMISED SELF-IMAGE

> "Hannah, Hannah, where are you? Hannah? Hannah?" The calling voice can be heard throughout the hall and dining area. The resident calls out again and again. The resident's name is Hannah, and she is calling for herself. Hannah cannot "find" herself. Perhaps she is experiencing an overwhelming sense of being totally lost, of being a nonperson. By calling out she may, hopefully, "find" herself.

Residents with an impoverished or compromised self-image are not able to grasp a peaceful quality of life. The world appears splintered, not "user friendly." Fears can become the basis of aggression, combativeness, and unresponsiveness that often lead to apathy, withdrawal, and depression. The resident often paces and has catastrophic reactions as his or her loss of abilities and dependency increase. Paranoia, delusions, and perhaps hallucinations appear to stem from an inability to feel comfortable with one's self. Residents with a limited understanding of or tolerance for others may exhibit a decreased ability or interest in socialization. For example, a resident's angry fixation centered on a specific person or object may precipitate an outburst of emotions. Visual, spatial perceptual, and auditory deficits can add to the difficulties and may limit the resident's responses and escalate his or her frustration.

Residents with a limited ability to feel safe and in harmony with themselves may use negative or abusive language that signals their loss of control. Verbalization may decrease, with limited attempts to communicate, or they might be able to express their inner sadness with comments such as, "I'm trash, throw me away," or "I'm crazy, there's a squirrel in my head."

There are times when residents have almost a complete inability to respond, as though their "sense of self" is gone. They appear to reject all of the caregivers' attempts to enter their world, except perhaps through food and drink. Awareness of the physical self and appropriate body movements or posture become limited.

> Shirley appeared not to have a self-image or inner picture of who she was. Each day she would sit in the family room in her geriatric chair. When the staff stopped to interact with her, she was not able to turn toward their voices or track their movements with her eyes. To look at Shirley, one would think that she was capable of a response because she had a bright, open-eyed look, but her face lacked expression. She was not able to "know" that an item was placed in her hand. Even a soft teddy bear or her own grandchild did not elicit an awareness or reaction. Further attempts to stimulate a response included actually getting into bed with Shirley and holding and rocking her gently. Soft stroking down her spine also was not met with a response.
>
> Perhaps, however, Shirley did have a sense of self. She would reach out occasionally and grab at people going by. Even when she had someone in her grasp it seemed as though she did not realize it. Holding someone's hand did not bring her any peace

because she would continue to grasp the person again and again. There appeared to be little that the staff could do to enable a quality of life for Shirley. There were a few times when Shirley would take the hand she grasped so tightly and slowly raise it to her lips. The staff often wondered if she was going to bite, but Shirley only would kiss gently the hand she held.

Somehow caregivers need to understand more about the "Shirleys" and their narrow, seemingly empty world and find an effective way to reach and nurture their inner beings.

DEPRESSION: OVERWHELMING SADNESS

Depression in the elderly is often misunderstood, undiagnosed, misdiagnosed, or left untreated. Depression frequently further compromises the wellness of persons with impairments that are physical, cognitive, or both. Depression may be experienced by residents with Alzheimer's disease. Possible causes leading to intense sadness can include anxiety concerning losses being experienced, awareness of having dementia or the diagnosis of dementia, frustration over not being able to express oneself, feelings of being unable to control changes and situations, mourning over past abilities and roles, changes in living situation, and perhaps sadness over changes in physical abilities.

Written on a piece of toilet paper in a hospital, a therapist found the following note at the bedside of a patient with dementia:

I am losing my memory.

I tried to commit suicide 3 times because you said you wanted to move on with your life.

But I don't blame you.

WHERE WILL YOU PUT ME?

Thank you for a wonderful life.

I'm doing my best to correct (my mistakes) everything.

Depression may also occur if the resident has experienced periods of depression in the past. Symptoms of depression may include a persistent sad or empty mood, difficulty concentrating, loss of interest in activities, fatigue and decreased energy, sleep disturbances, poor posture, neglect of personal hygiene, weight change, slowed physical movement in ambulation and self-care, increased memory difficulties, feelings of worthlessness and helplessness, crying, tearfulness, and focusing on chronic aches and pains.

Residents with a compromised self-image due to feelings of inadequacy or lack of acceptance are likely to exhibit signs of depression. The Christmas and holiday season, with all of its traditions, rituals, and memories, greatly affects the person with dementia, often leading to withdrawal or sadness or both. Also, a resident's fall or a change in the environment can trigger a depressed response, perhaps due to fear or feeling out of control.

At other times, the precipitating factors cannot be identified, and it can become impossible to know why residents become apathetic, often responding poorly to their food and showing a lack of interest in people or surroundings. Attempts to increase the frequency of pleasant events plus promoting activities in which the resident can be successful may be helpful.

Equally confusing is why the depression sometimes ends and the resident returns to active involvement. A specialist experienced in working with residents with dementia and depression should be contacted and encouraged to evaluate the resident. Physicians assessing residents' depression are encouraged to respond with appropriate interventions. Accepting depression as part of the journey into dementia is detrimental to the resident's well-being. If allowed to go untreated, depression can compound the effects of dementia, leading to increased anxiety, forgetfulness, and difficulties with maintaining personhood. Sometimes treatment of the depression fails, however, leading possibly to increased despair.

INTERVENTIONS AND SUPPORT OF PSYCHOSOCIAL NEEDS

Residents' conceptions of their emotional well-being and interaction with the social environment do not stay static. Too many variables pull at residents, varying their moods and responses. The unifying caregiving objective that becomes the primary basis for resident support is the focus on positive, nurturing care that will validate residents as worthy human beings.

Expectations for residents need to be realistic, and attempts must be made to never place them in situations in which they cannot cope. Flexibility and willingness to change care approaches and interventions are imperative. Caregivers can encourage a sense of belonging and security if they understand how their verbal and nonverbal communication affects the resident. Residents have increased confidence if their environment is perceived as being safe and supportive.

Self-esteem can be validated by awareness of the resident's life story and past roles, and by incorporating, if possible, a similar lifestyle (see Chapter 3).

> William, a former executive, was outfitted by his daughter in plain, dark blue sweat suits with crew necks and drawstring waists. When he wore these outfits, he would look down at himself, apparently not "recognizing" himself because he had never dressed in this type of clothing. His daughter had meant well and was trying to help the staff by making his dressing easier—William had been asked to leave two nursing facilities because of disruptive behaviors during morning bathing and dressing. When the staff became aware of William's past business position, they changed his clothing into a shirt, tie, and pair of slacks. His perception of himself was that once more he was a business manager. He often wore a conference-type name tag and was encouraged to be "in charge" of a team activity or project. By dressing and being supported as the leader he once had been, William felt a sense of purpose, dignity, and

Alzheimer's Disease: Activity-Focused Care

self-worth. He then was able to become an integral part of
his peer community.

Psychosocial aspects of care also can be addressed through the use of "normal-ization" activities (see Chapter 9). These are failure-free tasks, or "work," that promote a purposeful use of time and are similar to what residents with Alzheimer's disease would be doing if they were well and at home or on the job. Normalization activities are familiar and can be an important part of the daily routine. Activity modification and breaking an activity down into small tasks enable participation and contribute to a positive self-esteem. For example:

- Serving each other at a party combines a comfortable activity with the ongoing ability to respond appropriately in a social setting.
- Walking, vacuuming, or raking leaves are examples of activities used to reduce stress and anxiety. These tasks facilitate a positive avenue to address emotional and behavioral needs.
- If appropriate, "messing up" a resident's bureau drawer when he or she is not present allows the returning resident to feel needed "in keeping this house tidy" and being able to help and use time purposefully.

Equally important as normalization activities are service activities (see Chapter 9). Being able to focus on helping someone in need of one's service and assistance enables residents to experience being valued and appreciated.

As the resident with dementia becomes more confused about daily living and experiences decreased awareness, reality orientation should be used sparingly or not at all. This method of orientation communicates a focus on "real" information about events, time, places, and people. Residents are corrected if their "reality" is faulty. This approach can lead to escalated anxiety and aggression because the resident often becomes embarrassed and frustrated.

The key is in knowing the needs and memory recall of the residents. Communication with residents should allow dignity and promote self-esteem. One method is to use what can be called a "therapeutic fib." For example:

> Fred's perceived basis of reality is back in time when he
> managed a candy factory. He does not understand that he is
> now in an Illinois nursing home; in fact, he thinks the nurs-
> ing staff are his employees. He will approach a staffperson,
> excited and anxious, wanting to know if the shipment has
> gone to Michigan. Rather than explaining to Fred that he
> now is retired and lives in a nursing home, the staff respond
> with, "Fred, the shipment has been sent." He then will go
> on his way, satisfied that his company is doing a good job
> and that he is a successful businessman.

However, a therapeutic fib may not always be a wise intervention to use.

> Lillian wants to go home. Her anxiety makes bathing an
> upsetting challenge. If the staff say, "Lillian, let's shower
> and wash your hair, your daughter is coming," she does

indeed go willingly into the shower. However, after bathing she will collect her belongings, stuff them into a pillowcase, put on her coat and hat, and stand by the door for hours, waiting for her daughter to take her home. This "therapeutic fib" might have gotten her into the shower, but the price of Lillian's increased anxiety as she waited for her daughter's arrival was not fair to Lillian. Another approach to alleviate bathing fears needs to be tried.

The resident's feelings need to be recognized and not ignored. A hug or softly spoken words will show that you understand, and again will validate the resident as a person of worth. After you have responded to his or her feelings and a change of focus is needed, an activity can be introduced or the resident can be asked to help with something. This distraction technique often helps residents end a sad or angry response to their feelings because they then forget just what the concern was originally. For example, a distraction technique for Lillian as she becomes more anxious standing by the door might be to say, "Traffic is heavy today and your daughter might be late. Why don't you put your warm clothing here on the chair and (if appropriate) we can go to lunch together." Or, "Lillian, I was wrong, I am not sure when your daughter will be here. I am very sorry. Would you like to phone your daughter after lunch? I can help you make the phone call."

Bernie was wedged into Marcia's coat, which was much too small, and he would not give it back, even when offered another coat in exchange. His bony arms hung well below the cuffs and the coat stretched tightly around his shoulders. Marcia was in a rage as she recognized her coat and wanted it back immediately. A staffperson approached him and quietly said, "Bernie, I really like the color of that coat on you, but the sleeves are too short, so why don't you let me have it and I'll lengthen the sleeves." This combination of a "therapeutic fib" and distraction technique allowed Bernie to maintain his dignity, and he was able to make the decision to take the coat off to be "fixed." The staffperson then took Bernie to his own closet, where he selected a coat to wear.

Sometimes, residents' anxiety can lead to socially unacceptable responses. Stripping off clothes or incessant swearing are examples. Feelings often are expressed by residents' verbal or physical behaviors. If appropriate, caregivers may set limits, but usually attempts to intervene with behavior modifications do not work because of residents' inability to learn from an experience or event.

Louis had been a car dealer and always had prided himself on being able to talk easily with customers. As he developed word-finding problems, Louis became more and more agitated. His wife became exhausted and placed him in a nursing home. The nursing home used restraints to prevent his wandering and to hold Louis down when he exhibited aggres-

Alzheimer's Disease: Activity-Focused Care

sive behaviors. Becoming frightened, feeling unaccepted, and having increasing word-finding problems, Louis could only "unlock" swear words as a response to his situation.

Louis's wife then moved him to a nursing home with a trained staff specializing in Alzheimer's care. His vulgar language shocked the residents, families, and even the staff. It was decided to touch Louis gently on the shoulder and to say firmly, "Louis, swear words are not appropriate." Within 2 weeks the swearing stopped. It could have been the result of the verbal clues, but more likely the swearing stopped because Louis felt safe and accepted as part of the group. There continued to be occasions when Louis felt insecure and the swearing would return. Simplifying the environment, increasing the use of touch, and demonstrating acceptance were used as interventions and the swearing would stop again.

Residents often focus on the fact that they do not have any money in their pocket, purse, or wallet. When they have always "paid their way" in the past, not having money is demeaning and troublesome to them. Suggestions for decreasing residents' anxiety over money include

- Assuring them that the meal, the room, and so on, is paid for by insurance
- Creating a facility credit card of appropriate size and shape, with the resident's name and room number
- Having "paid-in-full" letters available with a fill-in-the-blank place for the resident's name (Figure 2-1)

Date:

To:

This letter is your notification that the rent for your apartment has been paid in full for the current month of _____.

Manager

Figure 2-1
Sample of a "paid-in-full" letter to decrease residents' anxiety about money.

- Using the same type of letter when the resident is concerned about not paying for meals, adding that the tip has also been included

BEING INCLUDED: RESPECTED CONNECTEDNESS

Residents also have a need to know. They are especially intuitive of feelings and have more insight into what is going on around them than they often are given credit for. For example, if there has been a death on the caregiving unit, residents often will search for the person who is "missing." They will stop at a doorway to a bedroom and peer in, apparently searching for someone. They will point to the empty chair at the table where the missing person usually sat. If appropriate, residents can be told quietly that their friend has died and that everyone is feeling sad, and then the caregivers can hug and assure the residents that all is well. The residents might continue to point again and again to the empty space, but in time they usually forget and stop. They appear to understand that they have been treated with respect.

The same response can be true when the resident senses that there has been a death of a family member. The family might choose not to share the information, but the resident "feels" the sadness and appears to miss the person who no longer visits or is mentioned in conversation. It is often more appropriate for the family to share the loss with the resident and then reminisce about happy memories.

Similar to residents' need to know is their need to participate in family events, if at all possible. For example:

> George had worked hard all of his life and achieved a number of special recognitions for his inventions. Two years after admission into a nursing home, the honorary fraternity that George had been invited to join in college decided to hold its annual meeting near the facility so they could honor George and his contributions to his field. George's wife was concerned about taking him to the dinner and presentation. George was prone to verbal outbursts and had limited tolerance for staying seated or in one place for any length of time. It was decided that a staffperson would join George and his wife and the three would attempt to attend the dinner in his honor. George's wife brought in his favorite business suit, shirt, tie, and shoes. George beamed after he was dressed and he saw himself in the mirror. The event went well. George was able to shake hands with the guests and murmur appropriate remarks. George enjoyed his dinner. At the time of his award presentation, George and his wife went forward to the stage. With his plaque in one hand, George, standing tall, went to the microphone. He was able to put words together that reflected his delight over receiving the award and graciously thanked everyone. George had indeed "risen" to the occasion, helped along by the familiar peo-

ple by his side, his sense of pride emanating from the apparel he wore, and the validation of his peers. George's wife was thrilled that George was able to participate in this special event of honor.

Josephine's granddaughter's wedding was to take place near the care center where she lived. Josephine's daughter, the mother of the bride, really wanted her to attend but felt that she had to focus her full attention on the bride. The care center's director was asked to bring Josephine to the wedding. It was decided that Josephine's tolerance for being away from the center, coping with crowds, and the overall stimulation of the wedding could be handled if Josephine went to just the wedding, not the reception. This decision was a good one, and the special event was enjoyed by all. Josephine's granddaughter was especially touched, delighted, and thankful that her Grammie shared the wedding ceremony with her.

Lenora's grandson was going to have a small, private wedding ceremony. The reception, however, was a big, fancy affair with a band, sit-down meal, and many family friends. Lenora was taken to the reception by a staffperson. Plans had been well made in advance for the party. Lenora sat at her daughter's table, which was set aside toward the back of the reception hall. This allowed Lenora to get up, walk, or pace undisturbed, in fact not even noticed. Lenora loved the party. Her only concern, which she voiced every 2–3 minutes was, "So honey, who's paying for all this?" Fortunately, she could be easily directed to another subject.

Taking a person with dementia to a special event or a wedding is a complicated decision and certainly is not appropriate for everyone. Again, it challenges the caregivers to understand the resident's psychosocial needs and to support them when appropriate. For more suggestions, see Chapter 13.

Residents with dementia have the same emotional needs as other people. They want to feel that they are accepted and "belong." Staff of day-care centers and nursing homes with specific activity-focused care for persons with dementia usually find that a well-run program will help to create a peer community that supports the residents' psychosocial needs to feel accepted and safe.

COUPLES WITH DEMENTIA: FINDING BALANCE

Finding the most appropriate way to deliver care when a husband and wife both have dementia is a challenge. Safeguarding the personhood of each while promoting their self-esteem is not easy at times.

Care considerations for finding the balance in caring for couples with dementia include the following:

1. *Balance.* Are the husband and wife cared for as spouses? Or, as individuals first and spouses second? This is a tough question, needing help from family members and each of the spouse's life stories. There is no right or wrong answer.

2. *Marriage history.* Study the couple's marriage history. Talk with the family before admission to find out about the marriage history and how it has been affected by the dementia. If the marriage has been stormy for years and continues to be, this will be helpful information in regard to whether being roommates is wise or courting disaster.

3. *LifeStory.* Each person is a person first, and part of a couple second, usually. At times there are spouses who seem to give up their own identity and needs to assist the other. Look at each one's history, especially his or her personality and how he or she coped in the past with difficult situations.

4. *Current abilities and needs.* Each person will require a thorough assessment so the staff are aware of abilities, needs, cognitive level, and physical and psychosocial wellness.

5. *Roommates?* This is often an extremely difficult decision. Again, the couple's history of marriage, past responses of caring for each other, and how the experience of dementia is currently affecting them are important components in the consideration of the efficacy of spouses rooming together on admission. Would being roommates be appropriate, therapeutic, or possibly confrontational? Look at sleep patterns, behavior triggers related to being in the same room or in very close proximity, understanding or lack of understanding of each other's current condition, overall tolerance that will be stressed by the move itself, any sexual issues that may be seen as positives or negatives, amount of hands-on or skilled care needed that might disrupt the other, unhealthy overprotection of one for the other that limits the other's ability to be as independent as possible, and, of course, family needs, concerns, and preference. Intimacy issues of one spouse being forceful and demanding sex requires considering each resident's needs and responses. There are times when sex between spouses works out all right for both, and, just the opposite, times when intimacy leads to the personal rights of one of the spouses being invaded. Another concern is when one of the couple seeks sexual favors with another resident, at times in front of the spouse. This can occur whether the couple is rooming together or not.

6. *Care goals.* What would be the plan of care for each? Can that plan be carried out if the spouses are living together or would that be impossible? Tangled up in this decision are "resident rights" and unwritten, though just as emotional, "couple rights." The couple's sexual activity may be considered during the decision making and goal setting, especially if it appears that one of the spouses is taking advantage of the other or is harmful to the other. There are times when the family supports the behaviors of Mother and Dad, although one of them is not achieving his or her potential. A situation like this is extremely difficult on staff.

7. *Decision time.* Usually the decision as to whether spouses should live together is relatively simple to make when there is a wide gap in their needs and

Alzheimer's Disease: Activity-Focused Care

abilities. When the decision is not as clear, an informed choice is made with input from the couple, their family, and the staff, with the realization that changes may have to be made in the future.

8. *Family support.* Placement of both parents touches the hearts of all who see or hear of this situation. There usually just do not seem to be any simple answers, or any answers at all, to all the decision making that needs to take place as part of the giving of care. Open communications with family members, providing opportunities to listen to their story, and an emphasis on the fact that they are not alone and that the staff are right there as partners can be helpful.

9. *Staff support.* Admission of a husband and wife with dementia to a health care facility may create strong feelings of sadness for the staff. The couple may be loving toward each other or hateful. The staff have to deal with either situation. For example, even though Charles and Elaina roomed separately at different ends of the care center, they spent the day seeking each other. On admission, their "finding" each other was often a negative experience, which was a major part of the reason for having them live separated. Both Charles and Elaina had severe word-finding problems. Several months after admission, they were able to stand face to face, perhaps with their arms around each other, talking intently while not using any comprehensible words. Even though they seemed to understand each other, the staff often felt tremendously sad as they observed the husband and wife. Charles and Elaina continued to room separately, because they appeared to benefit from and need time apart. Staff need special support while caregiving for a husband and wife. The decisions that have to be made can be difficult. At times, staff can be overwhelmed with the seeming unfairness of it all.

Difficulties can be encountered when the couple's marriage has experienced difficulties or has been focused on needs that do not appear to be fair as seen by a facility's caregivers. For example:

> Henry has very mild dementia and feels that he is living in the health care facility to "take care of my wife, Emily." Henry has been Emily's caregiver for a number of years, catering to her to the point that Emily chooses not to do anything for herself. Henry's daughter states that Henry's dad did the same thing for his wife, so Henry has seen this overprotective caring before.
>
> Emily's nursing needs involve assistance with dressing, toileting, bathing, and walking. She has Parkinson's disease and dementia. Emily lives in another part of the facility because of her care requirements. She is "picked up" by her husband each morning after breakfast and spends the rest of the day in his part of the building. Her husband immediately lays her down on his bed, where she spends the day, other than for the meals they share together.

This appears to be a pleasant story, both Emily and Henry seem content, but is it really all that pleasant? Staff were able to get Emily away from Henry for a few mornings and took her to activities such as exercise and music. She appeared to thoroughly enjoy herself. In fact, when her husband was not present, Emily would stand and walk around the activity area. At other times, when the staff would find Emily resting in Henry's bed and ask if she would like to come to activities, Henry would answer for her in the negative. Henry would then resume reading his paper as he sat in his easy chair beside the bed.

The same would be true if Henry and Emily were together in a public place. A compliment or comment made to Emily was always answered by Henry. For example, "Your new sweater is really pretty," comments a staffperson. Henry answers, "She's really sick today, she doesn't feel well at all."

The staff were puzzled. Emily appeared to enjoy activities, could walk, and could speak up independently when Henry was not present. If he was, she reverted to an invalid response. Are her abilities and rights as an individual being upheld? If staff asked Emily to join them for an activity in front of her husband, she would choose to say that she was ill and return to his room. Staff struggled with wanting to impose their goals on Emily for what they thought was her benefit. Was this right or wrong? When Emily was alone, attending activities and enjoying being on her own were also her goals. When Emily was with Henry, the goals changed. Although the staff "contracted" with Henry to share Emily and he signed the contract, he did not honor it. The agreed-on contract stated that Emily would attend morning activities on Monday, Wednesday, and Friday mornings. On other mornings, Henry and Emily could do what they wished. The contract caused staff more anxiety as they attempted to make Henry "live up to the contract." End result? Emily continues to spend the day in Henry's bed while he sits by her side, reading the paper and refusing to attend functions because he wants to care for his wife.

Each person that is part of a couple, as well as the couple itself, requires careful consideration. There are rarely easy answers in this challenging caregiving situation. Hopefully, a balance between the "I" and the "We" can be found that upholds both residents' cognitive, psychosocial, physical, environmental, and spiritual abilities and needs. For example:

> Bessie and Arthur have been married for 64 years. Arthur's cognitive abilities have diminished to a greater degree than Bessie's. Arthur and Bessie's family selected a large double room for them as they entered a nursing home. This allowed for their king-sized bed to be on one side of the room and a couch and visiting area on the other side. For the first year, Bessie and Arthur managed quite well with monitoring and reminders for their activities of daily living. During the second year, Arthur became more confused and required a lot more care. He needed assistance with dressing and toileting. The staff were able to handle the increased caregiving. Problems developed when Arthur began to wander at night, getting in and out of bed several times an hour. He would go over to Bessie's side of the bed and shake her, demanding that she get up and fix him breakfast. Bessie became exhausted but steadfastly refused to be moved away from Arthur. They had shared a bed for 64 years, and Bessie firmly stated that she wanted this arrangement to continue.

Alzheimer's Disease: Activity-Focused Care

The staff tried a "bed-check" under Arthur's side of the mattress. This pressure-sensitive device would set off an alarm whenever Arthur's body left the bed so the staff could come into the room and refocus Arthur away from Bessie by taking him out of the room for a snack. The problem then became one of the alarm awakening Bessie four to six times an hour. Again, Bessie was not able to sleep. Maintenance was called to help rewire the device so the alarm sounded at the nursing desk, rather than in the room. Bessie is now able to sleep. The next problem will be surfacing soon, when Arthur needs skilled care. Will or should Bessie move with him into this care area? Can Bessie's cognitive, physical, and psychosocial abilities be supported in the skilled-care area?

Again the question becomes, can there be a balance between the "I" and the "We"? The interdisciplinary team, involved family members, and, if possible, the residents themselves who share open and honest dialogue with each other have the most success with approaches, interventions, and overall caregiving support for couples with dementia. Questioning whether each resident's fulfillment of personhood is being respected and honored will help to enable a balance of compassionate caring and resident self-actualization.

DEVELOPMENT OF A PSYCHOSOCIAL SUPPORT GROUP FOR RESIDENTS WITH MODERATE IMPAIRMENT*

I feel bad when I forget. I never did before, it just started.
Know what helps? The family room, wonderful place,
everyone there saying "Hi, how are you." It feels like we are
with everybody, you don't feel alone.—Faye

A support group for residents with dementia living in a specific care unit or throughout a nursing home can provide an excellent opportunity to promote psychosocial well-being. The following information on the development, implementation, and observations of a support group for residents with moderate dementia is from the Care Center Support Group at Bethany Methodist Terrace, Morton Grove, Illinois. This group is for mid- to late-stage Alzheimer's residents who are living in a specific care unit.

Objectives

- To promote a positive self-image through validation of residents as they are today and renew their pride in life's accomplishments

*A special thank you to Lisa Storto for her creative planning and participation in this group.

- To encourage cognitive and emotional responses and to identify feelings
- To provide an arena of acceptance for initiating and increasing verbal responses
- To increase the responses, interactions, and meaningful relationships with program peers during the group and afterwards in day-to-day contact
- To decrease dependence on the staffpersons to be major facilitators of the group

Member Selection Criteria

- The resident should be able to express responses verbally without severe word-finding problems that limit interaction with group members.
- The resident's attention span should allow group participation for 25–30 minutes without leaving the meeting area or exhibiting disruptive behaviors or pacing.
- Members should be from the same care unit if there is more than one dementia unit in the facility.
- Permission for participation should be given by a family member.

A group of four to six women from the same caregiving area, within a nursing home, met in a private conference room area. They knew each other by sight, but not by name. The average mental status test score was in the moderate dementia range. The group met every other week for approximately 40 minutes. A small, quiet room, with a table to sit around, was used. The Alzheimer's coordinator and a social worker facilitated the group.

Focus Areas

Three areas were selected as focal points for the objectives: feelings, coping, and relationships. Each group meeting reflected these areas in unique ways, depending on the residents' participation.

Feelings

- Loss or grieving: for parents, friends, home, children, independence, privacy, health
- Depression
- Fears
- Joys and wellness
- Aging
- Forgetfulness

At times, sadness with appropriate tears was expressed. Generally the group was happy and content, and anxiety was not displayed. For example, Jenny showed anger and rage for "all those people" (her father's patients) because her father, a doctor, had died at a young age due to overwork.

Some residents expressed fear that they might "do something wrong" because of memory loss (e.g., "I put things away and I don't remember where").

Pride also was demonstrated. The facilitator asked Alice if there were any other famous people named Alice. She responded, "Not in my house."

Coping

- Dealing with memory loss
- Coping strategies: past and present
- Stress management: past and present

Each resident easily shared her own coping strategies. Susan would open her purse and hunt around within it whenever she was asked a question that she could not answer. She often stated, "The answer must be in here someplace." She used the same coping pattern for finding her name when she was asked to fill out a name tag.

Alice used humor to fill in the time gap as she prepared to respond to a question or game. For example, she exclaimed each time she was to move her game piece, "I chose this white one for purity." The "joke" also helped by giving her the needed clueing to move her piece.

When residents were asked what they did when they could not remember, Faye talked about going into the family room; Esther stated that she preferred to be alone and would go to her bedroom; and Alice said, "I sing," and promptly led the group in singing "You Are My Sunshine."

Relationships

- With self
- With family
- With friends
- With staff

The residents were usually social and friendly. They easily expressed compliments and support to each other. Often, they would hug or reach over and pat each other, always appropriately. They were especially kind and caring when a group member cried or showed sadness. For instance, Jenny said, "You have such pretty hair," as Alice looked in the mirror. In response to Faye's grief about feeling alone, Svea said, "That's not true—I love you."

Implementation

Sessions had a preplanned focus but were very flexible so the discussion could continue as members brought up different subjects or wanted to continue on the current subject.

A familiar greeting and start to each session was used, the same for each session. This ritual gave the needed clueing that the group had begun. The group shook hands and made name tags. As the session ended, the facilitators thanked each member and then stood up and gave them each a hug. The residents then stood and hugged each other.

Name tags were found to be tremendously important because the residents could call each other by name, and because they forgot that they had a tag on, they would beam with delight. Svea was especially touched and often would say, "My name was important in Sweden, but I don't hear it very much anymore."

Sessions were planned around a theme that was used as a springboard to discussion and participation. Sometimes the theme was used in a way that had not been planned. Examples of themes are (1) identification of self, (2) belonging, (3) having fun, (4) feeling useful, and (5) daydreaming (see Appendix 2-1).

Theme Facilitation Plan

1. Welcome: Introduce members; pin on name tags; sing a song, such as "Let Me Call You Sweetheart," if the participants are not relaxed.
2. Theme introduction and implementation
   a. Objectives: Outline goals or projected outcome.
   b. Steps and alternatives: Develop steps to access the theme with various ways to express the same focus or tools to redirect if needed.
3. Enable feelings and responses: Work with the actual moment that the resident is in and able to express. Use this time to enhance program objectives and to promote psychosocial well-being.
4. Appreciation, support, and closure: Each resident is thanked, hugged, and then escorted to the unit's family room.

Various mediums and props were used to support the theme or to encourage conversation. These included pictures, music, poetry, symbols, rituals, slides, videos, foods, objectives, animals, mirrors, and so forth. In addition, families were asked to make a LifeStory Book for the resident (see Chapter 3). Games were used to involve and increase participation in the group because the residents were very comfortable and familiar with activity table games in the family room. The support group's objectives and focus areas could be included and implemented in a game-like structure. See Appendix 2-2 for details on making and using a support group game.

Observations

- Morning support group meetings worked best because residents were usually the most alert and relaxed at that time.
- Having a planned theme with props was important when the group first met; in time, the residents preferred the support group game.
- Name tags pulled the group together and increased residents' participation in response to each other, which decreased the need to rely on the facilitators.
- The residents were capable of giving caring compliments to each other and enjoyed doing so. However, they were very shy and reluctant to receive the compliments from one another. In time, they became more receptive.
- Moods were very contagious. For instance:

> Carol had a tendency to whine about most everything. At times, she would continue during the support group. If she was not distracted and allowed to continue, the other resi-

dents became sad and faultfinding. However, Carol usually responded to the distraction of being asked to set up the game.

- Holding objects in the hands, such as questions written on file cards, game pieces, pictures, and poems, helped to focus the residents' attention.
- Greeting and ending rituals became celebrations.
- Reminiscing was used but at times it led to sadness and increased confusion.

> "Where is my mother? Have you seen my mother? I can't find her," said Svea. This often was stated when the group was reminiscing. The group members were confused by Svea's remarks and became anxious because they did not know how to answer her questions.

- Showing the group pictures alone generally received no more response than, "That's nice."
- If poetry is used, the poem should be very short and a copy in large print should be made for each member to hold while it is being read. Several residents were able to read the poems out loud to the group.
- Visitors, especially family members, disrupted the group. The group was too small for them to sit and observe without distracting their loved one.
- Do not move the conversation too quickly; allow plenty of time for responses. For example:

> Jenny was not able to respond directly to a remark or a question. At times, her reply took a full 5 minutes, and often it did not fit into the conversation. She would say, "When people tell you something and you forget it, it will come back."

- Generally, the use of fantasy, such as talking about taking a trip or how residents would spend a million dollars, did not work.
- Information from the support group could be shared with the staff and family members if it helps to clarify the resident's needs and approaches for support. This information was especially helpful when the resident had displayed increased anxiety or depression. The sessions were taped for study.

The residents in the support group did not know what the word "Alzheimer's" meant. They also were not aware that they were living in a nursing home. They thought that they lived on the same street. They were very much in touch with the embarrassment and concern about their memory problems; however, they did not connect the fact that they lived where they did because of their memory dysfunction.

It would be difficult to measure the carryover benefits of a support group for residents with dementia. Certainly during the group session, the residents were truly enjoying themselves as evidenced by their smiles, remarks, and ability to reach out to each other in loving ways. A group of this type would be especially meaningful for residents with dementia who are integrated throughout a nursing home and do not have the benefit of being with a peer community.

STAFF PERSONHOOD: A STAFF STATEMENT OF RESPECT

Personhood indicators for residents, a bill of rights for residents, psychosocial goals for residents. . . . What about the staff that are expected to deliver care that supports residents with dementia? If staff are expected to support their residents, then the staff also need support and affirmation. "Catching" staff "doing it right" is required. Care centers that do not treat their staff as having value and deserving of support will probably experience difficulty. The staff's psychosocial and personhood needs are as important as those of the residents.

As nursing home services director (1990–1995) for the Rush Alzheimer's Disease Center in Chicago, I worked with nursing assistants throughout the area. The nursing assistants often expressed their likes and dislikes about their working experiences and climate of acceptance. The "Staff Statement of Respect" evolved when they were asked how they would like administration and management to offer support and honor for them as persons and for their work. The comments are exact quotes.

To be involved in decision making

To be listened to

To be informed of changes in a timely way

To have promises carried out—otherwise don't promise

To stop "fixing things that ain't broke" and fix things that are broke

To have opportunities of pride

To receive compliments when appropriate

To have opportunities for growth

To develop team goals—why do we exist

To be involved in monitoring/evaluating performance

To be involved in monitoring/evaluating program

To have as much staff as possible and to have management really try to fill when short and when we are short stop complaining about what has not been done and talk about what has been done

To have regularly scheduled meetings with management

Staff empowerment requires commitment to the thoughts and feelings expressed in the preceding staff statement. All of administration must unite in respecting the nursing assistant, the activity therapist, and all the other hands-on staffpersons if the desired outcome is one of enabling staff to reach their highest potential (see Appendix 2-3). Refer also to Appendix 2-4. Staff who enjoy their work, who honor and respect residents with dementia, and who are honored and respected in return by management are the most efficient and caring facilitators for maintaining residents' personhood and psychosocial well-being.

HEALTH CARE PROVIDER AND STAFF ISSUES

Health care providers and their administrators set the tone of caring within their facility. If choices include the empowerment of staff and honoring them for their dedication and hard work, the care center thrives. The emphasis on the personhood of the residents and all within the facility can almost be "felt" as you walk through the door. Compassionate caring for staff and residents is not easy. At times, the compassion component fluctuates and brings to mind an up and down escalator. Monitoring the commitment to uphold psychosocial well-being can be implemented by using Kitwood and Bredin's (1992) indicators or Bell and Troxel's (1994) bill of rights, or both, as quality indicators. Measuring the outcomes is not an easy task; measuring quality of life has never been. There may be times that the facility's ethics committee and perhaps ombudsman are helpful when discussing difficult situations in which resident rights might be negatively affected or seemingly not upheld.

Ensuring positive outcomes starts with staff sensitivity training. Reading accounts written by persons with dementia, asking family members to tell their story about their loved one's journey into dementia, and doing specific sensitivity exercises with the staff are helpful. For example, each staffperson selects a resident he or she knows well and lists that person's abilities and challenges. The staffperson then goes into the daily living area where that resident lives and pretends to be that resident. The staffperson watches other residents, listens and observes the staff, hears the activities in progress, flinches at the banging doors or piercing door alarm, and takes in the entire scene for 15 minutes. The staff then gather to discuss their feelings and observations from their selected resident's point of view. The staff will have both positive and negative feedback. This simple experience will enable staff to be more sensitive to the needs of their residents.

Another way to help staff see the "total picture" is by requiring each staffperson to select a resident and prepare a comprehensive case study about him or her (see Appendix 2-5). The case study demands that the staffperson seek out staff from other shifts and from various disciplines. The study form is simplified, with questions under each heading that help staff who have difficulty reading or expressing themselves. The information does not have to be written down if it can be remembered. A group of staff peers and administrators are then gathered for the case study presentation. Asking the family members of the selected resident to attend is also suggested. If the staffperson becomes "stuck" during the presentation, a manager is there to help him or her along by asking questions or making comments. Invariably, the staffperson is nervous, but on completion of the case study, he or she is delighted in the outcome. The case study helps staff to pull together all their learning, and they almost always remark that they were surprised that they knew so much. It is a proud moment for all.

SUMMARY

Being valued, included, and supported, and finding the balance of psychosocial wellness and daily life, helps to promote the resident's personhood and actualization of well-being. As they enter the resident's life with compassionate caring, touch, simple words, songs, rituals, and routines, caregivers should learn and use supportive interventions that will enable a dialogue through social interaction. This often "unspoken" dialogue affirms the resident's sense of self and supports his or her longings for optimum emotional well-being. Finding the balance between promoting the resident's independence and offering respect-filled helpfulness is a challenge. Caregiving that upholds the resident's psychosocial well-being is a monumental responsibility.

REFERENCES

Bell V, Troxel D. An Alzheimer's disease bill of rights. Am J Alzheimer's Care Rel Dis Res 1994;9:3–6.
Kitwood T, Bredin K. Towards a theory of dementia care: personhood and well-being. Ageing Soc 1992;12:269–287.

SUGGESTED READING

Doernberg M. Stolen Mind: The Slow Disappearance of Roy Doernberg. Chapel Hill, NC: Algonquin Books of Chapel Hill, 1989.
Lustbader W. Counting on Kindness: The Dilemmas of Dependency. New York: The Free Press, 1991.
Moore T. Care of the Soul: A Guide for Cultivating Depth and Sacredness in Everyday Life. New York: Harper Collins, 1992.
Nouwen HJM. The Road to Daybreak. New York: Doubleday, 1988.
Rose L. Show Me the Way to Go Home. San Francisco: Elder Books, 1996.
Sabat SR, Harre R. The construction and deconstruction of self in Alzheimer's disease. Ageing Soc 1992;12:443–461.
Sacks O. A neurologist's perspective on the aging brain. Arch Neurol 1997;54:1211–1214.

Alzheimer's Disease: Activity-Focused Care

A2-1
Dementia Support Group Theme Facilitation Plan Example

THEME TITLE: IDENTIFICATION OF SELF

I. The gathering and welcome
  A. Tell residents about the group after breakfast.
  B. Have a room ready for 10 A.M.
  C. Gather the residents at 9:50 A.M. and bring them to the meeting room.
  D. Welcome residents with handshakes and expressions of pleasure that they are in the group or club.
II. Theme introduction and implementation
  A. Objectives
    1. Comfort and self-acceptance
    2. "Naming the self" or reality
    3. Value of naming; being "chosen" by being named
    4. Recognition of name changes through role changes (e.g., wife, mother, husband, father)
    5. How these names are different, how they are the same, positives and negatives
  B. Materials, equipment, and props
    1. Crayons, markers, paper
    2. Plastic name-tag holders
    3. Scrabble (Milton Bradley Company, Springfield, MA) letters or plastic letters
    4. Magnetic letters and a board
    5. Magazine cutout letters
    6. Words written on cards (e.g., *mother, wife, daughter, friend*)
    7. Hand-held mirror
III. Here and now: questions, feelings, and responses
  A. How was your name chosen?

B. Did a previous family member have it? Did you know her? Like her?

C. Do you have a nickname? What is it? Do you like it?

D. What is your maiden name? How did you feel about "losing" that name?

E. What is the ethnic, cultural, or religious significance of your name? Is it special, common?

F. What name do you like to use now? For example, Mrs. Jones or Sally?

G. How do you feel about your name when I say your name this way (say the name sternly, loudly, softly, questioningly, etc.)?

IV. Implementation of the theme

A. Use conversation, questions, and statements.

B. Residents should write out names for name tags and put them on.

C. Have letters available for making names.

D. Put names on file cards and have roles written on file cards that the residents can select.

E. Use the mirror and pass to each resident so she can see herself, if she chooses, and talk about her name.

F. Have single plastic, wooden, or paper letters available for selection in spelling out residents' names.

G. Use 3×3-in. sturdy paper or cut-up file cards and spell out all the residents' names by placing one letter on each square. End the session by inviting the residents to gather the individual letters needed to spell their name. Take the longest name, and lay out the letters side-by-side. As in the game Scrabble, the other residents each take a turn attaching their name by using a shared letter with another name spelled out or using a blank card to "attach" their name to the group.

V. Appreciation, support, and closure

A. Gather materials.

B. Collect name tags.

C. Thank and hug each resident for coming to the group.

D. Remind residents that "we will meet again."

E. Escort residents back to their unit.

VI. Observations and evaluation

A2-2
*Support Group Game**

The objective is to use carefully selected questions in a support group game as a safe arena to encourage residents' expression of feelings, concerns, joys, and coping skills. The group's facilitator uses residents' responses to validate the players, promote self-esteem, and encourage interaction between group members to increase meaningful relationships with peers.

Nursing home residents with dementia respond enthusiastically to table games. Adapted games often are used in small group activities. The residents selected for a support group game would require a sufficient attention span to sit down and play the game. The length of time can vary. It is important to select residents with similar verbal abilities and social awareness.

In the support group game, each player is given a game piece to move around a drawn daisy petal with dots on each petal. Color the dots on the petal to match each game piece. Using large dice with numbers one to three, the players take turns rolling the dice, moving their piece, taking and reading a card or having it read to them, and responding to the question on the card. There is no "winning" because the movement is just either way around the petal, so there is no right or wrong, just as there are no right or wrong answers.

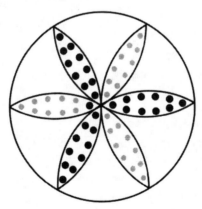

The support group game involves making cards (such as index cards) with questions in clear, dark print. Place the cards face down so they can be drawn. Having the residents hold their cards while answering helps to elicit a cognitive response.

---

*Adapted from UNGAME, Talicor, Inc., Brea, California.

The ability to answer also is increased when the needed response is at the end of the question.

The game can be made any size. A piece of oilcloth or plastic tablecloth can be used and then rolled for storage.

The following are suggestions for questions. By knowing your group, you can be creative and make your own questions.

Complete these statements:

- If I were free like a butterfly I would. . . .
- If I were sad like a lost puppy I would. . . .
- Being loved makes me feel. . . .
- Being alone makes me feel. . . .
- I cannot remember, and it makes me feel. . . .
- I love myself because I. . . .
- I wish I were 10 years old because. . . .
- I like to have friends because. . . .
- Sometimes I feel. . . .

A2-3
Staff
Empowerment
Considerations

Hands-on staffpersons are the backbone and essential component for the successful delivery of care to persons with dementia. Administration and management must offer staff respect and fairness. The following are considerations and suggestions for enabling the staff's skills, creativity, and holistic well-being.

1. Identify staff strengths and interests, then schedule an opportunity for them to use their skills. Ask the staffperson to identify the personal role model that led him or her to be who he or she is. Find common threads from the role model that the staffperson reflects today. Provide opportunities for the staffperson to build and expand on these strengths.

2. Study the current nursing assistant job description. Does it have room for creativity and opportunities for team interconnection and participation? Is there support for the nursing assistant to provide a holistic approach to resident care? If so, consider calling the nursing assistants *resident living assistants* (RLAs).

3. Create a job description that cross-trains staff so they can assist each other. For example, nursing assistants can be trained to implement and participate in activities.

4. Train staff on how to interact with family members. It is often taken for granted that staff have these skills, when indeed they can experience difficulties.

5. Provide ongoing educational opportunities on subjects that the RLAs select, using a variety of teaching and learning opportunities based on information with immediate application. Staff are more interested in skills than in principles.

6. Position an RLA as a team leader to run meetings, contribute to the training, and so forth.

7. Develop a mentoring system for new staff. Have each staffperson sign up to "teach" the new staffperson a skill that reflects his or her personal identified strength. For example, if Mary is especially capable of helping difficult residents to bathe, then Mary will demonstrate this skill to the new staffperson.

8. Understand why people fail, and develop approaches for thwarting failure. Reasons staff fail may include not understanding what is required, not being given a reason for doing what they are asked to do that makes sense to them, or not being asked for their opinion.

9. Involve RLAs or other hands-on staff in interviews of potential staffpersons.

10. Use RLAs to develop standards of caregiving. For example:

- Distraction and other interventions will be used to refocus residents' unwanted behaviors as soon as the behavior is noticed rather than waiting for its escalation.
- The resident's abilities will be considered and encouraged by active involvement in all aspects of care.
- Timing of caregiving activities will be considered in relationship with the resident's mood.

11. Staff will be major contributors to resident care conferences (see Appendix 5-3).

12. Have the RLAs and other hands-on staff evaluate their manager.

13. Use hands-on staff for all tours of the facility, both for professional visitors and family members inquiring about placement for their loved ones.

14. Recognize staff for their accomplishments, formally and informally.

15. Staff are treasures—treat them as such. Train them and position them as experts. Cultivate a relationship with staffpersons. Managers should be coaches, stewards, mentors, and designers. Empowerment is not something managers "give" to the staff; it comes from the staff themselves, from within.

A2-4
Administrators Walk in Assistants' Shoes *

Administration staff at The Wealshire Alzheimer's care facility in Lincolnshire, Illinois, were given an opportunity to "walk in the shoes" of their nursing assistants through an innovative program. Nursing assistants are dedicated staffpersons, the "heart and soul" of The Wealshire, and are called *resident living assistants* (RLAs). During the "RLA for the Day" program, 14 managers experienced firsthand the many facets of an RLA's job, one that calls for providing compassionate, hands-on care.

The managers' objectives for RLA for the Day were to gain sensitivity, insight, and knowledge into the RLA's role and involvement in all aspects of resident caregiving. The program was also an opportunity to offer personal respect to The Wealshire nursing assistants, supporting them as valuable team members. Managers expressed their interest in learning how the RLAs interacted with other disciplines and how they organized themselves to accomplish their many duties. "I want to learn caregiving skills so I can be more helpful," stated one manager.

The RLAs demonstrated how patience and understanding are the basis for their caregiving success. The managers were impressed that RLAs really knew each resident's likes, dislikes, and what it takes to involve the resident in daily life care activities. Assisting with showers, dressing, and toileting; helping with meals; and walking with restless residents took place throughout the day. Management rotated to various households at The Wealshire so they could join RLAs to work with residents with mild, moderate, and advanced dementia as well as those needing skilled healthcare. Each participant in the program interacted with residents receptive to care as well as those who resisted. Experiences ranged from delight in helping a frail resident walk to "wearing" a bowl of tossed oatmeal.

Benefits from the program have already been seen. During one icy morning when some of the RLAs traveling a long distance were late to arrive, managers, fresh from their RLA experiences, comfortably helped to serve, assist, and enable residents to enjoy their breakfast.

---

*Thanks to The Wealshire, Lincolnshire, Illinois, an Alzheimer's facility serving residents with a continuum of care.

The uniqueness of the RLA for the Day program reflects The Wealshire's philosophy of teamwork and respect, not only for the residents, but for all staffpersons. Where else could you find the chief financial officer, an administrative assistant, the director of housekeeping, or a nursing home's president, for example, actively engaged and wanting to learn from nursing assistants?

"I will be more sensitive to the RLAs' needs, feelings, and expectations from me as a supervisor," stated one manager after the program. Jennifer Loughney, director of operations at The Wealshire, wrote in her evaluation of RLA for the Day, "I have a better understanding and appreciation for all the RLAs, their work, and how important they are to the success of The Wealshire's mission supporting a quality of life for our residents."

A2-5
Form for Resident Case Study

Nursing home staff receiving training in caregiving of residents with dementia could be invited to prepare a case study of a resident on completion of their formal classes. The case study's objectives include empowering the staff's abilities to make choices, promoting problem-solving techniques, supporting creative caregiving skills, and providing staff with opportunities to experience pride in their accomplishments. A resident is selected by the staffperson to study and present to caregiving colleagues. The individual needs of the staffperson related to his or her reading, writing, and speaking abilities are taken into consideration. For example, a brief outline or notes under each heading may be used as long as the staffperson has the needed information to share orally.

The case study components are key areas derived from training modules, each containing detailed questions to trigger observations, approaches, and interventions. The areas transcend specific disciplines, so each staffperson must engage other caregivers for their insights, ideas, and experiences with the resident. Family members become involved as staff turn to them for background and current information. The summary includes goal setting as well as the opportunity to reflect on what the resident has "taught" the staffperson personally and what effect this has had on the staffperson's caregiving approaches and interventions.

Administrative, nursing, social services, activities, rehabilitation services, dietary, pastoral care, housekeeping, and maintenance staff find that preparing a case study helps them to focus on the resident's abilities. As members of the staff team, caregivers experience an increased willingness to be flexible and creative as they develop ways to refocus difficult behaviors and situations. Presentation of the case study to the caregiving staff team members offers the staffperson increased self-confidence, pride, and a sense of fulfillment.

The following is an example of a form used for a resident case study. The form has been reduced for publication; when using, leave spaces under each heading for the staffperson's remarks and notes.

CASE STUDY

Date: _____

Resident's name: _____ Age: _____ Admission: _____

Diagnosis: _____

Medications: _____

Cognitive Ability and Awareness
How does the resident respond to you? To surroundings? Can he or she follow one-step commands? Two-step? Does the resident know his or her name? Where his or her room is? Can the resident find the family room on his or her own? Can he or she perform a simple task? How is the resident's attention span? Does he or she use things appropriately? Does he or she appear alert? How can you give the resident clueing to help make him or her more aware and responsive? How does the resident feel about himself or herself? What expressions of intimacy does the resident use or respond to?

Activities of Daily Living
Can the resident perform any of his or her own hygiene? Brush teeth? Dress? Comb hair? Does the resident care what he or she looks like? How does the resident respond to care? Do you use clueing? What approaches from you are best? What does not work? What behaviors affect activities of daily living (ADLs)? If the resident dresses himself or herself, is it appropriate? How can you help him or her to be more independent in ADLs?

Eating and Feeding
Can the resident feed himself or herself? Does he or she eat well? Poorly? How do you set up the tray? Does the resident eat quickly? Slowly? Does he or she chew food carefully? Is he or she prone to choking? What behaviors affect eating? What can you do to help the resident eat more and be more independent?

Bowel and Bladder
Can the resident toilet himself or herself? Wipe himself or herself? Respond to clueing? Is he or she incontinent? What behavioral problems affect bowel and bladder functions? Does the resident give clues when he or she wants to go to the bathroom? Does he or she toilet in appropriate places? What can you do to help the resident use the toilet at appropriate times and places?

Behaviors and Staff Interaction
What are the positive and negative behaviors of your resident? Does he or she respond to touch? Is he or she loving? Happy? Sad? Depressed? Agitated? Anxious? Restless? Wandering? Pacing? Prone to outbursts? Combative? Prone to inappropriate sexual behavior? Paranoid? What do you do when a negative behavior is a problem? How do you encourage positive behaviors? Does the resident have mood swings? Why? How can you interact with the resident to help promote positive behaviors?

Mobility

Can the resident walk alone? With an assist? Not at all? Why? Does he or she walk safely? Bump into things? Sit correctly and safely? How much walking does he or she do? Too much? Too little? How about upper body movement? How can you help the resident maintain mobility?

Safety Risks

Is the resident a safety problem? Why? What can you do about it? Might the resident harm himself or herself? Other residents? You? Does he or she go off the unit unsupervised? What suggestions do you have to help keep the resident safe?

Activities Participation

Is the resident involved with activities? Large groups? Small groups? One to one? Which is best to encourage response and participation? How is his or her attention span during activities? Does the resident respond well to the staff? To the other residents? Can the resident sit quietly by himself or herself? Do tasks or activities independently? How can you involve your resident more in activities?

Speech and Communications

Is the resident's speech clear? Does he or she make sense? Use correct words? How do you encourage a response? Does he or she respond to nonverbal speech? Can you understand his or her nonverbal speech? What suggestions do you have to encourage speech and communications?

Relationships with Other Residents

Does the resident respond to others positively? Negatively? Does he or she ignore others? Have a friend? Appear happy with others? Unhappy with others?

Relationships with Staff

How does the resident respond to you? What can you do to encourage positive feelings toward staff? Decrease negative responses?

Family Support and Response

How does the resident respond to his or her family? How do they respond to him or her? Is the family realistic? Demanding? Helpful? How can you help the family cope with their loved one's dementia?

Conclusion and Goals

How is the program affecting your resident? What needs changing? How? What is going well and needs to be maintained? What goal can you set to reach in the next month with the resident? Within the next 3 months? How are you going to accomplish these goals? Is there any other information about your resident that you wish to share?

What have you learned by doing this case study? How has it helped you in your work caring for persons with dementia?

Name: _____ Position: _____

3

LifeStory Book: LifePreserver for LifeAffirmation

A LifeStory Book is a personal history of the past, a book of precious memories, a kaleidoscope of treasured friends and family, and a LifePreserver enveloping oneself with safe and nurturing wellness.

The LifeStory Book becomes not only a bridge to the past, but a connection to the present. It is in the bringing of the resident's former life roles and experiences forward, into the milieu of day-to-day care, that the links of the connection are strengthened. Each resident journeys through the experience of dementia in his or her unique way. This uniqueness may well be determined by the resident's "bridges" from the past, the connections he or she made throughout life between his or her experiences and himself or herself and others.

The LifeStory Book's multiple uses can vary from a distraction technique for refocusing difficult behaviors to a tool for enabling a sense of security when taken to the hospital or other "scary" or unfamiliar places. The book can be used, for example, in a one-to-one relationship, to establish "membership" in a club of peers, or for the resident's self-initiated "show-and-tell."

There are no rules for making a LifeStory Book or determining its contents. A book can be a handsome, computer-generated masterpiece or perhaps a collection of crinkled photographs taped on paper and stuffed in a folder. If the book is too "special," however (e.g., holds prized photographs or looks too expensive), it may be put on a shelf and used just for special occasions. Regardless of the format or quality of a LifeStory Book, the goals are the same. A LifeStory Book is to be used often, offering residents with dementia the gift of personal affirmation.

LIFESTORY BOOK INDICATORS: LIFEAFFIRMATION

Life is affirmed and validated when the feeling of positive connectedness with self and others occurs. The resident's emotional memory and memories from the past are usually retained long into the progression of dementia. Therefore, the goals of the LifeStory Book as indicators of the resident's LifeAffirmation include the following:

- Emotional support and security, plus a tool, if needed, for refocusing mood and difficult behaviors
- Promotion of holistic well-being, validation of life's journey, celebration of one's uniqueness, and a encouragement of reminiscing

- Opportunities for pride: adapting a LifeStory for focusing on today's abilities, not difficulties, and for enhancing self-esteem
- A look at personal history for connecting to today and the present precious moment (e.g., family background, traditions, customs, work experiences, hobbies, educational background)
- A frame of reference for daily living (e.g., personalization of care, overall living style, dressing preferences, favorite foods, tasks performed at work or home)
- Encouragement for meaningful activity and shared connections (e.g., enabling focus, increasing attention span, prompting verbal and nonverbal exchanges, promoting sequencing abilities, creating possibilities for a good laugh, increasing socialization opportunities and skills)
- Extends an invitation to family members and caregivers to nurture and hold the treasures of the resident's personal past throughout the Alzheimer's journey into the unknown

LIFESTORY BOOK: CONTRAINDICATIONS FOR USE

When is a LifeStory Book not appropriate to use? Residents experiencing a profound sense of loss might respond to their book with increased grieving and demonstration of depression. For example:

> Emily is unable to remember what she had for lunch today. But she has a keen memory of her wonderful marriage and shared years with her late husband, Alan. She has the tendency to stay focused on a subject, especially when it contains emotional aspects. Therefore, Emily can become transfixed on her loss and sadness over her husband's death. Just seeing pictures of Alan can facilitate 2- to 5-day periods of depression and agitation. Having family pictures in her LifeStory Book would have provoked these emotional moods even though she had appropriately grieved his loss 14 years ago. Emily's daughter realized the difficulties and sadness that a typical LifeStory Book would inspire. She decided to make a book featuring pictures of Emily and herself involved in pleasant activities at the health care facility where her mother now lives. Also included were pictures of Emily's new friends and favorite staffpersons. Affirmation and opportunities for reminiscing can still occur as the book is shared with friends and family.

A resident focused on looking for his or her mother, for example, can be distressed if her picture is included in the book. This possible response needs to be assessed because there are certainly times when having a picture of a loved one who has died with the dates of his or her life or a simple statement, such as "Mother passed away in the winter of 1973," can close the loop of searching and provide the resident with peace.

Any significant loss that fosters anxiousness, fearfulness, oppressive sadness, or could be the possible trigger of current phobias needs to be considered when using the LifeStory Book as a therapeutic modality. It is not just the loss of loved ones that may precipitate emotional distress. Other examples could include a favorite car that triggers a reminder that driving is no longer an option; a picture of work or coworkers that reminds the resident of premature retirement; or a beautiful holiday meal that reminds the resident that she can no longer prepare elaborate meals or use her gift of hospitality.

Family members or persons pictured in a LifeStory Book that may cause the resident to experience a response of anger, paranoia, suspiciousness, or blaming would be best deleted from the book. For example, the daughter who "has all my money," the son who "took my car," or the husband "who abused me." The timing for the anger or ill feeling may vary. The person that becomes the object of the anger one week might be a "good guy" the next week. If the feelings of anger are persistent, then remove the offending pages or pictures. Reintroducing them into the book at another time might work or it might not. Watch the resident for nonverbal displays of negative feelings and verbal responses.

The resident may experience or react to the book in a variety of ways that change from day to day or moment to moment. Caregivers are challenged to be aware of the resident's mood, needs, and ability to receive comfort when the book is used.

BOOK FORMAT SUGGESTIONS

LifeStory Books can be created in many different styles and formats. Books that are pleasing to the eye; can be dropped without falling apart; and have sturdy pages that will withstand pulling, tugging, and multiple page turnings are suggested. For example, a three-ring binder that uses file folders cut into pages or thick paper, often called *card stock*, is usually durable. The binder also allows pages to be added throughout the years. Page or sheet protectors can be used, but they often reflect light and cause a glare, making the contents difficult to see or read. Books that are "too" pretty, expensive looking, or fragile in construction will often be put up on a shelf and seldom used.

Favorite color or black and white photographs can be used. If photographs are one of a kind, the pictures should be photocopied by a good copier to retain their color and clearness. Drawings, maps, clippings, brochures, and just about anything that will affix to the book page can be used. Families should not part with treasured pictures, certificates, or mementos because there is a high risk that they could get lost or abused during the use of the book.

Residents seem to be able to read long into their journey of dementia. Therefore, phrases and captions under each picture or item in the LifeStory Book can be read by the resident or, if needed, by the caregiver. Large and dark lettering that is neatly done is recommended. Books appear to be the most meaningful when they are written in the first person (i.e., from the resident's point of view). For example, "I love my grandchildren, Caitlin, Nicholas, and Elizabeth."

Actually, a book is not the only option for connecting the resident with his or her life story. Other formats can include a video, posters, bulletin-board displays, multiple wall pictures, pictures and captions glued on large file cards and placed on a ring for easy access to each card, and mementos that have their "story" attached. Another option is a life story memory box of items from the past that have meaning. The family could identify the items and their significance by providing a listing inside the box lid.

LIFEAFFIRMATION: BOOK CONTENT RECOMMENDATIONS

Families are urged to be creative with their loved one's LifeStory Book. A letter to families that lists the many possible categories that can be included in the book is in Appendix 3-1. The best topics are the ones to which the resident would have the most positive response. These would probably include key life events, family members, places lived, work history, and favorite holidays. The book can start or stop during any period of the resident's life history. The choice may be dictated by the accessibility to pictures and knowledge that the family has of the resident.

> When Harry went to make his mother's LifeStory Book, he found that all her pictures and personal mementos had been thrown out by another family member who was not able to deal with his mother moving into a care center. Harry was very disappointed. He decided to switch the focus and make a LifeStory Book about himself, his work, family, and friends. He labeled the pictures from his mother's viewpoint. For example, "This is my son, Harry, coaching his son's soccer team in Chicago. George, my husband, was Harry's coach when Harry was a youngster." Harry's mother was still able to make connections to her past, through her son's pictures and story.

FAMILY SUGGESTIONS AND QUALITY INVOLVEMENT

The LifeStory Book has different meanings for each family. For some, it is a joy to create and provides a sense of being able to make a real gift to their loved one. The book can bring forth treasured memories and provide an opportunity to honor their family member. Collecting the pictures, writing down the oral history, and focusing on positive experiences can help make the book a caring gift of memories as the involved family members put the book together. Families with a number of siblings may find that it brings them together to make the experience one of healing family relationships.

For others, Alzheimer's disease is a journey into sadness and the book is never made. Family members should not be made to feel that they must make a book, because when they do not, their guilt compounds the difficulties they are already experiencing.

The LifeStory Book also connects the family to the staff and the care facility that makes the book an integral part of its program. It lets the family know that the staff really want to learn about their loved one's life experiences. The book becomes a symbol of the desired partnership.

Staff may need to offer family members assistance in using the LifeStory Book. For example, using the book to "test" their mother's memory of all her grandchildren's names is not appropriate. A book club might invite family members to attend so they can observe interaction between staff and residents that offers validation and honor to residents through their life story. Using the book's pictures and contents to validate the resident's past and current times can help families be more accepting of the challenge and struggle their loved one is experiencing.

For the family, the book can become a symbol of the wonderful person their loved one was before dementia took its toll, making changes that are often devastating for the family to accept. Families generally want staff to know the wonderful person their loved one was before changes from dementia.

GUIDELINES FOR STAFF USE OF BOOKS

Staff also need training on how and when to use a LifeStory Book. The overall goal for staff is increased sensitivity and understanding as they learn about the resident's life history and the ability to apply the information to the current caregiving experience.

Guidelines include the following:

1. Find the components of the resident's past that are still present, abilities that can be brought out into the current day's caregiving approaches and programs.
2. "Look" at the resident through his or her life story and find a deepening of acceptance for today's care challenges or difficulties.

> Jennifer was not able to control her bladder due to a physical problem. Her dementia made the situation more difficult because Jennifer could not figure out how to use an incontinence product independently. She was a very proud, cultured woman, and the problem of dribbling urine was overwhelming for her. She needed to have a shower daily because of the urine, but Jennifer would not let the staff near her. The care coordinator met with the nursing assistants to discuss the best way to help Jennifer with her problem while allowing her to maintain dignity. Jennifer's LifeStory Book was reviewed at the start of the staff meeting. The staff looked at the pictures and saw the lovely, self-confident woman she was throughout the years. Jennifer's husband had died many years ago, and she was able to raise three sons by entering the teaching profession. Jennifer's incontinence and her bathing challenge were then reviewed. The staff discussed several ideas. A nursing assistant then said, "Since Jennifer was and is today such a proud, private woman, could we 'contract' with her about our need to help her bathe on a regular basis and for the assistance she needs for toileting?" The staff wrote up a simple contract consisting of times for assistance and what would happen. The

contract was taken to Jennifer by the staff, and she made a few revisions and signed it. Jennifer was able to honor the contract when it was mentioned by the staffperson offering her assistance. Jennifer's LifeStory Book had "set the stage" for an excellent caregiving intervention that preserved her psychosocial well-being.

3. Use the LifeStory Book to distract the resident when there are difficult behaviors that need refocusing or moods that might respond to positive input, calling forth the resident by offering him or her validation as a person of worth.

> Joe became anxious late in the afternoon. It appeared that he was relating to his years at work and was worried that he would not be able to complete what he needed to do before the end of the day. Joe would start to pace, push against the door to leave, and become verbally angry with anyone in his way. The staff would open his LifeStory Book to the pictures of Joe all dressed up at his retirement party. At first, staff would have to walk alongside Joe as he paced, but when they would say, "Joe, look at you on retirement day, you were so handsome in that suit," Joe would start to relax. In time, Joe would sit down with the staffperson, have a cup of tea, and enjoy looking at his book. His anxious behaviors had been refocused by using his book to validate his past life experiences at work.

4. Use the book as a basis for assessment when determining approaches and care interventions. For example, the selection of a meaningful activity, the hair or clothing style preferred, the possible items or experiences the resident could relate to and, if needed, used as a distraction technique.
5. Use the book when developing the resident's case study (see Appendix 2-5).
6. Enable the resident to have easy access to his or her LifeStory Book instead of putting it away in a closet or bureau drawer.
7. Be sensitive to the resident's experience looking at his or her LifeStory Book and be watchful for any negative or hurtful responses.
8. Always empower the resident to "own his or her life's story" by asking permission to see the book.

HEALTH CARE PROVIDER AND STAFF ISSUES

"Where shall the books be kept? How can we protect them so they do not get lost?" These sound like simple questions, but the answers are not always that easy. A safe, but easily accessible place is needed. Being able to find the book quickly is often needed when the purpose of its use is refocusing behaviors. Families should realize that if one-of-a-kind pictures have been included in the book, they are taking the risk that the pictures might be lost or destroyed in some way. The bottom line is that the book should be used, not just put away to look at occasionally.

Staff can play an important role in making up books for residents who do not have family members or for whom the family is not going to create a book. It is important for the staff not to judge the family that does not make a book. Staff may not know or understand the dynamics of the resident's and family's relationship. If the resident does have a family, it is suggested that the staff tell them that they wish to make the resident a book and, if needed, seek their permission. The resident's story, therefore, may start from the time of his or her admission. Staff can gather pictures of events at the care center plus find pictures that reflect information in the social history. For example, if Phillip loves the garden in the summer, his book could be multiple pictures from a seed catalog with the names of the flowers labeled. The caption could say, "I love spring flowers, especially these bright yellow daffodils."

Confidentiality is also a staff issue. If the family has made the book and given it to staff to use, this information should be sharable. If the facility is concerned, the family could sign a permission-for-use form. If made by staff, the book should reflect information that is general knowledge, personal to the point that it reflects the resident's interests and abilities, but not so personal that it includes information that the family has not shared openly with the staff. If there is any question at all, the contents of the book can be reviewed with the family to receive their consent.

The bottom line is to have the LifeStory Book easily available and ready to use. Equally important is to have staff trained to understand the book's value and to use it appropriately to connect with the resident.

SUMMARY

A LifeStory Book's photographs, mementos, and words create a network of caring that surrounds the resident with dementia. The book can indeed be a LifePreserver for LifeAffirmation. The LifeStory Book, honoring the resident's past life activities of great meaningfulness, creates a framework for caregivers extending respect via activity-focused care. Connections are made with the joys of the past as they bring respect to today. Family members, friends, staff, and the residents themselves find in the book experiences of love, comfort, honor, security, and pride. The LifeStory Book extends the warm invitation to all persons to come together for the celebration of the resident's unique life gifts.

SUGGESTED READING

Bell V, Troxel D. The Best Friends Approach to Alzheimer's Care. Baltimore: Health Professions Press, 1997.

Kiernat J. The use of life review activity with confused nursing home residents. Am J Occup Ther 1979;33:306–310.

Kitwood T, Bredin K. Towards a theory of dementia care: personhood and wellbeing. Ageing Soc 1992;12:269–287.

Rose L. Show Me the Way to Go Home. Forest Knolls, CA: Elder Books, 1996.

Sheridan C. Reminiscence: Uncovering a Lifetime of Memories. San Francisco: Elder Press, 1991.

Zgola J. Doing Things: A Guide to Programming for Persons with Alzheimer's Disease and Related Disorders. Baltimore: Johns Hopkins University Press, 1987.

A3-1
LifeStory Book Letter to Families

The Wealshire
150 Jamestown Lane
Lincolnshire, IL 60069

January 1, 1999

Dear Family Member:

The Wealshire is asking for your assistance. As we seek partnership with you in caregiving for your loved one, we wish to know his or her life story. As you know, the person with dementia often lives in the past, in the "world of work." These years often represent a period filled with pride and meaningful experiences, many of which are retained as memories. The Wealshire staff wish to have the opportunity to learn as much as we can about residents' pasts so we can use the information as a basis of our approach to therapeutic caregiving. A LifeStory Book offers the staff insights into likes, dislikes, past interests, and names of key persons and family members. The life story information is then adapted for daily life interests and activities and provides residents with opportunities for companionship and reminiscing. The book can be used to help with the transition from home to The Wealshire because the staff will quickly "know" the new resident and be more able to build a relationship based on memories shared.

Caregiving at The Wealshire focuses on residents' abilities. Often, these abilities are enabled and strengthened with information from residents' LifeStory Books. We hope that you will consider making a book for your loved one.

Making a LifeStory Book
A LifeStory Book can be made from photograph albums, notebooks, or any durable booklet. We at The Wealshire suggest using a three-ring binder notebook so pages can be added at any time. Using thick, stiff paper or cutting up file folders for paper provides a sturdy page that will survive constant handling. Drawings, writings, pictures, maps, and so forth can be used. If you wish to include precious photographs, please photocopy them and keep the originals, placing the copies in the book. Persons with dementia can read for many years, so please write information in short sentences or phrases. Placing names under photographs is especially important. Use a dark pen, printing the words clearly and in large print.

LifeStory Contents Suggestions

1. Genealogy
   - Nationality, heritage, birth dates, family tree, siblings and their relationship to the resident
   - Use short phrases to note important memories about the family
2. Religion and spirituality
   - Background, interests in organized religion
   - Faith community: pictures of outside and inside the building, and inside the sanctuary
   - Current participation information, perhaps a worship bulletin
   - Use of or response to ritual, traditions, blessings, and prayers
   - Prayers used with their children (e.g., meal blessings or nighttime prayers)
   - Favorite songs and hymns, including both words and music
3. Personality
   - Happy? Liked people? Joker? Favorite joke?
   - Responses to others
   - Responses to life roles (e.g., father, mother, daughter, aunt)
   - General mood description
   - Where did the resident's name come from? Was it liked? Disliked? Any nicknames?
4. Childhood
   - Relationships with brothers, sisters, parents
   - Description of bedroom and childhood house, any moves
   - Schooltime memories (e.g., first day of school)
   - Friends and clubs
   - First kiss
   - Summer activities and vacations
   - Work history during the school years
   - Memories of parents, grandparents, aunts, uncles, and cousins
5. Education
   - Grade completed, kind of school, school names, degrees
   - Favorite subject, most disliked subject, extracurricular events, teams, clubs, etc.
   - Ongoing education via travel? Elderhostels?
6. Key life events
   - Dates (years) and description of events, for example:
     Graduations
     Marriage, children, grandchildren
     First home
     First car
     Deaths of family members, close friends, etc.
7. Places lived
   - Description of places lived, perhaps using a map. Liked or not liked? Why? Talk about specific rooms, the outside grounds, distances from school, shopping, etc. Use pictures if possible.
8. Close friends, neighbors
   - Was the resident a helper with others?
   - Names and attributes of best friends

Alzheimer's Disease: Activity-Focused Care

- Did the resident have special friends for sharing travels or vacation time?
9. Work history
   - First job, salary, travel, etc.
   - Memory of how that first dollar was spent?
   - At home, in the marketplace—worked alone, with others?
   - Specific kinds of work? What did resident like? Not like?
   - Depression-era memories? Effects on family?
   - Retirement information
10. Military history
    - Military history of the resident, significant family members
    - Memories of war, rationing
    - Where was the resident on key days (e.g., V-E Day, V-J Day, bombing of Pearl Harbor)?
    - Memories of peace
11. Favorite transportation
    - Did the resident drive? Own a car? What kind? Pictures?
    - Description of first car
12. Awards received
    - Any honors, major accomplishments
13. Involvement in clubs and groups, positions of leadership
    - What groups did the resident belong to? Fraternity? Sorority?
    - Did the resident hold any positions of leadership?
14. Volunteer experiences or service organizations
    - Description of services given
15. Politics
    - Interested? Not interested?
    - Favorite president? Why?
    - Most disliked president? Why?
16. Interest in literature and reading
    - Titles, passages, verses, poetry, scriptures
    - Favorite magazines, newspapers
17. Interest in music and creative arts
    - Instruments played, enjoyed, disliked
    - Kinds of music enjoyed, not enjoyed
    - Stage or choral performer? When? Describe
    - Theater or movie favorites
18. Recreational activities and hobbies
    - Inside and outside recreational interests, favorite hobbies
    - Team or individual sports played
    - Sports enjoyed on television
19. Animals and pets
    - Childhood pets
    - Pets the resident's children had
    - Recent pets
20. Travel
    - Locations of places visited, favorite places, maps, etc.
    - Recent travels? Where?

21. Favorite foods, recipes
    - Favorite foods
    - Like to cook? Bake? Barbecue? Describe
    - Favorite recipes? Include copies
22. Holidays, seasons of the year
    - Traditions, rituals for each holiday, types of decorations used
    - Special foods for the holidays

Thank you for your help.

Staff
The Wealshire

4

Communication: Understanding and Being Understood

Communicating, or exchanging information, can be considered an activity because an action or response is involved. Even when the outcome is silence or muteness, the body's position is still "speaking" to others. Language is just a simple part of making thoughts and needs known. Many factors, such as tone of voice, body positioning, facial expressions, and gestures, often speak louder than the words themselves.

If communication is an activity, then the reverse is also true—the activity of persons with dementia becomes their mode or tool of expression—of facilitated communication. For example, pacing, combativeness, excessive sleeping, or sitting with the eyes closed all can be an activity-focused message to the caregiver relating to the resident's fears, concerns, and frustration. The "whole" message must be responded to, not just the words. The caregiver's ability to understand the resident's communications requires careful listening, observation, time, and patience. Only then can the appropriate response be offered.

Language skills vary with each resident with dementia but invariably the ability to access words, sequence thoughts, and express needs is diminished almost to the point of muteness. Some residents with dementia lose their verbal skills early in the disease process. Others continue for years with sufficient vocabulary to be socially comfortable.

Communication is transmitted by both verbal and nonverbal responses. The objectives of the two types of response are

- To enable self-expression of thoughts and needs
- To enhance the self-image and sense of self-worth
- To honor memories and share memory fragments
- To facilitate maximum quality of life enjoyment
- To encourage understanding of others and the environment
- To foster socialization, community, and acceptance
- To promote a world view of safety and comfort

WORDS: BLOOMERS OR WITHERERS?

In a garden of words, pick your words carefully. Communication between the caregiver and the resident can be affected by "labeling." Sometimes, just the label

"Alzheimer's resident" may lead to certain expectations of difficult caregiving because of the resident's inability to understand communications and to follow directions. Another label connected with Alzheimer's disease is, "People with dementia are crazy or dumb." Labels may encourage a tendency to discount the need for interactive communication.

Words that wither self-confidence include *no, don't, can't,* and *stop.* When these words are said with a negative voice tone and body language showing anger, disgust, impatience, or exhaustion, the resident becomes very well aware of his or her dysfunction and inappropriateness. How very different to say, "Charlie, sit here with me," rather than, "Charlie, don't sit in that chair." Rephrasing negatives into a positive decreases the resident's emotional response of resentfulness or feelings of being manipulated.

Examples of words that bloom and give life to the resident in a positive sense include, "Thank you," "I really appreciated your help," "That's a lovely smile," "You have made my day," "How thoughtful of you to find my wallet," "Good job," "You're safe with me," "I'll be here today," "I was just going your way," and "Let's walk together to the activity room." Connection to the resident is made through a pleasant tone of voice, eye and touch contact, and words that "grow" the resident's self-esteem and personhood. Choose words that bless and encourage.

Throughout the disease process, residents with dementia continue to need to be asked about their opinions, feelings, and concerns. At times, it is the caregivers' own discomfort with "feelings" that denies residents the opportunity to express themselves. Talking about the residents while they are listening is never appropriate. It is often not easy, but the door to shared and positive reinforced conversation can be held open. Acceptance and trust between residents and caregivers can keep the dialogue going even when words are few. Select the most beautiful from the garden of words. Communication is when you care enough to say the very best.

COMMUNICATION: GUIDELINES FOR CONNECTING

Appreciating communication as a two-way street, residents and caregivers both seek to be understood and to understand. Verbal and nonverbal communications become the connecting bond, even when language skills, ability to access words, or conversation attentiveness are diminished. Guidelines for enabling the *COMMUNICATIONS* connection include the following:

C: Care enough to listen carefully. Be attentive, actively with full attention, as you endeavor to connect with what is being said. At times, you will hear only one or two words that are related to what you think the thought content might be focusing on. Listening is like being a detective: The answer develops from putting the word clues together with the emotional context. *Communications* is a broad term; words are often just the outside border of the jigsaw puzzle, calling to be understood and solved.

O: Openly display respect—the resident is an adult. Consider the climate of the communication milieu. Cultural differences, gender, age, emotional wellness, and cognitive abilities create the fundamental picture of the communication connection. Address the resident by name. The resident will assist you in identifying the name by which he or she wishes to be called. "Honey" or "sweetie" are usually not appropriate, but perhaps "Gram" or "Captain" might be because they are connected with the resident's life story. Identify yourself to the resident so he or she can put your face and words into context as much as possible. Promote the resident's social communication through opportunities that engage others in a nonthreatening activity.

M: Make eye and touch contact to attract attention. Locate yourself at eye level and with good lighting on your face, not from behind you, which would make your face appear in shadow. Again, identify yourself as you use a therapeutic touch to help the resident focus on you and what you are saying. Be sure that the resident can see and hear as well as possible. Realize that the eyes can reveal one's true feelings. Once you obtain attention and express your words, the most important aspect of success is allowing the resident enough time to respond. Caregivers have a tendency to be uncomfortable with silence and therefore they hurry into the delivery of words again without allowing the resident to think through the message and call forth the needed words to respond.

M: Monitor the feelings and emotional needs "behind" the words. Respect the resident's feelings, because they may be speaking louder and more meaningfully than the word content of the communication. Respond appropriately to the emotions being displayed. If the words sound sad, acknowledge their sadness, perhaps with, "Harry, that sounds so sad. May I give you a hug? Your words have made me sad, too." Or, if the words are upbeat, "Vivian, your words sound jolly today, I am happy as I hear them."

U: Understand the language of your posture, facial expression, voice tone, and word selection. Do the expression on your face and the words coming from your mouth "agree"? Do you look trustworthy? Safe? As residents with dementia lose the ability to use nouns and to engage words effectively, they appear to become more and more intuitive. For example, a staffperson arriving at work after a dispute with her child might still be angry, frowning, and working in punctuated movements. Residents easily pick up moods from persons around them and respond by becoming concerned, perhaps even thinking that they caused the gloomy mood they see. Lean forward, talk slowly and with a low-pitched voice, using simple, direct statements. Do not increase the volume of your voice if the resident does not appear to understand and you are sure that he or she heard you. Be aware that the resident's personal space is not being invaded. If the personal space is being invaded as perceived by the resident, he or she will probably start to look anxious, and try to back up or withdraw from the conversation. Continued invasion of this space may lead to a severe verbal or physical reaction. Relax during conversation, look friendly, and nod your head to responses.

N: Notice the resident's nonverbal communication. The word content of the communications might be empty, but the language of expression is usually full of meaning. The whole body communicates. How the resident speaks is at times more important than what he or she is saying or trying to say. The eyes often become a mirror of the resident's thoughts trying to be expressed. Challenges occur when the resident is parkinsonian and may therefore have little or no facial expression. Determining the thought and emotional content being expressed, therefore, becomes exceedingly difficult when words cannot connect you to the content.

I: Interject or identify missing words, if appropriate. The resident's train of thought may easily become stuck as words cannot be accessed and used in the conversation. These word-finding delays can sometimes be responded to in a way that allows the resident to save face. For example, the resident may begin, "Yesterday I, I, I, I . . . " and the words do not come forth. If you know that yesterday Betty's daughter had visited, you could respond with, "Betty, yesterday I saw that your daughter was here to visit." If you do not know what Betty might be referring to, the response could be, "Betty, you were just saying that yesterday, you . . ." and wait for a response. Be careful of asking questions about what is being said; very often the resident feels like he or she is being tested. Open-ended questions, for example, "What would you like for lunch?" actually lead to decreased ability to find words for responding because the choices are too vast. Offering a choice between two or three foods would limit the resident's embarrassment of not knowing what to say. If the missing word has truly disappeared, the use of humor may save the day. For example, "Betty, we must have thrown that word out with the old newspapers this morning."

C: Communicate by connecting with multisensory cues. Comprehension and communication responses can be enhanced by using props and cues related to the questions or conversation thought content. Asking Jim to sit down in the red chair while patting the chair with one hand and gently touching Jim to gain his attention and then pointing to the chair may enable Jim to figure out where to sit. Using pantomime, having objects that the resident can visualize along with the words and, if appropriate, using items that demonstrate taste or smell cueing, can provide residents with increased opportunities to comprehend the message and respond.

A: Assess for environmental distractions. Eliminate all elements of distraction, if possible. These include television, too many people present, excess motion in the area, lighting that is too bright or too dull, radios, intercoms, telephones ringing, vacuum cleaners, and noisy or loud conversations. Having areas available where the resident can focus on just the caregiver and himself or herself can help conversation to be successful. An outside stimulus can easily catch the resident's attention and lead to loss of thought content or listening focus (see Appendix 4-1).

T: Try therapeutic fibs, if appropriate. When the reality of a situation is hurtful or humiliating to the resident, the caregiver can contemplate the use of a "bent" fact, the therapeutic fib. First the mood or emotion of the inquiry from the resident is to be considered. Then the cognitive awareness and psychosocial need is evaluated. Telling a fib that angers, insults, or depresses a resident is not therapeutic. The goal is one of saving face and maintaining dignity during the difficult journey of dementia.

I: Ignore your need to be right, to argue, to confront. In other words, save your breath. Long explanations and even short ones generally do not work because the resident may have forgotten what the original question was. Often, this question is asked again, right after the answer has already been given. With short-term memory difficulties, the resident does not remember having just asked, for example, "What time is it?" The need to be right usually leads everyone to frustration and possibly tears of anger. Caregivers need to be the first to apologize when communications are not being understood. An apology and a hug may help to change the focus.

Alzheimer's Disease: Activity-Focused Care

O: Observe behaviors as communications. Increased agitation might be telling you that the resident has a headache. Pacing could be "words" saying that the toilet cannot be found. Ask yourself, "What is the resident trying to tell me?" when unusual behavioral responses are observed. Residents with dementia often communicate by getting the message across any way they can. If they need to demonstrate their needs through difficult behaviors, it might be their only option.

N: Nurture well-being through the communication connection. Knowing the resident's expressions of abilities helps caregivers to read the signs of pain, hunger, sadness, or loneliness. This is especially imperative for supporting the resident's caregiving well-being during the later stage of progressive dementia (see Appendix 4-2). Communicating by using touch, stroking, massaging, rocking, singing or humming, applying warmth or coolness to the skin, and using aromas or foods are examples of ways to connect with the resident through his or her senses. Equally important is awareness of the resident's "space" or possible intolerance to being touched. Caregivers are then challenged to find ways to promote communications and a sense of well-being by adapting approaches that do not violate personal space. Aromas, touch, and visual and auditory elements of communications become the ideal modality for reaching residents and facilitating their overall well-being.

S: Sensitivity sets the tone and mood for success. Sensitivity includes knowing the resident's life story and integrating it as a cornerstone for promoting communication's focus on dignity and abilities (see Chapter 3). The choice of words, the method of gaining the resident's attention, plus the knowledge of adapting language offers the maximum resident-caregiver connection. Words alone are just words—communication with another is an open door to holistic connection.

VOCAL AND SPOKEN COMMUNICATIONS

Meaningful words, nonsense or made-up words, singing, sounds, and shouts are components of verbal language that are used to communicate. At times, these components are mixed together, making understanding the resident a complicated challenge.

> Nona, having endured several small strokes that complicated her speech abilities and increased her confusion, became the "town crier." She sang the events of the moment, including people in her environment and what they were doing. Included also in this "Geriatric Rap" were significant memories from the past. This unique form of perseveration (repetition of words, phrases, or motions) became helpful if the caregivers wanted to assess Nona's mood or needs. However, the nonstop singing was tiresome to her fellow residents and puzzling for her family members.

Residents' abilities to understand verbal conversations also are affected, which leads to misinterpreted information, and at times inappropriate responses.

Caregivers should keep talking with residents, breaking down information into one idea at a time. Open-ended questions such as "Who am I?" or "What do you want for supper?" may lead to hurt feelings and frustrations. For example, stating who you are and not playing guessing games with residents helps to prevent their embarrassment when they cannot recall your name. Rationalizing, arguing, asking a barrage of questions, or using condescending words or a tense, annoyed tone of voice have the same effect.

Therapeutic fibs, or bent facts, are responses that allow residents dignity by not confronting them with the facts or with corrections of their misinformation.

> Larry is anxious to catch the bus to work. He asks everyone when it will be arriving. Rather than telling Larry that he is living in a nursing home and that he is retired, the staff tell Larry that the bus is late. They then use distraction techniques to give him a meaningful task so he feels like he is "working" and appreciated.

Therapeutic fibs can backfire. If incorrectly used, a therapeutic fib can cause the resident to be sad, angry, or frustrated. For example:

> Hazel informed staff that she was waiting for her daughter to come home from school. She became increasingly agitated as she looked out the window and at times banged on the glass. The staff knew that Hazel's daughter was very involved in Girl Scouts. Hazel was told that her daughter, therefore, was at a scout meeting. "What do you mean? I am her scout leader. I am not conducting a meeting. My daughter is not here," yelled Hazel. She then raced to the door, pounded on it, and demanded that she be taken to the scout meeting. The staff had not realized the history of Hazel being a scout leader for her daughter. The use of the therapeutic fib that was supposed to offer a meaningful explanation for her daughter's absence had obviously backfired. Hazel was angry and extremely disappointed that she had not been included at the Girl Scout meeting. She proceeded to cry because she thought that she had been a good and loyal scout leader. The staff were sad that they had caused Hazel to become so upset. They were able to distract Hazel from the focus on her daughter by asking her to teach them how to prepare the tables for supper as she had in the past for the scout's cooking badge. The successful participation in this meaningful activity helped to reconnect Hazel with her sense of well-being.

Assessment of a resident's hearing and vision is an important consideration in promoting good verbal communication (see Appendix 5-2). Hearing aids, unless they have been worn before the dementia, usually are not well received and the resident often will put them in the wastebasket. Glasses need to be kept clean and in good repair. A soft, stretchy band worn around the back of the head can help to keep glasses in place.

The activity of vocal and spoken communication involves:

Understanding the Resident	The Resident Understanding You
Words, especially nouns, are difficult to express.	Supply the word if you know it or give a choice between two words. At times, asking simple yes or no questions helps.
The resident talks around the subject when a needed word is not remembered.	

Examples:

Svea wanted to comb her hair. She said, "Where is that thing, you know" as she ran her fingers through her hair. The caregiver responded, "Here is the comb for your hair, Svea."

Bob was a new resident in the Alzheimer's unit. Louise approached as Bob and the unit director walked down the hall. The director said, "Louise, I want you to meet my friend, Bob." Louise looked at Bob and said, "Will you marry me?" Perhaps she actually was saying, "Welcome, I want to be your friend."

Understanding the Resident	The Resident Understanding You
Delays in responding or hesitates between words or sentences.	Wait for response; it may take a while to process what has been heard, so do not assume that you were not understood. Repeating the last few words said may help to continue the response or thought. For instance, ask, "Joseph, do you want a drink of water?" If there is no response, ask with the same words again. Do not say, "You must be thirsty, what can I get you?" He still might be trying to process and respond to the initial question. After restating the question two or three times, another approach can be tried. For example, "Thirsty?"
Answers a question or makes a comment after the subject is no longer being discussed or combines information from past conversations.	

Example:

Mary was driving her mother home from a party the day before Christmas. The car radio conveyed the news of governmental changes in a foreign country in which the king was dethroned. The holiday carol "Hark the Herald Angels Sing" was played. After the words "Hark the herald angels sing, glory to the newborn king" were sung, Mary's mother asked, "Who's the newborn king?" "It's Jesus," Mary replied. After a few moments passed, her mother asked again, "Who's the newborn king?" Mary gave the same answer, "It's Jesus, Mother." Mary's mother then said, "Oh, I thought they were trying out someone new." Mary's mother obviously had combined the information from the news bulletin with the Christmas carol.

Understanding the Resident	The Resident Understanding You
May repeat words, thoughts, or whole stories over and over and can lose the sequence of thoughts and confuse the order in which things happened.	
May become insistent about a certain topic or need.	Listen carefully to the meaning behind the concern, responding to the emotional tone.

"I want to go home," is an often heard remark in a nursing home. What really is being said? Does "I want my mother" have the same connotation? These remarks can mean, "I am lonely"; "I want my family"; "I want to feel loved, safe, and secure"; "I want to be needed"; and so forth. Caregivers should respond to the meaning behind the words, giving the resident extra attention and using touch or hugs of reassurance. Including the resident in an activity that the caregiver is doing helps to distract the resident with a meaningful task. If appropriate, ask and reminisce about the resident's mother or home. Tell about your family. Avoid explanations about why he or she cannot go home. Rarely is it wise to tell the resident that his or her parent is dead because the resident may respond to the explanation as though it is "news" and he or she is hearing it for the first time. This may lead to intense mourning and depression. A rare example of when reality was appropriately used and it worked follows.

Lenore, age 89 years, seemingly all of a sudden, started looking for her father. She questioned everyone, saying, "My father, have you seen my father?" Lenore continued her seeking questions for more than 2 days. She started to show signs of anxiousness and deep concern because she could not find her father and no one seemed to know where he was. Cognitively, Lenore was very alert, independent in activities of daily living, and seemingly oriented. Her search for her father puzzled the staff. After a staff team meeting, it was decided that Lenore needed to

Alzheimer's Disease: Activity-Focused Care

know the truth about her father because she was generally so well oriented. The next time Lenore approached a staffperson asking for her father, the staffperson took a deep breath and said, "Oh, Lenore, he died a number of years ago." The staffperson held her breath. Lenore answered with, "Oh, good, then I don't have to look for him." She smiled at the staffperson and went on her way. The staffperson was greatly relieved.

Reality orientation is often cruel and unneeded because the resident may forget the question soon after being distracted. Reality orientation may force the resident's confrontation with his or her memory dysfunction unnecessarily.

Understanding the Resident	The Resident Understanding You
Responds literally to words and signs.	Do not use sarcasm or double-meaning jokes.

Example:

A "wet floor" sign can be an invitation to do just that—urinate on the floor. Grace saw a sign on the door in her room. It said "Bathroom." She responded, "Do you suppose there is a toilet in there?"

Reverts to primary language and use of slang or "family names" for functions such as urination.	Ask families for a list of family words used and foreign words for various functions or basic needs such as water, food, toilet, etc.
Echoes words back to you or repeats sounds, shouts, or swear words.	Listen for tone or inflection of the words, watch body language, and observe what is going on in the environment. These sounds may be the resident's only method of communication.
Unable to initiate speech.	Show a positive response to all speech attempts, and sing with the resident to promote verbal confidence.

Example:

Wilbur, a former judge, quickly lost his ability to respond verbally in conversations. The family thought that he always had been proud of his oratory abilities and when word-finding problems affected his speech, he apparently chose to stop talking. Participation in an accepting community, encouragement to sing old familiar songs, and compliments for simple remarks encouraged Wilbur to once again attempt conversation. He started by first talking with staffpersons with whom he felt comfortable and accepted.

Understanding the Resident	The Resident Understanding You
Uses words unrelated to subject or each other, often lacking in meaning to the listener, but that appear to be meaningful to the resident.	Take seriously any attempt to communicate. Nod or smile, if appropriate. Listen attentively.
Loses ability to understand words. Does not turn toward speaker or know where the words are coming from. In time, just sounds are used or the resident is mute. Occasionally, a "window" seems to open and a perfectly understandable, appropriate response can be made.	Use simple sentences—one thought at a time. Have eye contact when conversing, use touch to attract the resident's attention, identify yourself often, use names instead of pronouns, continue social greetings, do not use childish talk, and show respect for feelings expressed. Write words or draw pictures to increase understanding. Limit environmental noise or number of people present.

NONVERBAL AND IMPLIED COMMUNICATION

Professor Rushmore, a resident with dementia, watched closely as Philip, a new resident, was admitted to his care area. The professor counted on the nonverbal language and messages he obtained from others. He was no longer able to speak in sentences, although at times he could put two or three words together. Most of the time, the professor was mute. He kept watching the nurse and the family members talking and filling out papers. In time, he walked over to the desk and announced, "It appears that the gentleman has arrived without his credentials." The staff was totally flabbergasted that the professor had put the needed words together that demonstrated his awareness and understanding of the event he was witnessing.

The old adage "Actions speak louder than words" is certainly true for persons with dementia. The tone of voice and body language of both the resident and the caregiver become the primary transmitters of language and understanding.

Edward wandered around the care center most of the day. He shadowed the caregivers while mumbling nonmeaningful sounds or words. Toward the end of the day, Edward and his nonstop sounds would be tiresome. Harriet, the nurse, was in poor humor one day and shouted at Edward, "Edward, you go to your room now. I am going to my room now to do my paperwork." She had her hands on her hips, her voice tone was stern, and her face looked like she meant exactly what she said. Edward stopped, straightened up tall, and said, "In the military, I was in solitary confinement, so I can do that standing on my head." He turned and left the area. Harriet was awestruck. She had never heard Edward speak meaningful words before and, furthermore, she had no idea he had been in the military. Obviously, Edward was responding to Harriet's "drill sergeant" tone and body stance and had understood fully within his frame of reference what Harriet had said. The family confirmed Edward's statement.

It appears that as the resident's ability to use meaningful words diminishes, his or her intuition and ability to "read" another's feelings increases. Sensitivity to the emotional climate intensifies. A caregiver who appears tense and nonaccepting is "sized up" by the resident immediately. The resident often responds to this person with increased anxiety, which may lead to combativeness or other catastrophic reactions. Caregivers with calm, clearly visible faces that show acceptance and caring will facilitate the resident's positive response and focus.

The activity of nonverbal or implied communication involves the following:

Understanding the Resident	The Resident Understanding You
Observe and look for meaning in the resident's facial expression and eyes. Is his or her mood sad, happy, withdrawn, or embarrassed? Watch for the appearance of tension in body posture, gestures, voice tone, and noises. Are his or her hands open or in fists? Observe behaviors such as pacing, combativeness, etc. Watch for physiologic reactions such as pallor and sweating.	Be aware of your body position, placement of hands, facial expressions, tense or relaxed shoulders, and tone of voice. Use an accepting, caring sound in your voice and keep eye contact on the same level as the resident's eyes. Do not stand over the resident and do not grab or touch from the back or where the resident cannot see you.

Example:

Simon had been a prisoner in the extermination camps. When touched from the back or out of his visual field, he reacted swiftly with clenched fists, turning quickly and hitting the person who touched him. Being touched from the front was almost as threatening to Simon until he was able to trust a few staffpersons. Touching residents needs to be done with discernment.

Understanding the Resident	The Resident Understanding You
Relies totally on nonverbal clues.	Use items for visual clueing (e.g., soap and towel to communicate bathtime or a sweater held up to "ask" if the resident is cold).

LANGUAGE OF TOUCH

The use of a caring touch can convey love, acceptance, and self-value. Touch is a component of communication. Touch can become its own language. The question becomes, how does the resident "hear, see, and feel" the touch language? Is the message one of: caring and compassion? assistance and functional aid? safety and security? intrusion? manipulation? irritation or annoyance? anger?

A pat on the shoulder, holding hands, and hugs usually promote residents' positive quality of life. Touch should be used cautiously at first because there are a few residents who dislike having their "territory" entered and prefer not to have physical contact. These residents should have their responses of hypersensitivity respected. The boundaries and location of touch can vary widely by culture, society, and age. Gender, cultural, and age-related factors are to be considered for using the language of touch wisely, effectively, and with empathy. Individual variations must be respected.

Touch, used with sensitivity, with purpose, and in a timely way, can affect both the resident and the caregiver. Both need to agree on what the language of the touch is imparting and saying. Touch talks.

ASSESSING COMMUNICATION IN LATE-STAGE DEMENTIA

Access to words and the clarity of their understandability diminishes during the late stage or terminal-care period of dementia. Sentence fragments, sounds, utterances, or jargon may be used. Stretched sounds, such as a syllable, cry, call, or sung words, may occur continuously, interfering with eating and sleeping.

Muteness may occur, and eye contact and movement tracking are often lost. Communication becomes the focal point or responsibility of the caregiver. Picking up the slightest changes in the pitch, loudness, or use of sounds may be meaningful and reflective of the resident's needs.

A late-stage Alzheimer's communication profile (see Appendix 4-2) provides a tool for evaluating a resident's verbal and nonverbal abilities. The profile includes listing observations of how the resident uses his or her body to "tell" caregivers information he or she cannot relate with words.

ASSESSING THE ENVIRONMENT FOR PROMOTION OF COMMUNICATION

The visual, tactile, auditory, and olfactory elements of the environment affect the communication connection. Another consideration is how the environment promotes the social aspects of communications. Certainly, there are environmental structures, items, or situations that cannot be changed. Awareness of how the environment affects the resident is the starting place. For example:

> Mildred can eat her supper and focus on the conversation with
> her two tablemates. Mildred tracks the conversation best if she
> maintains visual contact with their faces. The two ladies are
> soft-spoken, so conversation is difficult to maintain. When

Alzheimer's Disease: Activity-Focused Care

Jonathan finishes dinner early and rises from his table to turn on the nearby television at full volume, Mildred's attention seems to automatically swing to the television. This ends not only her attempts to converse with her tablemates, but also her ability to continue to eat. Mildred's attention becomes focused on the television set, not on her plate.

A communication and environmental assessment (see Appendix 4-1) lists considerations that may impede reciprocal communications. Making changes in the environment that are possible can enhance resident care.

HEALTH CARE PROVIDER AND STAFF ISSUES

Being able to understand residents with Alzheimer's disease and having them understand holds staff and residents together in mutual respect. Training with a strong emphasis on sensitivity assists staff to relate to residents' experience of dementia. Difficulties arise when staff are not willing to make the effort to connect. When they hold the resident in high regard and as a person of worth, no matter what his or her language skills are, staff are the most effective. Activity-focused care requires the staffperson to become resident-centered, listen, use nonconfrontational suggestions, and concentrate on the resident's abilities.

Issues, therefore, include the following:

1. Staff sensitivity and willingness to connect through communications.
2. Staff awareness and understanding of the effects of their nonverbal communications.
3. Staff skilled in "reading" the nonverbal language of the residents.
4. Staff concentrating on their English-speaking abilities and pronunciation of words, if English is the major language of the facility. Certainly, only English should be spoken in the presence of English-speaking residents.
5. Staff willing to use touch as a caring modality, especially with residents experiencing word loss and decreased communication skills.

Health care providers offering staff constructive criticism of their communication skills and, if needed, English as a second language classes, will find an overall decrease in resident anxiety. Resident awareness of the emotional climate in which they live demands staff that are attuned to a language of empathetic caregiving.

SUMMARY

Invariably, the responsibility for open, shared communication that enables a climate of acceptance falls on caregivers. The ability to accept residents' limitations and continue to converse with them in an adult, supportive way is a challenge. The caregiver's personal feelings of loss and sadness can be overwhelming, complicating the acknowledgment of communication as being a difficult and often exasperating task. It is hoped that communication skills and efforts will become an intriguing puzzle, instigating participation from both the caregiver and the resident. The ability to communicate verbally and nonverbally is more than just words and gestures for residents with dementia. All attempts by the residents to communicate are their methods to hold up before the caregiver a mirror of inner feelings and attitudes.

SUGGESTED READING

Bell V, Troxel D. The Best Friends Approach to Alzheimer's Care. Baltimore: Health Professions Press, 1997.

Gruetzner H. Alzheimer's: A Caregiver's Guide and Source Book. New York: Wiley, 1992.

Kovach C (ed). Late-Stage Dementia Care: A Basic Guide. Washington, DC: Taylor & Francis, 1996.

Mace N (ed). Dementia Care: Patient, Family and Community. Baltimore: Johns Hopkins University Press, 1990.

Rau MT. Coping with Communication Challenges in Alzheimer's Disease. San Diego: Singular Publishing Group, 1993.

Robinson A, Spencer B, White L (eds). Understanding Difficult Behaviors. Geriatric Education Center of Michigan. Ypsilanti, MI: Eastern Michigan University, 1989.

A4-1
Communication and Environmental Assessment Form

Area Being Assessed: _____

1. Visual environmental factors
   a. Lighting: too much, too little, sources, consistency
   b. Glare: floors, surfaces, furniture, mirrors, windows
   c. Cueing: way-finding? confusing rooms or hallways? labeled items, rooms, or objects?
   d. General visual mood: pleasant? cluttered? overstimulating? understimulating?

2. Auditory environmental factors
   a. Noise: from where? controllable? intercoms? radio? television? equipment? heater or air conditioner? overheard conversations? alarms? doors opening? doors closing? staff?
   b. General auditory mood: pleasant? jarring? boring? overstimulating? understimulating?

3. Olfactory environmental factors
   a. Occasional: pleasant? unpleasant? overpowering? recognizable?
   b. Ongoing: pleasant? unpleasant? overpowering? unrecognizable?
   c. General olfactory mood: pleasant? unpleasant?

4. Tactile environmental factors
   a. Surfaces: interesting? variability offered?
   b. Contrasts: surfaces? doorways? seating and floor?
   c. General tactile mood: dull? overpowering? inviting to touch?

5. Social environmental factors
   a. Spaces: private? small group? personalized?
   b. Cueing elements: season of the year? way-finding? personal belongings? special events? props? multisensory cueing?
   c. Furniture: couches? chairs in groupings? along the wall? small dining tables?

d. General social mood: meets residents' abilities? inability needs? orientating? disorientating? access to residents with similar communication skills? staff appear friendly and approachable?

6. Action plan
   a. Elements to be eliminated: _____
   _____

   b. Elements that can be changed or adapted: _____
   _____

   c. Unchangeable elements and suggested intervention for reducing effects that limit communications: _____
   _____

Name: _____ Date: _____

A4-2

*Communication Assessment Profile Form for Residents with Late-Stage Dementia**

Late-Stage Alzheimer's Communication Profile

Name of resident: _____ Room: _____

Hearing: _____

Vision: _____

Prefers to be called: _____

Responds to caregiver voice: Low: __ High: __ Soft: __ Authoritarian: __

Reassuring words to use: _____

Names of key family members or friends: _____

_____

_____

Supportive environmental considerations: _____

_____

_____

Verbal Abilities and Strengths

	Yes	No	Describe
Uses single words			
Uses phrases			
Repeats words			
Makes sounds			
Sings			

Response to:	Describe
Singing or music	
Touch or massage	
Rocking	
Silence	
Environmental noise	
Other resident noise	

Nonverbal Responses

	Yes	No	Describe
Facial			
Postural			
Arms			
Hands			
Legs			

How does the resident "say"

Pain: _____

Hunger: _____

Wet: _____

Tired: _____

Bored: _____

Alzheimer's Disease: Activity-Focused Care

Overstimulated: _____

Lonely: _____

Inabilities or Problems
Cannot make needs known: _____

_____

Cannot understand spoken words: _____

Outbursts or profanity: _____

Communication Goals or Intervention and Approach
1. _____

2. _____

Staff name: _____ Date: _____

5

Daily Living Care Activities

Caregivers' attitudes, approaches, and hands-on involvement in daily life care activities are the essential components supporting residents' quality of life. There is nothing more personal than the giving or receiving of basic care (e.g., dressing, bathing, and toileting). The ease with which these tasks are carried out sets the mood for both the caregiver and the resident.

Activities of daily living (ADLs) are an integral component for promotion of the resident's self-esteem. All aspects of ADLs need to enable residents' abilities, reduce their inabilities or challenges, and provide assistance that promotes successful involvement and completion of the task (see Appendix 5-1). ADLs provide the opportunity for one-to-one meaningful interaction for enabling the resident's strengths and abilities. ADLs are familiar, overlearned activities that provide opportunities for success.

If appropriate, the focus needs to support doing care "with" the resident, not just "to" the resident. Independent, assisted, or dependent participation in the basic care task becomes the resident's activity at that specific time of involvement. Redefining or "framing" daily care tasks as an activity encourages creative problem-solving approaches. For example, a caregiver might allow Jim the 3 hours he takes to dress himself in the morning because dressing is his activity at that time. This allowance releases expectations that Jim should take only 15 minutes to dress as well as concerns or annoyance that he is being slow on purpose.

DEMENTIA FACTORS AFFECTING DAILY CARE ACTIVITIES

The cognitive, physical, psychosocial, and emotional well-being of persons with dementia is affected by the progression of the disease. These factors, combined with responses to or from the environment may limit or challenge residents during the daily living activities of personal care. Focusing on the remaining abilities of residents calls for caregiver sensitivity, awareness, and compassion.

Cognitive Factors

- Has limited attention span, is unable to complete the activity or task, and does not understand the benefits of the activity or the expected outcome.
- Takes long periods to complete a simple task.
- Is unable to accurately report or describe pain.
- Has communication problems or verbal limitations.

- Has limited ability to follow directions or cues but may be able to mirror the caregiver.
- Is unable to problem solve or express needs or both.
- Reacts to a lack of needed clues in the environment for orientation. For example, resident may dress quickly during the night, thinking that it is time to prepare breakfast. The bright lights outside the bedroom "tell" him or her it is morning.
- Has problems with sequencing tasks (e.g., dresses in layers with three or four blouses or dons underwear on top of clothing).
- Does not understand what is expected or how to do a task (e.g., holds a toothbrush and uses it on the hair).
- Has poor body image or awareness of his or her body in space.
- Has perceptual dysfunctions such as lack of depth perception, knowing right side of clothing from wrong side, disturbed body scheme as to where the clothing should be placed.
- Has sensory deficits that decrease cognitive understanding (e.g., does not realize that whiskers are attached to the face or thinks that the face in the mirror is his face and therefore shaves the mirror). The resident may be unaware that shoes go on the feet or may not know where the feet are in relationship to the rest of his or her body.
- Is unable to be responsible for safety (e.g., dresses inappropriately for the weather, wears shoes on the wrong feet, brushes teeth with cleanser, or scalds skin in the shower because the hot water was turned up instead of down).

Physical Factors

- Is unable to move or use body or extremities because he or she does not remember how (apraxia)
- Has poor body scheme (i.e., understanding the parts in relationship to the whole)
- Has dysfunctions due to disease or limited use, such as rigidity of the trunk or extremities because of parkinsonian-like symptoms; may experience decrease in endurance and strength, limited range of motion, or pain, or all three, caused by prolonged inactivity
- Has balance or mobility problems due to medication
- Experiences a decrease in fine motor coordination
- Exhibits an overresponse to presence of an illness
- Has an undifferentiated grasp reflex that does not let go

Psychosocial and Emotional Factors

- Has demonstrative responses to needs for privacy, modesty, and dignity.
- Is depressed, too sad to be interested in the process or outcome.
- Emotional responses include embarrassment, fear, paranoia, anger, frustration, combativeness, depression, loss of control, and so forth.
- Has negative responses to being ordered to do a task.
- Reacts to excessive environmental stimulation—real, perceived, or imagined.

- Has prejudices against the caregiver, or those of another culture, race, or gender.
- Fears falling, especially if the caregiver is of small or fragile stature.

Environment-Related Factors

- Inappropriate caregiving area (e.g., room size, temperature, lighting, sound, color)
- Care equipment is unfamiliar, frightens, confuses
- Lack of storage space to have caregiving items immediately available to use
- Unsafe equipment or surroundings perceived by the resident as dangerous

USING A SENSORY PROFILE

John is wearing glasses. Three basic assumptions are often made: (1) He can now see, (2) the glasses are clean and properly adjusted, and (3) the glasses John is wearing are his. In reality, the glasses might not be the right prescription, they might be smudged and ill fitting, and they just might not be John's glasses. Residents with dementia require caregivers to monitor their sensory needs, provide needed supportive aids, and ensure aids' applicability as enablers, not as deficits.

Sensory processing is the interpretation of sensory stimuli. For example:

- *Tactile*: interpretation of light touch, temperature, pain, and pressure as experienced through the skin
- *Visual*: interpretation of stimuli through the eyes
- *Auditory*: interpretation of sounds, discrimination of background noises
- *Gustatory*: interpretation of tastes
- *Olfactory*: interpretation of odors

Using a sensory profile (see Appendix 5-2) allows the caregiver to assess the resident's responses as perceived through the senses. Equally important is how this information is integrated into cognitive, physical, and psychosocial awareness. Agnosia, the inability to interpret sensory input, can greatly affect successful self-care or caregiver assistance with ADLs. For example:

> Sam appears angry most of the time. He demonstrates his frustration by ripping up activity supplies, writing curse words on scraps of paper, and being combative during bathing and dressing activities. He has a hearing deficit and was admitted to the facility wearing two hearing aids. Several months after admission, Sam probably threw out or misplaced one of his hearing aids. His wife was informed and she began the process of ordering a replacement.
>
> During the period that Sam wore just one aid, his agitated behavior decreased. He no longer was difficult to bathe and dress. He stopped destroying objects and ceased other displays of anger. It became apparent that the presence of two hearing aids provided too much "noise" for Sam and was

the source of his frustrated behavior. Apparently, Sam could not sort out or interpret the sounds he heard into meaningfulness when he had input from the two aids. His hearing ability with one aid did diminish somewhat, but he could still follow and participate in conversations. The staff found that rotating the hearing aids (using the replacement aid as well as the remaining aid [e.g., the right aid one week, the left aid the second week]) provided the needed intervention for reducing Sam's difficult behavior during ADLs.

ADLs could be misinterpreted by the resident as aggressive or abusive care. Acting out, combative, and difficult behaviors often occur during the resident's caregiving morning period of bathing and dressing. For example, if the resident has limited ability to understand the nature or reason for the task, rubbing the resident's hair dry, combing snarled hair, brushing teeth, clasping a tight bra or pant waist, pulling up elastic hosiery, or pulling a sweater down over the head and eyes of the resident may be interpreted by the resident as physically abusive. This response is heightened when the resident is hypersensitive to touch or dislikes to have his or her personal space invaded.

A sensory profile of each resident allows the caregiver to be more sensitive during ADLs. Approaches are then incorporated that provide positive communication by using the functional and supportive sensory responses. Sensory information about each resident can be shared in the plan of care and in individualized daily staff assignment sheets. Adapted interventions, in response to the sensory information, may help to enable the resident's ADL abilities.

ACTIVITIES OF DAILY LIVING GUIDELINES

Providing care to residents with dementia requires assessing abilities and inabilities at the time of caregiving. What went well or poorly yesterday or this morning might not elicit the same reaction or response at this moment. "Success" may need to be redefined. For example, the fact that a resident's plaid shirt and pants clash may not be an appropriate reason for insisting on redressing, especially if it leads to combativeness. Activities of daily living guidelines provide helpful suggestions and an ability-focused framework that can assist staff as they offer the resident support, interaction, and creative interventions for enabling successful, basic, personal care.

1. *Timing*: "Know" the resident. Watch for signs of agitation or preoccupation with a real or imagined "something" that would indicate the need to delay care. Be aware of what time of day is best for the resident's bathing or other ADLs. Schedule flexibility may be needed. Residents are sensitive to being rushed.

2. *Monitoring*: Use the giving of care as an opportunity to check on the resident's physical well-being (e.g., skin integrity, bruises, blisters). ADLs can provide infection-control opportunities. Watch and anticipate the resident's need for help.

3. *Consistency*: A familiar caregiver, comfortable with the resident, using a routine approach, is often the most successful. The resident often feels comfortable

when the daily care routine is structured and familiar. Usually, male residents are less agitated when cared for by men.

4. *Focus on abilities*: Involve the resident in ADLs as much as possible, even if it is just to hold a washcloth. As the resident holds the cloth or empty bottle of shampoo, thank him or her for helping you. Always be ready to take over or help with the parts of care that cannot be done independently. Do not scold or degrade the resident if he or she is not able to participate. (Rarely is the resident difficult just to be obnoxious to the caregiver.) Place the ADL items to be used on a contrasting color so they are easily seen. A flexible approach may be needed. Learn names or terms, routines, and preferences used by the resident in the past for ADLs such as toileting and bathing habits. Avoid arguing. Allow choices when possible (e.g., hold up two dresses and encourage a response). Focus on the resident's self-image by using information from his or her LifeStory Book (see Chapter 3). Residents respond well to "Would you please help me with. . . ?" and "Please show me how to. . . ." Use as much praise with the resident as possible—praise that is real, not phony.

5. *Clueing and task breakdown*: Each ADL has many steps and each step needs to be taken one at a time. Modifying or simplifying the task facilitates the resident's participation and promotes success. Have all of the needed items, such as clothing and soap, ready and available. Place the ADL items in the position and order in which they will be used. Talk with the resident as though he or she understands every word, and tell him or her what you are going to do and continually say thanks for his or her help and cooperation. For example, say, "Unbutton your blouse, (pause) pull it off this shoulder, (pause) slide your arm out, (pause) pull it off the other shoulder, (pause) slide your arm out. Good job. You did that very well, thanks for your help." If ADL items are to be handed to the resident, offer them to the resident to grasp at the level at which they will be used. Multisensory clueing, using as many of the resident's senses as possible, will help to orient the resident to the task and enable successful participation.

6. *Nonverbal input*: The caregiver's attitude should be kind and nondemanding. Body positioning and voice should be positive. Positioning and voice should relay a message of acceptance and not of demands that the resident perceives as manipulative. Touch must be supportive and caring, not forceful. Be aware of issues relative to the culture, gender, age, and physical size of the caregiver as related to the resident's perception of being comfortable and acceptant of care. Realize that a resident may have a lack of facial expression due to parkinsonian-like facial masking. Masking can present a problem for the caregiver, making it difficult to know if the resident is pleased and accepting or becoming angered. Watching arm and hand positioning is helpful in this situation. Be aware that the resident is often watching the caregiver's nonverbal communications; therefore, try not to show frustration, anxiety, or fearfulness.

7. *Distraction*: Use of singing, food, talking, not talking, holding items in the hands, etc., may divert the resident *from* becoming upset or anxious during ADLs.

8. *Cultural issues:* Issues around personal privacy needs, style of dress, hairstyle, use of accessories, type and amount of makeup, race, and gender of the caregiver may affect ADLs in a positive or negative way. See the resident's LifeStory Book (see Chapter 3).

The preceding ADL guidelines, combined with an understanding of how dementia influences the resident's responses, helps both the caregiver and the resident. Each ADL task, "framed" as an activity, then can be evaluated and performed. Residents may find participation a challenge and may need assistance to engage actively "with" the caregiver.

HANDS-ON CARE STRATEGIES

Caregiving for the resident with dementia requires an ongoing awareness of the resident's needs. Offering too much assistance may "institutionalize" the resident, making him or her assume dependency as the expected response to care. This "learned helplessness" may soon become the expected response, by both the resident and the caregiver. An equally sensitive issue is when the caregiver assumes too much from the resident. This may lead to the resident responding with anxiousness, frustration, combativeness, and perhaps depression due to feelings of inadequacy and failure.

Hands-on care strategies, combined with ADL guidelines, are methods of facilitating optimum resident participation. As with other care interventions, they may be successful one time, but not the next. They become a tool for calling forth the abilities of the resident to be actively involved in daily care. The following are examples of hands-on care strategies.

1. *Rescue strategy*: One caregiver starts the daily living task with the resident. If opposition is met, whether in the form of verbal or physical anxiety or aggression, a second caregiver arrives on the scene. The second caregiver sends away the first, for example, "Helen (first caregiver), just leave Jennifer (resident) and me alone, we are old friends," or, "Helen, you are needed someplace else. Jennifer will help me and show me what to do." Therefore, Jennifer feels "rescued" and will almost always calm down and let the second caregiver take over.

2. *Hand over hand*: The caregiver places one of his or her hands over the resident's hand and offers assistance while guiding the resident's hand into and through the task. This strategy is also used as a reminder of the task when the resident has stopped in the middle of the activity; hand-over-hand movement may help the resident start again.

3. *Mirroring*: The caregiver models the expected response hoped for from the resident. For example, the caregiver pretends to brush his or her teeth so the resident can reflect back, or "mirror," the activity by brushing his or her own teeth. Drinking from a glass may be the clueing needed for the resident to take a drink independently. Residents will sometimes watch other residents (e.g., at mealtime) and then copy (mirror) what they are doing.

4. *Chaining*: The caregiver initiates the ADL activity, enabling the resident to then take over independently. For example: Placing a hand over Harry's while he holds the fork, sticking it into the macaroni, and then starting the movement toward the mouth may be all the cueing Harry needs to be able to continue the process and eat the bite independently and, hopefully, several more after that.

5. *End chaining*: The caregiver carries out the completion of the task and does not initiate its reimplementation because the resident is now able to take over. For

example: Mildred appears to have lost interest in and perhaps the ability to brush her teeth. The caregiver, placing the toothpaste on the brush, dips it in water and then places it in Mildred's mouth. The caregiver's hand is then withdrawn, leaving the brush sticking out of Mildred's mouth. This may be all the clueing needed for Mildred to respond. She then lifts her hand to her mouth, enabling her to move the brush back and forth over her teeth by herself. She responded to the "end" of the task and was able to continue it.

6. *Bridging*: The caregiver provides a sensory connection with the resident by having the resident hold in his or her hand the same item the caregiver is using for the ADL task. This sensory bridging appears to the resident to feel as though he or she were doing the task for himself or herself. For example: Stephen would respond to the caregiver trying to give him a shave with anxiety, aggression, and pushing away the caregiver's hands. The caregiver got another electric razor and placed it in Stephen's hand so he could see, feel, and hear the razor. With his own electric razor, the caregiver successfully shaved Stephen, using the sensory bridging strategy. Stephen responded with pride, as though he had shaved himself.

BATHING AND HYGIENE AND ORAL CARE

Participation Challenges

- Cognitive, physical, and psychosocial factors due to dementia.
- Unaware of odors or need to bathe or brush teeth.
- Fear of falling; many older persons have been bathing themselves while standing at their sink for years to avoid climbing in and out of bathtubs and showers.
- Perceives water as hurtful because of misinterpretation of the senses (agnosia).
- Inappropriate response to water temperature.
- Perceived invasion of a personal space or area (e.g., brushing teeth).
- Perceived or real pain (e.g., bleeding gums, water in the face).
- Embarrassment that resident cannot bathe himself or herself or remember how. Residents often will say, "I'm clean," or, "I had a shower today already."
- High risk for falls due to poor orientation, limited judgment, medications.
- High risk for skin tears.
- Fear and negative responses to issues related to dignity and undressing before others.
- May be experiencing an illness at the time of bathing.

Participation Assistance

Use ADL guidelines and the resident's sensory profile (see Appendix 5-2) and focus especially on doing "with" the resident instead of doing "to" the resident. Being dressed and, therefore, clothing, is very much a symbol of having it "all together." When the ADL task involves undressing the resident, he or she often experiences combativeness or increased anxiety. It is as though taking off clothing and being undressed is frightening because residents already sense that they are "un-dressed" in their cognitive skills. Therefore, staying dressed in their clothes helps them to feel competent, and being undressed heightens their feelings of being vulnerable.

Bathing

- *Know* the resident.
- Take the half hour before bathing the resident to build rapport and trust, talking with him or her quietly about the coming bath, how he or she will be assisted, etc. If it appears that the information is not being well received, back away for a while, if possible. Then return to the resident and try again.
- Look at lifelong habits, the time of day, preference for a bath or a shower, and frequency of bathing. A shower is often faster, but a tub bath can be more relaxing.
- Be aware of safety issues: use a bath mat, grab bars, and a chair or stool in the shower. Do not leave the resident alone while he or she is bathing. Have a call light or phone within reach. A strong grab bar outside the bathtub or shower is helpful for the resident to hold on to while receiving assistance with drying. A shower bench is a good safety feature, as is a bath bench, which allows the resident to be seated outside the bathtub then slid along over the bathtub. A bath bench may be helpful, especially when the resident is fearful of slipping or falling. Prepare the room so it is pleasant and safe.
- Provide hygiene care in the appropriate place, if possible. For example, wash face and hands in the bathroom rather than at bedside. Be sure the room is warm and, if possible, also the towels.
- Try bathing the resident while he or she is seated on the toilet if stepping into the bathtub or shower is too upsetting.
- Have plenty of towels available: one for the face, one for the upper body, and so on.
- Start bathing the resident's head and work down, assisting the resident from the front, where you can be seen, rather than from the back, which may startle the resident.
- If the resident is totally against a shower or tub bath, try a bed bath. A no-rinse soap can be used. Towels can be moistened in hot water, placed in a plastic bag, and taken to the bedside to be used. Uncover just the part of the resident that is being bathed.
- Monitor the resident's skin for rashes, bruises, or reddened areas.
- Do not rush the resident or show anxiousness; go slowly.

> Raye would become anxious and aggressive if she knew she was on the way to the shower. Raye was asked if she would like to go for a walk, and she just "happened" to arrive at the shower. She was usually more accepting of being bathed, especially if the caregiver had a snack available.

- Use a handheld shower head that can be directed to the one part of the body being washed at a time. The shower water can be dispersed to a softer stream when the shower head is put into a stocking or a washcloth is placed over it. Give the resident a washcloth to hold over his or her face so the water does not go into his or her eyes or mouth.
- Use only soap or shampoo containers made of plastic.

- If privacy is an issue, start bathing with some of the resident's clothing on (such as bras and panties). When these become wet, the resident usually will allow them to be taken off. A towel placed around the shoulders or over the lap, even in the bathtub or shower, may decrease anxiety caused by embarrassment, fear of being nude, or having the water hit the skin. A large beach towel or a bath towel can be wrapped around the resident and held in place during the entire bathing period. Bathing can be done by reaching down from the top of the towel or up from the bottom, while maintaining the resident's need to be covered. Use privacy curtains when available.
- If needed because of catastrophic reactions, wash one part of the body per day (e.g., Monday the neck and shoulders, Tuesday the back, Wednesday the arms) in addition to daily basic bathing.
- Consider alternatives: Perhaps a family member present and assisting with bathing would help to reduce the resident's anxiety.
- Style the resident's hair for simple and quick shampooing and drying. Sometimes washing hair is easiest in a beauty parlor atmosphere, if available. Try bridging to facilitate hair care. For example, tape six to eight strands of yarn on the table in front of the resident. While the resident braids the yarn, the caregiver braids the resident's hair.
- If possible, direct warm air on the resident during bathing and drying by using a heat lamp (best if placed in the ceiling). Towel racks for warming the towels are especially nice but could be a safety hazard if the resident were to lean against them or touch them for an extended period.
- Make the bathroom as "homelike" as possible: Be aware of too much or too little light, and try to personalize the typical institutional-looking shower or bathtub room. Beach towels with attractive colors and designs will make a drab room look cozier and help to absorb sound from bouncing off the tile walls. A fake window can do a lot to make a bathroom look more homelike. The window frame can be made of wood with room to slide in various scenes, depending on the season of the year. A good source for a window frame is to take the mirror out from behind the frame of a windowlike mirror. If this is too difficult, soap over the mirror or cut up a poster of an attractive scene into pieces to fit within the frame over the mirror.
- Use a bench to set the resident's clothing on during bathing or to use as a seat for dressing.
- If the bathtub has a hydraulic chair, use verbal reassurance and touch to decrease the resident's anxiety. If possible and tolerated, keep the chair up after the bath and dry the resident as much as possible. While the chair is in this same position, put on the resident's stockings, panties or shorts, and pants and shoes, so that when you bring the chair down, the resident can stand or be stood and the clothing can be pulled up into place.

> Connie always scratched and pinched during ADLs, especially bathing. It took three or four aides to give her a tub bath. A new approach was tried. One staffperson came to Connie's bedside, spoke softly, touched her gently, and sang an old song as a distraction technique. Connie was given a folded washcloth for one hand and an empty plastic

shampoo container was placed in her other hand. She then was asked to hold these items to "help." The singing continued as Connie was transferred out of bed and to a bath blanket in the wheelchair. She also was reassured constantly that she was a great help and the caregiver greatly appreciated the assistance. This reassurance continued during the transfer into the hydraulic bathtub seat. The water already had been run in the bathtub and the room was well lighted and warm. Another caregiver came in to help with the actual bathing. Connie was told what was going to happen each step of the way, in between the singing and the "thank yous." All washing was done from Connie's front, with the caregiver positioned at her eye level. A wet washcloth was moved slowly up her body as the washing of her face and back took place. She was asked to help and she responded by washing her own face for the first time. Her hands continued to hold items, so she did not scratch or pinch. The staff remained relaxed during the bathing so Connie would not become anxious. Having just two caregivers, rather than three or four, appeared to decrease her fears. Bathing, drying, and dressing continued in the same pattern, with singing, "thanking," and keeping her hands busy.

Shaving

- Shave the resident at a bathroom sink, if possible, using an electric razor. Put your hand over the resident's hand on the razor, if appropriate, and guide it to his face, or let the resident hold one razor while you shave him with another. The resident's mood and the timing of this activity are important factors. Sometimes, splashing on after-shave lotion is the needed clueing that interests the resident in shaving and should be done at the beginning of the task. See Hands-On Care Strategies, especially bridging and chaining.

> Donald was adamant that his "barber" always shaved him. In fact, while checking with his family, the staff found out that Donald indeed had gone to the local barber for all his shaving needs. He refused to shave himself and pushed the staff away when they tried to shave him. A creative experiment then was attempted. A male orderly, Louis, unfamiliar to Donald, was dressed up as a barber. Shaving equipment and lotions were placed on a tray and covered with a white towel. The "barber" then was introduced to Donald. Donald said, "That absolutely is not my barber," however, and the scheme did not work. If the staff could have thought quickly, they might have said, "Donald, your barber is on vacation, so he sent Louis." However, the staff thought it had been worth the try.

Oral Care

- Have the resident's teeth cared for as much as possible during the early part of the dementia process so that the resident is able to understand what is going on and will be more cooperative.
- When dental care is needed, encourage the dentist to be realistic as to the resident's ability to cooperate with the treatment. Short appointments can be made.
- It is best if the dentist is all set up, ready to help the resident so the resident does not have to wait. The dentist needs to assess and be aware of the resident's ability or inability to carry out any dental requests, with or without assistance. For example, the dentist evaluates the resident's ability to follow through with flossing or to cooperate with removing prostheses.
- Yawning in the resident's face or asking the resident to say, "Ah" may help to facilitate the resident to open his or her mouth.
- Use a child-sized toothbrush to decrease the resident's fears of having a foreign object in his or her mouth.
- Use children's toothpaste that can be swallowed, especially if the resident does not understand how to spit out the paste or rinse his or her mouth.
- Apply toothpaste to the brush, if needed, to simplify the task.
- Standing behind the resident to assist with brushing may be acceptable as it is generally the same strategy the dentist uses. This also allows the caregiver to gently use the forefinger to pull the cheek away from the teeth for facilitating brushing.
- Oral swabs soaked in mouthwash, can be used if a brush is rejected.
- A washcloth, soaked in mouthwash, may be the only acceptable means of oral care.
- The caregiver can try "mirroring" the oral care by carrying his or her own toothbrush and demonstrating in front of the resident.
- If removing the resident's dentures is a problem, the bridging strategy may work. Give the resident a set of "generic choppers" in the typical denture cup and while the resident is handling and poking around these dentures, the caregiver can often bridge the activity successfully by reaching into the resident's mouth carefully to remove the dentures. The resident may think that he or she is the one removing the dentures.
- Announce that you are from the dental office, wear a white laboratory coat, place a white towel at the resident's chin and throat, tell the resident to "open," and see what happens.
- Set up a monitoring system to check a resident's mouth after mealtimes if he or she is at risk for removing partials or dentures while or after eating and wrapping them in the napkin.

DRESSING AND DISROBING

Participation Challenges

- Cognitive, physical, and psychosocial factors due to dementia
- Poor balance; possibility of falling when stepping into or pulling on pants
- A fearful response when clothing is pulled over his or her head

- Desire to wear the same outfit all the time, even after sleeping in it
- Taking soiled clothing from the laundry bag to wear
- Layering clothing inappropriately (e.g., wearing three blouses or placing a slip over the top of an outfit)
- Wearing unsuitable clothing for the environment or weather
- Undressing at inappropriate times or places
- Negative response to issues concerning dignity and undressing in front of others
- Embarrassment or humiliation due to not being able to do the task himself or herself
- Feeling rushed by the caregiver

> James hated mornings, especially getting up and getting dressed. He would become physically and verbally abusive during ADLs. A caregiver made a clever discovery. He offered James a piece of gum and found that the resident could not be verbally abusive and physically combative while chewing gum. The gum focused James' attention, and the ADL tasks could proceed calmly. Certainly, gum chewing is not recommended for all residents, but it should be considered and tried if appropriate.

Participation Assistance

Dressing
Use ADL guidelines. Encourage participation but know when to assist or take over because of the resident's anxiety or lack of capability. Realize that day-to-day responses can vary. Simplify the bureau drawers and closet, using labels to name items, if helpful. Dressing may be simplified if just the appropriate clothing for the current season is available. Hang a total outfit (e.g., a blouse and slacks that go together) on one hanger. The number of outfits in a closet may need to be limited if layering is a problem or if the resident becomes frustrated if there are too many choices. A lock for the closet may help to curtail inappropriate dressing or layering. Other suggestions are as follows:

- Have a chair available for dressing if the resident's balance is compromised.
- Use clothing at least one size larger than usual for dressing ease. Clothing made of 100% cotton does not retain urine odor when washed. The smell will cling to polyester garments. Remember to dry-clean jackets, especially those worn almost constantly by men.
- If possible, use an undershirt or a chemise in place of a bra, if the bra is rejected.
- Over-the-head shirts and blouses seem to work best because both arms can go into the sleeves at once. The resident does not have to reach around toward his or her back to place the second arm into the sleeve, as with shirts that button down the front. A resident may become combative or fearful when the slip-over-the-head top is covering his or her eyes. Talking with them at this time may help.
- Use slip-on shoes with hook-and-loop closures if lacing or tying is a problem.
- Outfits with elastic around the waist help to make dressing easier for both the resident and the caregiver.

- Jogging or sportswear outfits can be very attractive and comfortable, if acceptable to the resident who might not have worn this type of outfit in the past.
- Use thigh-high instead of calf-high stockings for women, but only if the tops are loose enough not to restrict circulation. Using queen-size stockings, even if the resident is small, helps to have more room in the top of the stocking. Pantyhose can be especially puzzling for residents with dementia. If the resident insists on pantyhose, but becomes tangled in the legs, use two pairs, each one with a leg cut off (i.e., one pair is put on over one leg, then the other pair is put on to cover the other leg).
- Encourage the use of cosmetics, costume jewelry, ties, and so on, if they were worn formerly by the resident.
- Do not rush the resident; use food, singing, objects in his or her hands, and so on, to decrease anxiety. Caregivers can wear a "fanny" pack and fill it with snacks, costume jewelry, scarves, ties, or puzzle pieces made out of cereal box fronts. By wearing the pack, the caregiver has access to items when distraction is needed.
- Be flexible, reasonable, and not overly concerned about matching colors and tops and bottoms.
- If a resident refuses to keep shoes on it might be that he or she needs more sensory input on the bottom of his or her feet to continue ambulation. With shoes on, the gait may become less stable and the resident may be more fearful.
- Residents' clothing needs to reflect their former life roles and style. Choosing clothing in familiar styles and colors previously worn may help the resident to feel more secure.

> Bill wore his heavy blue winter coat 24 hours a day. He was willing to take it off for bathing and dressing, but then it went right back on over his clothing, even with his pajamas. Wearing a coat to bed, meals, and throughout the day was barely acceptable by the nursing home's standards, but to Bill, it represented a feeling of security and being in control. The staff respected his needs and eventually Bill was able to go without his coat. The staff found a service that could clean the coat in less than an hour. Another approach could have been to have a duplicate coat for Bill to wear while his was being cleaned.

- Use praise and give the resident thanks for his or her helpfulness during the dressing procedure. If clothing selected by the resident is not what the caregiver had in mind, do not argue, and give in if at all possible.

Disrobing
First, look at the meaning behind the resident's disrobing (e.g., the need to use the toilet, wanting to go to bed, feeling bored). If the resident is seated, a lap board can be positioned close to the body with both of the resident's arms and hands on top, thereby limiting access to pants or skirts. Restraint protocols should be con-

sidered. Avoid putting shirts or pants on backward, because they would not fit correctly or be comfortable. Overalls may be an attractive piece of clothing that may stay on due to the complexity of the strap fixtures. Try jumpsuits or other one-piece outfits. If a zip-up-the-back one-piece outfit is used for a resident who insists on disrobing, it could be considered a restraint if he or she cannot remove it independently or on command. Therefore, the use of this kind of outfit needs to appear in the resident's plan of care. A man's belt can be slid around to the back of the pants, and suspenders may help to keep pants and skirts on. Use blouses that open down the back for women. After attending to the possible reasons for disrobing, use distraction activities or increase monitoring or both. A bridging strategy can be used by placing six to eight shirts on a teddy bear, telling the resident that the bear needs to be stripped, and hoping that undressing the bear will bridge the resident's focus on undressing himself or herself.

FINDING AND USING THE TOILET APPROPRIATELY AND INCONTINENCE

Participation Challenges

- Cognitive, physical, and psychosocial factors due to dementia, such as inability to interpret body toileting needs.
- Difficulty in locating the bathroom or finding the toilet within the bathroom.
- Becoming distracted by mirrors in the bathroom, perhaps thinking that someone is watching him or her.
- Perceptual dysfunctions in seeing the toilet seat as someplace to sit down, especially if the seat and floor are both white or the same color.
- Parkinsonian-like rigidity that causes difficulties in getting through the narrow bathroom door, sitting down on the toilet, or standing up from a seated position.
- Increased susceptibility to physical problems (e.g., urinary tract infections, bowel impaction, urine dribbling, prostate problems).
- Side effects from medications, especially diuretics.
- Need for constant monitoring of the resident's skin.
- Toilets self in inappropriate places such as bureau drawers, closets, wastebaskets, etc.
- Inability to wipe or care for himself or herself after toileting.
- Decrease in the ability to be continent due to the use of restraints (i.e., a restraining belt used in bed at nighttime will prohibit the resident from using the bathroom independently).
- Difficulty or lack of understanding of how to remove clothing to use the toilet.
- Fear of falling, especially when getting out of bed if the bed is too high to place his or her feet on the floor while the resident is in a seated position.
- Responding negatively when asked if he or she needs to use the toilet because he or she does not understand the question. Residents also may say no when they are fearful or embarrassed because they cannot remember what a toilet is or how to use one.

Participation Assistance

Use ADL guidelines. Inabilities to control the bowel or the bladder do not necessarily occur together. Most often, urine incontinence precedes bowel incontinence. In addition, suggestions to assist residents include

- Assess for any medically related complications that could be contributing to urine and bowel continence difficulties. Offer and urge residents to drink fluids throughout the day.
- Assess abilities and problems; monitor food, fluid, and fiber intake for optimum support of excretion.
- If possible, decrease medications with side effects of constipation, excessive urination, etc.
- Do not overuse laxatives or enemas. High intake of caffeine, impaction, diabetes, prolapsed uterus, or just the progression of the dementia may be causing the incontinence.
- Use knowledge of past toileting routines and habits as a guide for clueing or scheduling the resident's trips to the toilet. Remind or take the resident to the bathroom or both on arising, then every 2–3 hours, before and within 30 minutes after each meal, and at bedtime. Reminding or accompanying the resident every 4–5 hours during the night is usually adequate.
- Flushing the toilet might trigger the memory of previous usage.
- Show the resident where the toilet paper is. If excessive amounts of toilet paper or other items, such as paper or cloth towels are used, remove them from the bathroom. Place small amounts of toilet paper on the roll or be available to hand the paper to the resident.
- Use a picture of a toilet or signs saying "toilet" or "washroom" on the door of the bathroom, or signs pointing the way to the toilet. If the resident interprets words literally, the words selected for the bathroom sign are particularly important. For example, a washroom might be a place to do personal washing, a restroom might mean a place to take a rest or nap, a bathroom a place to take a bath. If the resident is looking for a toilet, a sign saying "toilet" is helpful. Some men respond well to military terms such as "head" or "john."

> A picture of a toilet was placed on Scott's bathroom door. He had been having problems remembering where the toilet was located. However, he interpreted the picture as the real toilet and would urinate on the sign. The picture was replaced with the words "Men's Toilet" without the picture. Scott was able to understand and to use the toilet in the bathroom appropriately.

- Respect residents' dignity by not teasing, blaming, or embarrassing them when they soil themselves or relieve themselves inappropriately. Using the words "had an accident," meaning that the resident has soiled himself or herself, is degrading. Saying to the resident that you will assist him or her helps the resident to maintain his or her self-esteem.

- Use the words for urine or bowel movement from the resident's past, especially those words that the resident used with his or her children.
- If English is a second language for the resident, learn the foreign words that are familiar.
- Encourage activity, routine exercise, and mobility.
- Change clothing immediately when wet or soiled. Even though the resident has seemingly already gone to the toilet, sit him or her on the toilet again.
- Protect the resident's privacy as much as possible. Stand out of eye view, if possible, when he or she is toileting. If not, cover the resident's lap with a towel.
- Simplify bathroom and toileting procedures by using one-step commands (e.g., undo your belt, open your pant button, unzip the zipper, slide the pants down to your knees).
- Dress the resident in clothing that is easy to put on and take off.
- Watch for signs of the resident's need to use the toilet (e.g., increased agitation, pacing, talking, yelling, pulling at clothing, moving from one foot to another while standing, bending over from the waist).
- Realize that if a resident is asked, "Do you want to go to the toilet?" chances are he or she will "go" right there and then. "Let's go freshen up" might work. "It's your monthly" might help a woman understand the need to use the toilet.
- If the resident is on the toilet and wants to stand up without having urinated or defecated, offer a glass of water, or give him or her something to do with his or her hands, such as looking at a scrapbook or untying a tight knot in a tube sock.
- When adult incontinence products are needed, do not call them diapers—diapers are for babies. The brand names for these products will be unfamiliar to most residents and the use of brand names can increase anxiousness and decrease their willingness to use a product or keep one on. Naming the incontinence product with a familiar name may assist residents' acceptance. For women, call the product "padded panties," "panties," or "briefs," and for men, call the product "supporter shorts," "shorts," or "briefs."
- Cut a hole in the front of the product if a male resident is incontinent of feces only so he possibly can continue to urinate independently.
- If the resident takes the padded panties or supporter shorts off constantly, try placing one on frontward, another one on backward. Snug-fitting underwear can be used over the product to discourage removal. Suspenders on the padded panties or supporter shorts often eliminate the resident's ability to take them off, especially when they are worn under an undershirt with a shirt or blouse on top.
- Use washable shoes if urine is being dribbled.
- Assess the bathroom environment. It should be free from clutter, as homelike as possible, and warm.
- A black toilet seat may help men to urinate when they are told to "hit a bull's eye."
- A night-light should be used during the night.
- There should be grab bars for getting on and off the toilet safely.
- A washable rug should be placed around the base of the toilet if the toilet seat and the floor are the same color or tone.
- Usually, changing the color of the toilet seat will make the resident suspicious and reluctant to use it.

Alzheimer's Disease: Activity-Focused Care

- Remove the wastebasket if it is confused with the toilet, or have a basket with a cover.
- Place a cover, such as a patterned towel, over the sink if it is being used for a toilet.
- Decorate a radiator or heating device that may look like a urinal with brightly colored designs.
- Be sure the resident's feet will touch the floor for optimum comfort when seated on the toilet.
- If a raised toilet seat is needed because of difficulty sitting on a low seat, assess its use. It might be just "different" enough to prevent use of the toilet altogether.
- Most residents will benefit from a consistent approach and routine for personal care that upholds their self-esteem, dignity, and sense of adulthood.

> Jonathan disliked having his shorts changed. He felt embarrassed and responded by pushing away the caregiver and making a fist. Mary Kay, the caregiver, found that if she told Jonathan before they started the task that she was pregnant and would he please be careful, Jonathan was always a gentleman. She no longer experienced any problems changing him.

HEALTH CARE PROVIDER AND STAFF ISSUES

ADLs are the backbone for all aspects of caregiving. When staff are trained to understand the "activity" part of ADLs, the caregiving can become more resident focused, rather than staff-timetable focused. Certainly, there are days when keeping up with residents' basic ADLs is a real challenge. Staff shortages, the presence of illness, such as the flu, or the need to focus one-to-one with a difficult resident can compromise time used for engaging the residents in ADLs and the need to just "do it."

Assisting residents with ADLs can be a "thankless" job. A great deal of work can go into an ADL task only to receive a negative reception by the resident; in fact, at times, a response of combativeness. Another example of possible caregiver frustration is when a lot of time has been taken to dress a resident and do his or her hair and then it seems that minutes later the resident has changed clothing and messed up his or her hair in the process.

Nursing assistants are called to share caregiving information concerning each resident with the charge nurse and report to the resident's plan-of-care conference. Nursing assistants are the staffpersons who truly know how much the resident is capable of doing independently, what assistance a resident requires, and how much (see Appendix 5-3). In preparation for the resident's care-plan conference, an ADL report form should be completed by each nursing care shift due to the changes that may occur to the resident throughout the day and evening.

One of the challenges is for one shift of caregivers to pass on helpful information to the other. Also important is how a new employee or floating staffperson to a resident area where he or she is not familiar can obtain the information needed for caring for a resident (see Appendix 5-4). This form can be kept in several places for easy access (e.g., on a clipboard with the assignments and on the inside of the resident's closet door).

Facilities surveyed with state and federal regulations may find conflicts around the tasks of ADLs. Deficiencies are usually based on resident dignity (e.g., the resident who dresses in the layered look with four blouses or a slip on top of a dress). A resident who does this often and takes great pride in dressing independently can have the layered look and its acceptance as part of her plan of care. Another way to be proactive about the sometimes bizarre dressing combinations worn by residents with dementia is to have a policy and procedure that provides residents with support when they choose to dress themselves (see Appendix 5-5).

There also should be a policy and procedures that describe the carrying out of ADL tasks that may need to occur in inappropriate places. For example:

> Arnold did not like to be shaved. It had been 4 days since his last shave, and he was looking scruffy. Margaret, the caregiver, had been trying to shave him all morning. Arnold always had a ready excuse or just said a firm no. At approximately 10:30 A.M. when Arnold was enjoying a second cup of coffee, Margaret asked him again about shaving, talking him into it by saying that all ladies would think he looked mighty handsome. Arnold said yes. Margaret grabbed the shaver and started in, right in the dining area during mid-morning. Not a very dignified place to have a shave. But almost all of the residents were out of the area at an activity, Margaret knew that if her supervisor saw what was going on she could explain it and the reason would be accepted, and, most important, Arnold had said "yes" and was cooperative.

Obviously, performing ADLs in public places is almost always inappropriate. But there are times when "you do what you have to do" (see Appendix 5-6).

Providing the resident with a consistent approach and support during ADLs requires all staffpersons to have shared information about what works, what does not work, and how to get the job done. The basis for success is the use of the resident basic care information form that can be updated as needed, usually at the resident's plan-of-care conference (see Appendixes 5-3 and 5-4).

Health care providers can help family members and all persons coming into the facility to understand the emphasis on accountable caregiving for daily life activities. Offering education opportunities helps staff to know how to facilitate ADL caregiving by using guidelines, strategies, and various problem-solving techniques. It is also helpful to advise family members on the type, style, and favored fabrics for their loved one's clothing. This information is best when delivered before admission. Education can also help caregivers, family members, and visitors to understand how having Alzheimer's disease or related dementia affects residents' acceptance and participation in all aspects of ADLs.

SUMMARY

The teamwork, support, and acceptance required each day to make daily care activities manageable call for an open, flexible approach and a good sense of humor.

Alzheimer's Disease: Activity-Focused Care

Framing the caregiving as the resident's activity can allow spontaneity to be an integral ingredient for increased participation. Daily care tasks bring about an intimate partnership between the caregiver and the resident. Acceptance of this partnership often requires reestablishing priorities and redefining success. Understanding how ADLs can be misinterpreted by the resident as being physically abusive can help caregivers to realize the great sensitivity their caregiving must reflect. By focusing on ADLs as activities, both the caregiver and the care receiver can reduce expectations that limit responses or lead to agitation in favor of comfort, safety, and satisfaction.

SUGGESTED READING

Beck C, Baldwin B, Modlin T, Lewis S. Caregivers' perceptions of aggressive behavior in cognitively impaired nursing home residents. J Neurosci Nurs 1990;6, 3, 169–172.

Calkins MP. Design for Dementia. Owings Mills, MD: National Health Publishing, 1988.

Gwyther L. Care of Alzheimer's Patients: A Manual for Nursing Homes. Washington, DC: American Health Care Association; and Chicago: Alzheimer's Disease and Related Disorders Association, 1985.

Heacock P, Beck C, Soudeer E, Mercer S. Assessing dressing ability in dementia. Geriatr Nurs 1997;18:107–111.

Kovach CR (ed). Late-Stage Dementia Care: A Basic Guide. Washington, DC: Taylor and Francis, 1996.

Making bathing pleasant for your patients. J Gerontol Nurs 1997;23:(entire issue).

Rader J. Individualized Dementia Care: Creative, Compassionate Approaches. New York: Springer, 1995.

Rader J. To bathe or not to bathe: that is the question. J Gerontol Nurs 1994;20:53–54.

A5-1
Daily Life Tasks: Resident Abilities, Challenges, and Assistance Needed

Tasks	Abilities	Challenges	Caregiver Assistance
Cognitive	Is able to respond to cueing and task breakdown; responds to physical needs (e.g., toileting and hunger); understands "helping" as cue to encourage participation; skills needed are long remembered tasks or rituals; task involvement provides opportunities to promote communications, verbal and nonverbal	Cannot remember where bathroom or bedroom is; is unaware of need to wear clothes, brush teeth; is distracted by mirrors or being watched; misinterpreted sensory information and awareness due to agnosia; confused responses (e.g., lipstick on eyebrows, slip on top of dress); uses utensils inappropriately; is confused, cannot make choices; is unable to interpret body needs; cannot sequence or follow through task; cannot remember familiar tasks or steps; has short attention span	Learn familiar names for bathroom, toilet, etc.; do not manipulate resident; use flexible approaches; consider timing, learn resident's schedule; allow choices; use cueing (e.g., singing or pictures); use familiar caregiver; break down task and simplify instructions; give a knotted sock to hold while on the toilet; give items to hold during activities of daily living to help focus attention; talk to resident as though he or she understands every word; have resident hold a tooth brush or electric razor while you brush his or her teeth or shave, or

Tasks	Abilities	Challenges	Caregiver Assistance
			have resident perform task; hang total outfits together; label drawers; lay out clothing in sequence; give praise and encouragement
Physical	Is generally active; gross and fine motor skills maintained; responds to affirming touch; changes in well-being are a signal for impending illness; able to "mirror" caregiver	Is unaware of body odors; shows inappropriate response to water falling on the body, understanding water temperatures; tends to have poor balance; tends to have trunk rigidity; has decreased motor planning (e.g., bringing food to his or her mouth, ability to sit down); has decreased body image	Select time of day when resident is most physically able; ensure adequate lighting; call incontinence products "padded panties" for women and "supportive shorts" for men; use suspenders to help keep incontinence products in place; use familiar bathing choices (i.e., shower or bathtub); provide caregiving in appropriate places (e.g., brush teeth at bathroom sink); use clothing at least one size too large; use cotton clothing, polyester retains urine odor; use cotton undershirt rather than a bra; check vision and hearing needs; use pants with elastic waist; buckle belt in the back if disrobing is a problem
Psycho-social	Has increased sense of dignity; task is familiar and comfortable (i.e., combing hair, bathing); is able to respond to appropriate clothing; has pride in appearance; is able to enjoy compliments	Is easily embarrassed (e.g., "I've had a shower today"); is depressed; shows fearful responses due to lack of understanding; has need for feeling safe (e.g., wearing the same clothing constantly); is fearful when clothing is put on over	Respect dignity, privacy; if too upset, bathe one body part a day; redefine success (e.g., wearing mismatched plaids); use singing as a distraction to reduce anxiety; provide a homelike setting to reduce fears; dress resident in familiar clothing

Alzheimer's Disease: Activity-Focused Care

Tasks	Abilities	Challenges	Caregiver Assistance
		the head; is anxious; perceives invasion of personal space	style, jewelry, etc., of former lifestyle; offer clothing choices

A5-2
*Sensory Profile**

Resident: _____ Date: _____

Auditory
Hearing: _____ Right ear: _____ Left ear: _____

Hearing devices and tolerance: _____

__ Functional hearing   __ Distracted by noise (e.g., television)
__ Hypersensitive   __ Hyposensitive
__ Eye tracks to noise source   __ Oblivious to noise

Describe response to:
Loud noise: _____

Unexpected noise: _____

Background or foreground noise/music: _____

Quiet: _____

Male voice: _____

Female voice: _____

Foreign accent: _____

Yelling or screaming: _____

Other: _____

_____

Visual
Sight: _____ Right eye: _____ Left eye: _____

Visual devices and tolerance: _____

__ Functional sight   __ Avoids eye contact
__ Eye tracks to sound   __ Eye tracks to movement
__ Squints   __ Stares
__ Eyes closed   __ Watches others

Figure ground discrimination: Yes: _____ No: _____

*Reprinted with permission from C Hellen. Eating: Mealtime Challenges and Possibilities. In M Kaplan, S Hoffman (eds), Behaviors in Dementia: Best Practices for Successful Management. Baltimore: Health Professions Press (in press).

Describe response to:

Bright lights: _____

Diminished lighting: _____

Blinking lights: _____

Darkness: _____

Other: _____

_____

Taste

__ Hypersensitive   __ Hyposensitive

__ Functional sense of taste   __ Mouth/taste defensive

__ Taste discrimination for nonedibles   Yes: ____ No: ____

Describe response to:

Sweet/sour/salty taste: _____

Rough/smooth texture: _____

Thin/thick texture: _____

Hot or cold foods/drinks: _____

Oral temperature sensitivity: _____

Other: _____

_____

Smell

__ Hypersensitive   __ Hyposensitive

__ Functional sense of smell

Describe response to:

Strong odors: _____

Pleasant/unpleasant odors: _____

Other: _____

_____

Touch

__ Normal response to touch   __ Tactile defensive: (specific body part)

__ Hypersensitive   __ Hyposensitive

__ No response   __ Grabs at others

__ Touches everything in environment   __ Holds on too tightly

Describe response to:

Standing or sitting near others: _____

Being messy: _____

Grooming/hygiene/clothing: _____

Water: _____

Heat/cold: _____

Wind: _____

Other: _____

_____

Name/Position: _____ Date: _____

A5-3
Nursing Assistants' Care Conference Activities of Daily Living Report Form†*

Name: _____ Date: _____

Circle appropriate score: 1, 2, or 3 in each category (1 = supervision only required: resident performs 75%; 2 = minimum assistance required: resident performs 50–75%; 3 = maximum assistance required: resident performs <50%) Cross out comments that do not apply. Add comments if needed.

A. Toileting

1. Cares for self at toilet, experiences no incontinence or uses incontinence products independently or needs supervision; asks to go to the bathroom; responds to verbal reminders or to help finding the toilet; cleans self; has rare (weekly at most) incontinence difficulties; has appropriate attention span

2. Responds to minimal assist and sensory cueing; soils or wets while asleep more than once a week; has intermittent attention span

3. Needs maximum assist but cooperates with resident living assistant (RLA); soils or wets while awake more than once a week or total assistance; has no bowel or bladder control; limited cooperation or noncooperative with RLA

---

*The Wealshire Alzheimer's care facility, Lincolnshire, Illinois, prefers to call nursing assistants *resident living assistants* because of their holistic caregiving based on activity-focused care.

†Courtesy of The Wealshire, Lincolnshire, Illinois.

B. Eating

1. Cares for self at meal-time or needs supervision; responds to verbal cueing; has appropriate attention span

2. Needs reminding to continue eating; has intermittent attention span

3. Requires maximum assistance for all meals; leaves table more than once during meal; has limited attention span or needs total assistance; limited cooperation or noncooperative with RLA

C. Bathing

1. Cares for self or needs supervision with RLA standby; responds to verbal cueing; has appropriate attention span

2. Washes hands and face only; responds to sensory cueing; has intermittent attention span

3. Does not wash self but is cooperative with RLA; has limited attention span or needs total assistance; limited cooperation or noncooperative with RLA

D. Grooming: Hair, Teeth, Shaving

1. Cares for self; always is neatly dressed and well groomed or needs supervision; grooms self adequately with verbal cueing; has appropriate attention span

2. Responds to sensory cueing; has intermittent attention span

3. Does not groom self; cooperates with RLA; usually remains well groomed; has limited attention span or needs total assistance; noncooperative with RLA

E. Dressing

1. Cares for self; selects clothes, dresses, and undresses or needs supervision; responds to verbal cueing; has appropriate attention span

2. Selects clothing, dresses, and undresses with minimum assistance; responds to sensory cueing; has intermittent attention span

3. May select from two items of clothing; cooperates with RLA; has limited attention span; may need total assistance; noncooperative with RLA

F. Communication: Understanding and Being Understood

1. Is conversational; makes needs known; understands or has minor difficulties; loses train of thought; has noticeable vocabulary loss; is persistent in making needs known;

2. Minimal difficulties; is less aware of verbal mistakes; searches for words; repeats thoughts; responds to sensory cueing; responds to short sentences; makes needs known by sub-

3. Maximum difficulties; has limited vocabulary; has difficulty making needs known; makes repetitious words or sounds; has limited attention span or is mute or makes

responds to verbal assistance; follows conversations; has appropriate attention span

stituting words and motions; has intermittent attention span

incoherent sounds; is nonresponsive except to touch or sound

G. Social Interaction/Activities

1. Active participant; selects own activity; initiates conversations with others or looks for others to initiate activity; responds appropriately within group setting; is accepted by peers; enjoys variety of activities; has appropriate attention span

2. Minimal difficulties; displays varying tolerance for others; is avoided at times by peers; needs sensory cueing or urging to participate; involvement increases with one-step-at-a-time activity; has intermittent attention span

3. Maximum difficulties; needs activities simplified; responds well to music; usually is cooperative; has decreased tolerance for others; is ignored or avoided by peers; has limited attention span; limited responsiveness or nonresponsive to others; may be uncooperative

H. Challenging Behaviors

1. Shows appropriate coping with emotions and responses to others or situations or both; is easily redirected

2. Minimal difficulties; displays difficult behaviors that respond to refocusing and redirecting; triggers can be identified; can provoke others; may use physical force on others; has intermittent attention span

3. Maximum difficulties; difficult behaviors require maximum staff intervention to redirect; provokes others; identification of triggers difficult; is easily provoked; has limited attention span

I. Safety

1. Can respond appropriately to emergency stimuli and unsafe conditions

2. Minimal difficulties; needs physical cueing, repetitive verbal cueing, or monitoring assistance in responding to emergency stimuli and unsafe conditions

3. Maximum difficulties; needs total assistance in responding to emergency stimuli and unsafe conditions

J. Orientation/Awareness

1. Is aware of self, others, and surroundings; responds to reminders; is aware of memory loss and disorientation; asks for

2. Minimal difficulties; becomes lost easily; asks for help again following assistance; needs multisensory cueing; is easily dis-

3. Maximum difficulties; needs ongoing reminders and redirection; is often unaware of surroundings; usually responds to name and

assistance and uses verbal cueing; responds to way-finding cues; has appropriate attention span

tracted; is often unable to finish tasks; has intermittent attention span

familiar faces; has limited attention span

K. Motor Coordination and Mobility

1. Mobile and coordinated; responds safely to physical limitations, balance, moving from one floor surface to another, getting in or out of a chair

2. Minimal difficulties; nonrhythmic gait; has increased balance problems; moves slowly or too quickly; often has difficulty remembering or using adapted equipment; may need stand-by assistance

3. Maximum difficulties; has limited self-propulsion of wheel chair; may need wrap-around walker monitoring; needs RLA assistance to ambulate; may not be ambulatory

Total score: _____ Signature: _____ Date: _____

A5-4
*Resident Basic Care Information Form**

A consistent caregiving approach for residents with dementia requires all staffpersons to know what is expected, what works, and how to complete the task with the least amount of resident anxiety. With three shifts of staffpersons involved with nursing care, as well as the assistance of other health care professions, having a consistent approach is a challenge. The resident basic care information form can help to provide uniformity of care. The form can be kept on a clipboard, at a nursing station if one is present, or taped to the inside of the resident's closet door, medicine chest, or any other place that supports the resident's rights to dignity. Updating the form can occur during the resident's plan-of-care conference, which takes place at least every 3 months.

Resident: _____ Room number: _____ Date: _____

Toileting
__ Self   __ Supervise   __ Assist
__ Before meals   __ After meals   __ Every hour
__ Every 2 hours   __ Every 2 hours while awake

Incontinence Product
__ Self   __ Supervise   __ Assist
__ Full product   __ Liner   __ Other

Eating
__ Self   __ Supervise   __ Assist
Mealtime location: _____
__ Cut up food   __ One utensil
__ Breakfast   __ Lunch   __ Dinner

Bathing
__ Self   __ Supervise   __ Assist
__ A.M.   __ P.M.   __ Nights
__ Shower   __ Whirlpool/bath

---

*Courtesy of The Wealshire, Lincolnshire, Illinois.

Hair Wash	__ With bathing	__ Before beauty shop	__ At beauty shop only

Oral Care	__ Self __ Dentures (upper) __ Partial upper	__ Supervise	__ Assist __ Dentures lower __ Partial lower

Shaving	__ Self __ Razor	__ Supervise __ Electric razor	__ Assist __ After-shave lotion

Hair and Face Washing	__ Self	__ Supervise	__ Assist

Glasses	__ Yes	__ No	

Hearing Aid	__ None	__ Left	__ Right

Elastic Hose	__ Thigh high	__ Knee high	

Dressing	__ Self	__ Select clothes and resident can dress self	__ Select clothes and assist resident to dress

Sleeping/Naps	Preferred rising time: _____	Preferred bedtime: _____	Preferred naptime: _____

Specific Family Requests (care, activities): _____

_____

Additional Instructions: _____

_____

A5-5
Sample Dressing Policy and Procedures: Supporting the Symbolism of Clothing

It is the policy of this care center to enable residents with dementia by involving them actively in all activities of daily living, supporting their choices whenever possible, unless their safety or the safety of other residents or staff is challenged. Therefore, clothing choices made by residents will be honored and understood as supportive of their abilities and a symbol of their need to feel in control.

Examples of Clothing and Appliance Challenges or Problems

1. *Inappropriate layering of clothing*: Combining clothing by wearing one item on top of another inappropriately
2. *Inappropriate clothing selection*: Based on the time of day, temperature, season, colors, type of clothing, ownership of the items, placement on the body
3. *Incomplete dressing*: Resulting from stripping off all or some of the pieces of clothing, including situations when redressing has taken place leaving out one or more basic clothing items (including dressing without underwear), the removal of shoes for comfort or increased ability to receive sensory awareness for integrating body movement, and incomplete dressing due to the long period needed to complete the task
4. *Refusal to wear or use or inappropriate wearing or use of clothing or appliances*: Wearing the same clothing item constantly beyond acceptable sanitary standards; refusing to change clothing at bedtime; taking off glasses, dentures, hearing aids constantly or not allowing them to be put on
5. *Situations of imminent safety risk to resident or others related to clothing or appliances*: Wearing glasses, dentures, clothing that is not resident's or wearing items incorrectly

Discussion

Caregivers' attitudes, approaches, and hands-on involvement in daily life care activities are the essential components supporting residents' quality of life. There is nothing more personal than the giving and receiving of basic care. The ease with which these tasks are carried out sets the mood for both the caregiver and the resident. Independent, assisted, or dependent participation in the basic care task becomes the resident's activity at that specific time of involvement. "Success" may need to be redefined from the resident's point of view. Success occurs when the resident feels connected to the task and experiences a positive sense of accomplishment even though the final results may not be the same as those preferred by the caregiver.

Resident Cognitive Factors

- Has limited attention span, is unable to complete the activity or task and does not understand the benefits or the expected outcome; is easily distracted
- Has limited orientation to self and situation
- Takes long period to complete a simple task
- Has communication problems or verbal limitations
- Has limited ability to follow directions or cues; inability to make decisions; poor memory for the task
- Has problems with sequencing tasks
- Does not understand what is expected or how to do the task
- Has poor body image or awareness of his or her body in space
- Has perceptual dysfunctions
- Shows poor judgment, is unable to be responsible for safety

Resident Physical Factors

- Has sensory deficits
- Is unable to move or use body or extremities because he or she cannot remember how
- Has dysfunctions due to disease or limited use, such as rigidity of the trunk or extremities because of parkinsonian-like symptoms; may have limited strength or endurance
- Has balance or mobility problems due to medications
- May have limited range of motion, impaired gross or fine coordination or both
- May exhibit motor restlessness

Resident Psychosocial/Emotional Factors

- Shows demonstrative responses to needs for privacy, modesty, and dignity
- Emotional responses include embarrassment, fear, paranoia, anger, frustration, combativeness, agitation, depression, loss of control, withdrawal
- Reacts to excessive environmental stimulation—real, perceived, or imagined
- Reacts to a lack of needed cues in the environment for orientation
- Has prejudices against the caregiver or certain races, cultures, or genders

Procedures

1. The appropriate wearing or use of residents' clothing and appliances will be addressed by all staffpersons 24 hours a day.

Alzheimer's Disease: Activity-Focused Care

2. The primary caregiver will use the following skills and guidelines to meet the residents' clothing and appliance needs:
   - Verbal and nonverbal communication skills
   - Choosing appropriate, simple clothing that is within the resident's ability to manage
   - Tasks simplified and broken down into basic steps and presented to the resident one step at a time
   - Timing based on the resident's responses
   - Consistent approaches and interventions
   - Necessary cueing
   - Decreasing extraneous stimulation
   - Appropriate distraction techniques when necessary
3. The primary caregiver will attempt to work with the resident to meet his or her clothing and appliance needs. If rebuffed or to avoid confrontation, the caregiver will retreat from engaging the resident at that time.
   - The caregiver is to attempt care again every 20–30 minutes for 2 hours.
   - After 2 hours, the caregiver reports the situation to his or her superior.
   - A plan is to be developed that can include
     Waiting until 2–6 hours have gone by
     Introducing another caregiver to attempt the dressing or appliance task (rescuing strategy)
     Postponing the task when judged by management to be in conflict with the resident's current abilities to tolerate
   - The clothing or appliance confrontation and results will be documented in the resident's chart.
4. Clothing and appliance issues that require a specific approach or intervention or both are to be included in the resident's plan of care.
5. Family education is important to help families be partners in caregiving in these situations. The family needs to understand that the *outcome* of self-dressing efforts is not as important as the acknowledgment and celebration of the successful *attempt* to dress. Acceptance of less than conventional results is necessary by both staff and family members, and changing the situation should only be attempted by the preceding methods after the resident's effort is validated, and an appropriate approach is worked out at a later time.

A5-6
Sample Staff Support Policy and Procedures: "Do What You Have to Do"

It is the policy of this care center to recognize the difficulties in caring for persons with dementia. Trained staff, specializing in dementia care, are required to follow all guidelines and regulations involved with their job description and overall resident care.

It is the policy of this care center to support staff trained in caring for persons with dementia who find that they cannot carry out their caregiving tasks in the traditional way. Following procedures and with permission from the caregiver's manager or supervisor or both *and the resident*, the care will be delivered in an alternative or nontraditional way—where and how care needs to be adapted for success.

Examples

- Shaving in the hallway or dining area
- Hair combing in the activity area
- Eating a meal in a public area
- Being fed while walking through the hall
- Having an eye examination in the dining area
- Putting on shoes in the kitchen
- Medications delivered in a public area

Procedure

1. All care performed in nontraditional or alternative settings *will only be carried out with the resident's cooperation.*
2. *Resident dignity is upheld at all times*: Care that involves any invasive procedure or any elements of nudity will take place only in privacy.
3. All caregiving procedures will be attempted three times during the course of 1–3 hours before consideration of an alternative or nontraditional place or method is considered. Medications will only be attempted over 2 hours.

4. Caregivers must receive permission from their manager before attempting nontraditional or alternative delivery of caregiving.
5. If the alternative or nontraditional caregiving procedure continues to be the only way the resident accepts the care, the procedure will be described, with its therapeutic benefits, on the resident's plan of care.

6

Eating and Mealtimes: An Activity of Consequence

Eating is not just "eating." When viewed as an activity, one can begin to see it as a process to be entered into, involved with, and purposefully carried out. The activity of eating then can be taken apart and looked at to understand its various stages, what can be successful, and what can go wrong. Changes then can be made to modify this activity, enhancing all that goes well and solving what should be changed. The primary goal is good nutrition. Residents with dementia are often a challenge at mealtime when they exhibit difficult behaviors. Creative interventions can be used to redirect residents and enable them to focus on the meal.

The eating activity is also a barometer of the resident's well-being. Subtle changes in the resident's approach to the meal and actual food intake can signal changes in physical, cognitive, and emotional health. An alert staff, familiar with the resident, can almost sense these changes as they are being played out at mealtime. Therefore, eating becomes a valuable tool to predict need and change.

Mealtimes are opportunities for connecting with the resident. His or her long-term memory may be triggered by the sharing of a meal, the communion of long-held and honored memories, traditions, and rituals. Most celebrations, special events, and holidays always involve a meal. A tablecloth, electric candles, attractive dishware, or soft music may help the resident to access these memories and feelings of mealtime communion with those now sharing the food.

Weight is easily lost when dietary support is not available or does not reflect the changes in the resident's well-being. Increased physical activity can reduce weight as well as just not eating enough food or the right foods. Making each bite count helps to maintain weight when the resident experiences altered absorption and metabolism during the later part of the disease process.

The crucial consideration in the entire food intake process is flexibility. Everyone and everything that has anything to do with this basic care component should be studied and assessed time and time again, using creativity and problem solving to make necessary adaptations and changes. Eating is the most important activity of the resident's day.

EATING: HOW DO YOU PROMOTE SUCCESS?

Ongoing resident assessment, flexibility in all areas of food service and delivery, and trained staff or family members that are creative and can adapt interventions become the significant elements of eating and mealtime success. Success is also demonstrated when staff are sensitive to the experience of dementia and have confidence to use creative methods for encouraging residents to eat. Staffpersons are an integral part of how nutritional well-being success is promoted.

Honor the Resident's LifeStory and Obtain the Resident's Eating History

Family members are usually the best resource for obtaining a listing of the resident's likes and dislikes, but it is usually appropriate to ask the resident himself or herself. The resident can often respond to simple questions such as, "Harry, do you like chicken or beef?" If you want to be sure, ask the question again at another time to see if you obtain a similar response. It is important to realize that sometimes residents forget that they did not like a certain food and may enjoy eating it now. The opposite can also be true: favorite foods can be disliked at any time. It is helpful to know what "style" eater the resident was (e.g., did the resident like his or her big meal at noon or at night? Did the resident "graze" and just pick up food as he or she walked?). Referring to the resident's LifeStory Book (see Chapter 3) will also provide a key to the resident's likes and dislikes. Pictures or descriptions of family celebrations where food is present or favorite recipes will be helpful. The resident's past life experiences will be helpful in designing creative mealtime approaches and interventions if they are needed.

Focus on the Resident's Remaining Abilities

Bringing the resident into the meal and making it possible for him or her to interact with the food helps the resident connect with this meaningful activity. Ongoing assessment and monitoring of the resident's cognitive, physical, and psychosocial abilities relating to eating and mealtime will enable participation when the focus is on residents doing as much as they can for themselves. Even when a caregiver is required to feed the resident, the resident can still be involved. Staff, trained to understand and respond to the difficulties residents with dementia experience during mealtimes, are able to be sensitive and help facilitate residents' remaining strengths and abilities. Certainly, great patience and flexibility are required of all staffpersons.

Use a Sensory Profile

The entire activity of eating is affected by the senses: how the food looks, the aromas, the textures and taste, as well as the sounds surrounding the mealtime. Each person responds differently to the various tastes as well as to preferences of hot or cold foods (see Appendix 5-2). The resident's response to touch can also affect his or her eating success. If the resident is hypersensitive to touch around the face, mouth, and lips, for example, a rubber-coated spoon might not be so offensive to him or her.

Implement Behavior Intervention Tools

A resident experiencing difficult behaviors that interfere with appropriate meal-time intake or participation requires the staff to identify possible causes or antecedents. Approaches or interventions that can refocus or decrease the unwanted responses can then be tried. A behavior profile (see Appendix 8-1) and a behavior observation form (see Appendix 8-2) are easily used and can become a basis for planning appropriate interventions.

EATING AND MEALTIME INTERVENTIONS AND FACILITATION

Task Simplification and Sequencing

The task of eating has multiple steps. As Alzheimer's disease progresses, it becomes more and more difficult for the resident to feed himself or herself. When problems occur, understanding how to simplify the process of eating, the number of utensils, the meal setup, and perhaps the food is required. Sequencing involves serving one part of the meal at a time and is used in conjunction with simplifying the food served and mealtime activity.

Mirroring

Residents with dementia are often able to copy or mirror the eating process by watching their tablemates or staff. For example, when the caregiver takes a drink of milk, the resident might reach for his or her glass and also take a drink. The objective is to obtain the resident's attention and imitate the activity using motions and also words and then encouraging the resident to do the same for himself or herself. Residents are usually striving to fit in and to respond appropriately. Their intuitive skills help them to process their environment and their remaining social skills combine to make mirroring a successful intervention.

Multisensory Cueing

Auditory, visual, olfactory, tactile, and gustatory cues are combined whenever possible to enable residents' awareness, attention span, orientation, and participation in the cued task. An example is the appetizing aroma of onion soup, combined with an attractive soup crock and pleasant encouragement for the resident to enjoy his or her favorite soup, prepared just for him or her.

Hand Over Hand

When the resident's focus and attention span limit active participation in the eating process, the caregiver can place his or her hand over the resident's hand and guide it from the food, up and into the resident's mouth. The resident, therefore, may feel a sense of accomplishment and connection to the activity of eating.

Chaining and End Chaining

Chaining is an intervention in which the caregiver places a hand over the resident's hand and starts the activity of scooping the food and directing the utensil up toward the resident's mouth. The resident is cued to the process and can then take over and finish the task. This may be needed for each spoonful of food, or the chaining may have a carryover effect, and the resident is able to eat several bites independently before chaining needs to be resumed. End chaining is when cueing is provided at the end of the task. For example, the caregiver scoops up a spoon of applesauce, inserts the spoon into the resident's mouth, and then withdraws his or her hand, allowing the spoon to remain in the resident's mouth. When the resident becomes aware, perhaps even annoyed, that there is this "thing" in his or her mouth, the response may be that he or she raises his or her hand to the spoon. The contact with the spoon may be what it takes to reconnect the resident to the eating process, and he or she can continue feeding himself or herself. If this intervention is successful, but after several bites the eating process stops again, end chaining can be restarted.

Bridging

Bridging is an intervention of sensory connection that helps residents focus, increase attention span, reduce anxiety, and encourage cooperation. During the bridging intervention, a resident holds in his or her hand the same object as the one that is being used for the task. This links the resident to the task. This sensory experience connects the resident from the task, to the caregiver who is actually performing the task, and then back to the resident. An example is a resident who is not able to respond to eating interventions and requires spoon feeding. The placement of a spoon in the resident's hand to be held while the feeding process is occurring will often help the resident to be more centered and focused on eating. Therefore, a connection may be felt by the resident, as though he or she were feeding himself or herself. The activity of eating is bridged, from the resident holding the spoon, to the caregiver, and back. A similar bridging connection can be made when residents hold a sandwich piece, a plastic cup, or an unbreakable tumbler.

Mouth Opening and Swallowing Facilitation

To encourage the resident to open his or her mouth, place your fingers, with your palm up, under the resident's chin and in a firm motion press up quickly and remove your fingers. To encourage the resident to open lips, gently but firmly place your thumb under the lower lip and index finger above the upper lip and squeeze firmly, but not hurtfully, and then release. To encourage the resident to swallow, gently stroke the resident's throat, on both sides of the neck, in an upward motion, from the base of the neck to the jaw, while saying firmly, "Swallow."

EATING BEHAVIORS EXHIBITED AND PROBLEMS ENCOUNTERED

Key Considerations

- Difficulty attending to the task of eating
- Overeating or undereating
- Motor problems: getting the food to his or her mouth, chewing, and swallowing

Residents sometimes refuse to come to the meal, or they stand up, sit down, or leave during the meal. They may call out, bang on the table, and throw or push food away. Food often is taken from another's tray, played with, eaten with fingers, or put into pockets and purses. Hidden food that has spoiled sometimes is eaten. Too much food can be put in the mouth, the resident may forget how to chew, and can choke as swallowing is attempted. A piece of meat that is too big may lead to choking, or a bite of food can be chewed with no attempt to swallow.

Residents can gorge themselves or may eat too fast or too slowly. At times, residents refuse to eat totally or refuse to be fed, often grabbing at the hands of the feeder or moving his or her head from side to side to make his or her mouth a moving target. Lack of motor planning, mobility, or understanding of how to get food to the mouth, how to chew, and how to swallow can limit food intake or self-feeding. Perceptual and cognitive problems may make food unrecognizable as something to eat. Nonedibles sometimes are consumed, including plants and dirt. Paper napkins and foam cups also are eaten at times.

Occasionally, a resident will gain weight. This usually is seen after admission, especially when the resident comes from a home or a facility that has not understood how to monitor and feed residents with dementia. Sometimes the socialization of eating with a group encourages residents to eat more than they did at home. If the activity program is using high-calorie food for parties or snacks, residents will gain weight if they are not active or mobile. Overeating can be the cause of increased weight, especially if the resident is clever in finding candy and cookie stashes. Weight gain, within reason, if it does not affect mobility and activity or cause significant transfer problems, can give residents a "cushion," as in time they invariably lose weight and become very thin. It is important to weigh the resident every 2 weeks to monitor weight gain and loss and respond via the plan of care as necessary.

The most common problem is weight loss. It can be caused by increased pacing and activity without appropriate food intake. A person who wanders may need up to 600 calories more per day than a less active patient.

During the final months of a resident's life, the following has been observed: The resident eats less and less, refusing food when it is fed to him or her. At first, the resident can be persuaded or enticed to eat by having something sweet at the tip of the spoon, such as ice cream. At this stage, he or she is still willing to drink. Chewing and swallowing become problems, so the food consistency is changed from regular to soft to chopped to pureed. In time, all food with bulk is refused, and the resident often picks out small pieces or particles from his or her mouth. For a while, the resident still is willing to drink, so high caloric drinks, protein shakes, instant breakfast mixes, and food supplements can be used. Pureed food also can be put into the drink, and the resident may like it at room temperature, warm, or cold. In time, the resident will not drink and will refuse to let any substance into his or her mouth. This usually precipitates death unless tube-feeding or other methods of feeding are used.

POSSIBLE CAUSES OR ANTECEDENTS OF EATING PROBLEMS: COGNITIVE CHALLENGES

Key Considerations

- Limited attention span
- Poor judgment and decision making
- Communication challenges: understanding and being understood
- Perceptual challenges

A short attention span and not understanding what is expected can lead to eating problems. Too much food on the tray or too many little dishes of food items can be distractions or, if handling choices is too difficult, the resident may just stop eating. The activity of eating, therefore, might be just too complicated with too many steps. Utensils may be used incorrectly or not at all if they are not recognized as part of the mealtime equipment or how they are to be used is not understood. Boundaries can be forgotten and food eaten from another's tray. Food may not be recognized as food (agnosia), which can lead to eating nonedible items such as napkins and sugar packets. Food is played with at times if the resident does not understand what it is or forgets how to get it into his or her mouth. Poor judgment may lead to the resident's pouring his or her beverage, such as juice or coffee, onto the meal. The resident may also not be able to judge if the food or drink is too hot or if the food is spoiled. Misjudgment may lead to eating pieces of food, such as meat, that are not appropriate and too large for one bite, and this may lead to choking. Overstuffing the mouth can also occur when the sensory information that the mouth is full is not comprehended.

Mealtimes may be a start, stop, start again process as the resident appears to remember how to eat and then, in the middle of the meal, forgets, then once again remembers and resumes eating. The resident may overeat or undereat if he or she does not comprehend the body's triggers of being hungry or being full.

Residents with limited communication skills may not be able to express their food likes or dislikes verbally. Usually, they are able to demonstrate their intent and feelings through nonverbal facial responses, noises, pushing the food away, or just not opening their mouth.

Visitors or strangers in the eating area can cause distraction. A television or radio can be equally distracting, taking the resident's focus away from his or her plate and the process of eating.

Alzheimer's Disease: Activity-Focused Care

POSSIBLE CAUSES OR ANTECEDENTS OF EATING PROBLEMS: PHYSICAL CHALLENGES

Key Considerations

- Physical dysfunctions, affecting body movement and coordination
- Presence of chronic physical problems
- Perceptual dysfunctions
- Weight loss or gain

A resident challenged with poor ability to motor plan as to how to hold a utensil and then lift the utensil to the mouth will experience eating problems. The inability to move purposefully, called *apraxia*, may limit the resident's ability to eat independently. Once the food is in his or her mouth, the resident may do any or all of the following: (1) chew one bite incessantly, (2) not chew at all and swallow the food, (3) pocket the food in the side of the mouth, (4) clamp the mouth closed, or (5) not be able to initiate the physical movements for swallowing.

Assess the resident by using a sensory profile (see Appendix 5-2) to help determine taste likes and dislikes as well as tolerance for food in the mouth cavity. If the resident has chronic pain, work with his or her physician to use medications on a scheduled basis rather than when the resident requests, because many residents often cannot respond to or ask for assistance when they are experiencing discomfort.

Residents may not be able to sit down during mealtimes due to their need to pace. They may also leave the table during meals because of restlessness or due to a short attention span. Some residents fall asleep during mealtimes and have to be wakened, perhaps by a spoon placed back in their hand to start the process again. If the resident is not physically comfortable, he or she will have difficulties eating. Examples include wet clothing or incontinence products, ill-fitting dentures, missing glasses, onset of an illness limiting the interest in or ability to eat, or the loss of the sense of hunger or thirst due to the dementia.

Chronic disabilities, such as a stroke, arthritis, back pain, or sensory deficits, may only increase the difficulty residents with dementia have during mealtimes. Parkinson's disease or parkinsonian-like problems can sometimes cause the resident to appear stubborn or unable to carry out the mechanics of eating. This Parkinson's connection is due to an "on-and-off" cycle that is related to the timing of medications and the resident's response to the medications. The on-and-off cycle may affect the resident in such a way that perhaps he or she was able to feed himself or herself at breakfast, but due to the medication timing and resultant rigidity or tremor, the resident cannot feed himself or herself at lunchtime. Parkinson's can also cause the hand to tremor and shake, making it difficult to get liquids to the mouth if heavy utensils are not used. Chewing and swallowing can also be affected. "Masking" of the resident's face due to muscle rigidity can also deceive the caregiver as to the resident's wish for more or less food, especially when accompanied by a loss of verbalization skills.

Perceptual problems with depth, one-side neglect, or poor eyesight can limit eating, as can tremor, rigidity, or restricted grasp due to muscle or joint limitations. Being unable to judge the resident's biting down force or his or her ability or inability to release a clenched-jaw response mandates the safety requirement that plastic utensils not be used.

POSSIBLE CAUSES OR ANTECEDENTS OF EATING PROBLEMS: PSYCHOSOCIAL CHALLENGES

Key Considerations

- Anxiousness or fearfulness, or both
- Negative responses to other residents, staff, or family, or all
- Flat affect, depression
- Mood and "old-learning" mind-set responses

Residents' activity just before meals is important. If a stimulating exercise or dancing program has just taken place, it is more difficult for residents to quiet down and focus on the meal. It is equally difficult for them if they are hurried to the table or are seated at the table long before the meal arrives. The presence of a resident who is constantly noisy can agitate the others.

Some residents are very concerned about their place at the table and are willing to defend it or they may become combative if someone is sitting in their seat. Residents who sit too close or at the same table with someone they do not like can become agitated. If they do not like the person assisting them, residents may stop eating or strike out.

Residents who are depressed or apathetic may not want to eat or eat very little during mealtime. Some residents become aware and upset that their meal is not quite like that of their neighbors, perhaps because of varying dietary restrictions or levels of food consistency at one table. Being the last one to be served at the table often results in anger and fear that they will not be fed, and they may even try to leave the table.

Another cause of not eating is that residents may think that their families are coming. An empty chair brought to the table beside the resident helps to assure him or her that there is a place for the family member.

Some residents' responses to eating and mealtimes, which can lead to problems, appear to derive from old learning, like old tapes they are replaying in their minds, things they have said to themselves or heard said to them throughout the years. For example:

1. *"I'm on a diet."* Residents, especially women, who dieted for many years or have a past association of being too fat, may refuse to eat all of the food placed in front of them. This often does not hold true when it comes to desserts. Even when these residents are frail and their health is compromised, they will stick to their diet mind-set. Many of the high calorie and nutrient dense foods are sweet, however, and if they are served as the main part of the meal, they can be refused. Placing high-nutrient candy bars in candy-store type paper cups or wrappers and then into an empty box of candy from a recognized manufacturer often works when other foods are refused.

2. *"I'll eat just part of this meal and save the rest for later."* Residents with a Depression-era mentality may not want to eat all of their meal because they are concerned about where the next meal will come from. Sometimes, a meal ticket with the three meals a day listed on the ticket may help them to feel assured that they will be fed again. At times, residents will continue to want to store food, putting it in their pockets and purses. In their room, the food is often placed behind

the drapes or in the tissue box. However, spoiled food is not always recognized by the resident and can be eaten and cause illness. A room food search should be performed on a regular basis for residents who hoard, but it must be done when the staff are sure that the resident will not return to the room and find his or her room being searched.

3. *"I can't eat until everyone is served."* Very often, women are anxious that everyone be served before they can sit down to eat. Mothers appear to continue their role of being sure that there is enough food for everyone before taking a plate for themselves. This "mother martyr" mind-set may lead to the resident's not eating, because just as the last resident is served it seems as though the earlier or faster eaters are ready for dessert or to have the table cleared. Assure the resident that there is plenty of food. It is best to place these residents, when they are finally seated, with their backs to other residents so they are not as aware of the mealtime's activities. At times when the resident might insist on eating last, having a microwave available for heating up the food is helpful. At other times, the resident may refuse to sit down but will stand up and eat at the kitchen counter.

4. *"You're not eating; here have some of mine."* Generally, no one likes to eat in front of people who are not eating. It can be an uncomfortable feeling for the resident when the staff or family are standing around. Persons with dementia continue to have the "gift of hospitality" and they worry about anyone not joining in the meal. Staff and family should be seated during mealtimes, therefore, to eliminate this stress (see Appendix 6-1). Seated staff and family should have a cup of coffee, juice, crackers, or any other food item, with them when they join the residents so they can appear to also be eating. At times, staff may need to eat a complete meal with the resident to encourage the resident to eat.

5. *"I can't eat, I don't have any money."* Some residents, especially men, will not go to the dining room or eat because they have no money. They can be told that the meal is paid for, but they sometimes still think that they should pay. The best answer, "It's covered by insurance," usually is accepted. Receipts or meal cards to be punched can be used. A facility credit card can be made up on heavy stock with the resident's name and used to "pay for" meals. The resident can also be told that the food is part of the "club" membership; therefore, he or she is required to eat at the club on a regular basis. Another suggestion is to have a "fill-in-the-resident's-name" letter that states that the resident has qualified to receive three meals a day, which have been paid for through a certain date. Some residents who have a Depression mentality will eat if they are told that the food has already been paid for. They do not wish to see food wasted.

6. *"This food is poisoned."* Fear of being poisoned can be very real to some residents with dementia. This reaction can easily occur when the resident's medications have been placed into food or drink. If the food being served looks different from that of other residents seated at the same table, the resident may become suspicious. When this occurs, the food can be served in a foam take-out box or a sealed container. Assuring the resident that the food has been specifically ordered for him or her may be helpful. Changing the eating area may help to decrease the resident's fears. If needed, the resident can be taken to the staff dining room to be served and allowed to eat there with a staffperson.

7. *"I am a volunteer, I don't eat here."* Give the resident a volunteer contract that defines the benefits of being a volunteer, which include free meals because he or she has worked hard and deserves to be fed.

8. *Decision to give up.* At times, residents may declare that they want to die or they want to just give up, which may include disinterest in eating. Sometimes, moving the resident to another part of the facility to eat may help. Having a beloved staffperson eat with the resident may encourage eating. Also helpful may be taking the food away from the resident when he or she resists eating and returning it a few minutes later as though it had never been served. The important caregiver response is to never give up.

POSSIBLE CAUSES OR ANTECEDENTS OF EATING PROBLEMS: ENVIRONMENTAL CHALLENGES

Key Considerations

- Overall ambiance: supportive or stressful?
- Dining area components
- Eating equipment: dishes, silverware, and so forth

The resident's "world" that surrounds him or her and how the resident perceives it becomes a major factor for enabling a resident to eat and enjoy food. The resident may experience stress because of an environment distraction he or she cannot control. The mealtime's general mood does not only derive from the persons in the area but from the look, sounds, and smells of the environment as well as the functional components such as furniture, utensils, dishware, lighting, glare, heat, room size, table setup and size, and appropriate chairs. If these components are incompatible with the resident's needs, eating problems may occur, including the possible escalation of overall behavioral problems or increased confusion, or both. For example, tables that seat more than four to six or tables that are close together because of limited space may lead the resident to feel trapped or overwhelmed.

An environment that calls forth residents' abilities and competency requires an ongoing assessment that focuses on residents' responses to eating. This assessment needs to be part of all resident plan-of-care assessments.

THE HUMILIATION OF BEING A "FEEDER"

Most of us cannot imagine having someone feed us, putting food into our mouths at a rate unnatural for us or in a sequence that does not appeal to our palate. Certainly, residents with dementia may experience this humiliation. Being labeled as a "feeder" adds to the diminishing of personal self-esteem. Thinking that the resident does not know what is going on and therefore that feeding him or her is all right is unfair and sometimes a projection of the caregiver's need to get mealtimes over and done with. Judging the resident's awareness of the possible humiliation due to being fed cannot be totally assessed. Careful observation of the resident's face and body posture during the feeding process can be a clue as to his or her feelings.

Being fed cannot be pleasant. For example, having food pushed into one's mouth before the last bite has been chewed and swallowed, or not being given time for relaxation before the next bite arrives. Residents can feel diminished and sad over the loss of their independence and dignity when they have to be fed. This lowering of self-esteem could initiate feelings of infancy because of the feelings connected with dependency. Residents may be remembering feeding their own children and the ultimate joy when the child was able to eat independently. These memories may compound the resident's humiliation. Depression is often a natural result.

Feeding a resident occurs only after all mealtime interventions and facilitation techniques have been tried. How the resident is fed is crucial to the resident's self-esteem. Meals are to be a social occasion. Therefore, the following suggestions are important if maintaining the social context of the meal and diminishing the resident's humiliation are to be achieved with sensitivity.

1. Never refer to the resident as a "feeder." Say instead, "Susie needs assistance with eating."

2. The caregiver should identify himself or herself to the resident and ask for permission to be of assistance. If possible, ask the resident about how he or she wishes to be fed (e.g., seasoning likes or dislikes, size of food pieces, sequence of food being placed in his or her mouth, how much food wanted in a spoonful or forkful, whether resident wants one kind of a food at a time, drink preferences, when a drink is helpful or not, whether resident would like to have foods mixed together). Asking these questions can be made more "natural" if the caregiver shares information about his or her own food preferences. Residents with limited ability to respond to questions can often give a "yes" or "no" answer when asked to make a decision between two choices. At other times, the caregiver can observe the resident's nonverbal language carefully when asked a question or in response to the eating activity. Caregivers can use mealtime with residents as a time of meaningful connection and an opportunity to support residents' dignity and self-esteem. Eating, even when being fed, is the residents' activity and therefore deserves to be one of offered and shared respect.

3. Talking with the resident during the meal is important. Residents are not a piece of furniture or an object; therefore, conversation is usually helpful to put the resident at ease. Talking over or around the resident to others is not only distracting but impolite if the resident is to be respected.

4. Bibs are for babies, and although they may be important to safeguard the resident's clothing, they can be called aprons or clothing covers. These clothing protectors should never be placed on the resident without first asking permission. For example, "You have such a pretty blouse on today, would you like this apron to protect it? I'm sure neither of us wants food spilled on it." Do not put clothing covers on a resident until the food is in front of him or her and he or she is ready to be fed. Coming up behind the resident and pulling a bib down over his or her face is not acceptable.

5. The food should be placed in front of the resident, not in front of the caregiver who will assist by feeding the resident. The caregiver should be seated where he or she can maintain eye contact with the resident. Because mealtimes are a

social event, the caregiver should have food or drink so he or she can also eat during the resident's mealtime. Proper table manners should be used. The caregiver should use silverware appropriately, keep elbows off the table, and not whistle or chew gum.

6. After the meal, the caregiver can ask the resident if he or she has had enough, if the resident wishes to have his or her hands or face washed, where the resident would like to go, or what the resident would like to do. The caregiver who just stands up, carrying away the tray or dirty dishes, and leaves the resident, not to return, is communicating a nonspoken message; perhaps, "Good, that's over for now." The caregiver who asks permission to leave the resident and offers a pleasant response to the mealtime experience can help to reestablish the resident's compromised feelings of being dependent and of little worth. "It was fun being with you at lunch today, see you tomorrow." With a few kind words, the caregiver returns respect to the resident.

INCREASING FOOD CONSUMED AND NUTRITION: APPROACHES AND INTERVENTIONS

Key Considerations

- Monitoring residents' eating, food intake, and unique needs
- Providing flexibility in food presentation and allowing as much time as needed for meals
- Understanding ways to promote eating
- All staff, volunteers, and family members trained to support residents and their eating

Mealtimes that enable residents to enjoy their food, consume the needed nutrients and fluids, and be as independent as possible require creativity and flexibility. Success requires addressing the residents' cognitive, physical, and psychosocial well-being as well as understanding the effects of the environment on mealtimes. The goal is for residents to experience their highest functional capacity while enjoying their food and drink.

Staff Approaches and Interventions

Staff attitude is the cornerstone for successful mealtime intervention. If they have the attitude of "Hurry up and eat, let's get this over with," the residents will not receive the nutrition they need. If the staff see mealtime as an all-important resident activity and that they play a vital role in its success, residents' ability to enjoy their meals and to eat the needed allotment of calories and fluids is greatly increased. Fostering the correct staff attitude takes staff training that is based on sensitivity and creativity. Certainly, each resident is a unique individual, but it takes a special staffperson to keep up with the many changes in mood and abilities that the resident may exhibit during the mealtime activity.

Staffpersons sitting between anxious or combative residents can reduce stress. Noisy residents should be removed from the group if at all possible. Even at times when staffing is short, the decision to take the one resident who is calling out, crying, or screaming away from the rest of the residents to be fed in his or her room is a good decision. Yes, the other residents will receive their meals and their needs met slower than usual, but at least they will eat. If the noisy resident remains in the area, all the residents may be affected and perhaps no one will eat or enjoy their meals.

Certainly, all assigned staff should be present at mealtime, including the activity therapist. All staff must be trained and knowledgeable in the Heimlich maneuver. Mealtime is also an opportunity for managers and non–hands-on caregiving staff to be present and assist the staff. This is especially true as the progression of the dementia increases and more and more residents need one-to-one feeding. Volunteers and family members are also helpful, and they also benefit from training.

The staff message to the resident at mealtime needs to be one of welcome, familiarity, nurturing, pleasant dining, and personal well-being.

Food Setup

If at all possible, remove the resident's plate, silverware, and other items from the tray. It is best to have a placemat on the table to help define which food is the resident's. The food must be prepared carefully: meat should be cut up into appropriate-sized pieces, and bones, fat, gristle, and garnishes removed. Assess all residents' feelings about having the meat cut up for them, as many would be offended if not permitted to do it for themselves. This decision may be altered depending on the softness of the meat. The milk carton must be opened and, if possible, poured into a tumbler, not a foam cup. Place silverware in the position in which it will be used if the resident is strongly one-side dominant and does not scan over to the other side of the plate. If not used appropriately, the knife should be removed because it seems that when there is a choice of an eating utensil, the knife is chosen. This is probably because the knife is picked up with his or her dominant hand to cut the food and then the resident forgets to put it down and starts to eat with it. Present just one utensil if simplification is needed, probably a spoon. If the resident, perhaps due to arthritis, has difficulty grasping the silverware, the handle can be enlarged. A soft, sponge-like tube from a hair curler can be slipped down the utensil handle, allowing the resident to increase his or her grip. Weighted silverware will enable a resident with tremor to eat with less food falling off the fork or out of the spoon. If possible, prepare the total tray or the plate away from the resident and then present it ready to eat. Help staff to be sensitive as to how the resident might feel if they reach over and onto the plate and start to cut up the food in front of the resident. The message of helplessness is certainly one that the resident may already be feeling, and he or she does not need it reinforced.

If the resident thinks that there is too much food in front of him or her, put half of it on a plate, serve it, and when that food is finished, place the remaining food on a clean plate and serve the resident again. At times, a resident cannot focus on an entire tray of food and may do better with one food item at a time (e.g., the main dish first, then the salad, then the bread and butter). This restaurant-style meal service approach can be done with staff training and acceptance. Staff set up a work table, one staff member serves the juice or water, while another prepares the first course. The first course is then delivered to the table. While the residents are eating, the next course is prepared and served after the dishes from the first course have been removed. The restaurant approach continues throughout the meal, allowing residents to focus on what is to be eaten at that time and not being distracted, for example, by the dessert arriving at the same time as the chicken.

Residents, Eating, and Food Approaches and Adaptations

Residents may require or benefit from an escort to the dining area at mealtime. The dining area should be prepared to provide multisensory cueing that the room's next activity is eating (e.g., using aromas such as coffee, cinnamon toast, soups, bread baking, and pasta sauce). Some residents like to stay in the same seat for each meal, some do not. Having assigned seating usually does not work but is worth a try when you are trying to group residents for socialization or for the assistance they require.

The meal should be monitored constantly and individualized as much as possible. One approach or way of delivering food is not effective for all residents in the dining area. Each resident is an individual and requires a resident-centered plan of care for mealtime. A simple checklist chart can be used by the staff to help each caregiver to know each resident's specific mealtime abilities, challenges, and needs for assistance.

Residents should be encouraged to eat independently for as long as possible. Independent eating includes eating with the fingers. A resident may need to be reminded to eat, to chew, or to swallow (see Hands-On Care Strategies in Chapter 5). Refer to the facilitation techniques described in Eating and Mealtime Interventions and Facilitation. Staff must remember that eating is an important activity and residents will require a great deal of time for successful mealtime engagement.

The main-dish meat, with or without the vegetables, made into a sandwich can be a successful finger food if utensils cannot be used. Milk and soups should be served in a cup with a large handle or perhaps two handles. Sipping from a straw can be too difficult for the resident to experience success. A damp washcloth under the plate can prevent it from sliding. A plate guard is helpful but can be a source of fascination and may result in the resident's not eating. The key is that the food must not be taken away too soon, as the resident has a tendency to start and stop eating many times throughout the meal.

A consistency-as-tolerated order from the physician allows changes in diet to be made as needed. A resident may eat "regular food" at first, then does better on soft food or chopped meat with regular vegetables. Soft foods can be used when the resident does not remember how to chew. These can include cream soups, egg dishes, stews, and pasta casseroles that are easier to move around in the mouth and swallow. As chewing and swallowing become more of a problem, pureed foods help to limit choking and aspiration. A thickener can be added to liquids to help prevent choking. Food supplements or pureed foods should not be used prematurely. Pureed food can be made more attractive for residents when it is sculptured. This is a process performed in the kitchen after the food is pureed, in which it is shaped in molds, frozen, and then prepared so it arrives at the table looking like the food item it once was. For example, pureed pork can be sculptured to look like a chop or pureed peas can look like the real thing. Using sculptured pureed food takes time and labor in the kitchen. If the pureed food is rejected, it can be put into milk or high protein drinks. Often, it is the metal of the spoon that the resident does not allow in his or her mouth with the food. The spoon may feel foreign to his or her lips or tongue and possibly repulsive if the metal hits against his or her teeth during the eating process. Try a rubber-coated small spoon when the resident starts to keep his or her lips closed or before placing the pureed food into a liquid.

It is especially important during this time that the resident is positioned comfortably with his or her head forward to protect his or her airway, especially if most of the eating involves liquids. Other positioning suggestions include having the resident's hips against the back of the chair with his or her upper body upright as much as possible. The resident's arms resting on the table or on a lap board can help to support his or her upper trunk. The chair needs to be close enough to the table to accommodate comfortable eating. Tables should be at appropriate heights for the residents using them.

Liquids can be frozen on sticks, and frozen pudding and gelatin on sticks are popular. At times, the resident will not open his or her mouth wide enough for a spoon to enter. A feeding syringe then can be considered, if part of the agreed-on plan of care. A resident who drinks his or her meals may be reintroduced to soft or chopped foods with success.

Weight loss and weight gain can be tracked and the therapeutic effects studied. Residents weighing more than their recommended body weight should be allowed to maintain that weight unless it interferes with ambulation. Doubling breakfast can help weight to be maintained if the resident starts to lose pounds.

The resident's nutrition and hydration is everyone's job. A nutrition or snack cart that is used two or three times a day between meals helps to ensure that residents are receiving the calories and fluids required for wellness. Items on the cart can include juices and water, snacks of sweets as well as fruits, cheese, or small sandwiches. Prepare the cart or tray so it is easy to handle and has all the needed items such as cups, napkins, and spoons. Especially effective is to have a resident work along helping the staffperson.

Feel free to experiment with the choice of foods. Residents sometimes forget that they did not like a certain food. They sometimes are able to make a choice and therefore can have a selective menu for the main meal. They seem to eat better when they have chosen the main dish. Having a substitute food handy is important. Honey drizzled over food can create a taste interest. The resident's favorite meal should be noted and then portions of that meal should be doubled if the resident is losing weight. Very often, this meal is breakfast.

The meal should be a gracious social event, and it can be, but a lot of thinking, planning, and creative approaches are needed to make it a success.

DIETARY DEPARTMENT: FOOD MODIFICATIONS AND MEALTIME SUPPORT

Key Considerations

- Availability of a variety of foods
- Finger foods for residents not using utensils
- Flexibility in number and size of meals
- High-calorie, fortified, and nutrient-dense foods available when needed

The dietary department plays a major role in the care of residents with dementia. The dietary staff need to observe the various eating behaviors, understand the resident's physical and cognitive problems, and support the resident's likes and dislikes. When the resident begins to lose weight, the dietitian plays a major role in advising the kitchen on foods. The following are suggestions for the dietary department:

1. Provide finger foods such as chicken nuggets, cheese squares, fruit gelatin squares, sandwiches, vegetables, fried potato pieces, or fruits in chunks (see Appendix 6-2).
2. Prepare soft food that does not require extensive chewing, and stay away from stringy foods such as green beans and corned beef.
3. Use boneless foods, including chicken breasts.
4. Use food carts to maintain food at proper temperatures, especially when one item is served at a time.
5. Deliver food at the designated time so that residents do not have to wait for their food or feel rushed to the table because the food has arrived.
6. Be willing to provide a change of food when requested by the staff who are feeding the resident and take it to the dining area as soon as possible.
7. Maintain flexibility in the size of food portions, doubling portions of favorite foods if needed.
8. Supply small meals if the resident is losing weight and is unable to eat enough at regular mealtimes. This extra feeding can lead to problems with the other residents feeling left out. It is usually possible to provide the resident enough calories and good nutrition with the three regular meals each day and with healthy snacks. These snacks can include peanut better and jelly sandwiches or crackers, cheese squares with or without crackers, milkshakes, fruit, vegetables, and some dry cereals. Residents, of course, almost always enjoy ice cream, cake, and cookies.
9. Use nutrient-dense foods and snacks, offered to the resident between meals (see Appendix 6-3).
10. Add protein and calories by including eggs, cheese, butter, peanut butter, honey, or cream in foods if appropriate. For example, omelets made with cheese, vegetables, or meats, or a combination, can increase calories, protein, and fiber.
11. Serve double-strength milk to drink and add it to cereals, potatoes, meatloaf, soups, cakes, and cookies.
12. Serve fruits in heavy syrup.

DINING ENVIRONMENT AND EQUIPMENT SUPPORT

Key Considerations

- A visually, auditorily, and physically comfortable environment
- A balance between overstimulation and understimulation
- Dishes, glasses, and silverware reflective of residents' life history and capacity to use appropriately

The balance between overstimulation and understimulation appropriate for mealtimes should be assessed before and during the meal. Residents are looking for a place to eat that is pleasant and one in which they feel welcomed.

Being seated and staying at the table for the meal can be problems. Residents who absolutely refuse to sit down can eat their meal from a cup as they pace, refilling the cup as needed. They also do well with their meal in a sandwich. A geriatric chair can be used, if there is a physician's order and the resident can tolerate being seated with a tray in front of him or her. A chair that is very heavy will keep some residents at the table. At times, you can seat wandering residents with their backs to the wall and put the table in front of them, but this also can lead to anxiousness because they may feel trapped. (Note: The heavy chair or the table that cannot be moved by the resident will be considered a restraint.) Residents should be spaced so they have their individual "territory." Various eating areas can help. For example, there may be areas that can hold large groups, small groups, or where someone can be seated alone but still be in the dining area or totally apart from the others. An L-shaped dining room allows for the highly distracted resident to eat apart from the others. An L-shaped room is also lovely to have for family meals. If possible, have several sizes of tables in the dining area (e.g., square tables that sit four plus some tables for two). This also allows for fulfilling individual needs.

A kitchen unit in the eating area is ideal. A microwave and refrigerator allow substitute foods to be prepared quickly before the resident loses interest in eating. Food that becomes cold can be reheated. Extra food can be readily available when the resident wants more than what was on his or her tray.

The ambiance and environment for the meal is important. The television should be off and soft music can be played if deemed appropriate for the present mealtime. Small square tables help to define "territory" and can be moved easily to provide desired groupings. Round tables appear to increase confusion over which foods belong to each resident because residents have a tendency to reach into their neighbor's tray. Glaring lighting or too much sunshine coming through the windows can be distracting. Some residents do better facing a plain wall or looking into the room rather than out the window. A comfortable room temperature should be maintained throughout the meal.

Dishes can be more effective if they are simple in style and plain in color, without a pattern or bold design. The color should contrast with that of the tray or table. If the edges of the plate curve up, the food will probably stay in place, rather than being pushed off the edges during eating. Mugs for soup and beverages are often easier to handle than bowls, especially when the handle is large and extends away from the cup for an easier grasp. No plastic utensils should be used no matter how sturdy because of the possibility of a piece being bitten off. Rubber-coated children's silverware can help protect teeth if the resident bites hard on the utensil. The bowl part of an iced tea spoon or baby spoon can be turned over to place food within the resident's mouth during feeding if his or her tongue or lips do not respond to taking the food from a utensil.

MEALTIME ASSISTANCE: ACTIVITIES INVOLVEMENT AND OTHER STAFFPERSONS

Key Considerations

- Preparing for mealtime with an appropriate activity and necessary environmental changes

- Using knowledge of individual residents to enable maximal food intake while providing for their social needs
- Participating in the delivery of food to residents and in their dining

The activity therapist needs to apply knowledge of the resident's attention span, interaction with other residents, distractibility, fine motor skills, motor planning, and spatial-perceptual disabilities to mealtime. The therapist uses this information to set up a seating plan that groups residents. The groups can be based on friendships, types of foods eaten (pureed, regular, etc.), or the amount of help needed during the meal. For example: some residents can handle the whole tray in front of them, some need one item at a time, some can feed themselves totally, some need help less than 50% of the meal, some need help more than 50% of the meal, and others need total feeding assistance. Residents' names can be color coded according to their needs and a seating chart can be made so that there is a consistent plan for each meal. This chart also will show any change in the arrangement of tables that may be needed. Staff should be aware that a seating plan may often not work. The staff will be required to be flexible and "go with the flow" if at all possible and serve residents where they have seated themselves.

Menu selection can be implemented by the activity department. Residents can usually choose which of the main entrees they would prefer. The staff can make up a menu selection form and invite the resident to check off his or her choice and sign his or her name. The form is then given to the dietary department. At times, the choice made the previous day is not what the resident wants at the time of the meal, especially when the resident has no memory of having made the selection. The dietary department should be flexible and send up enough of everything in case the switch needs to occur.

The activity before the meal often sets the mood and therefore should be stress-free and quieting. Stimulating exercise or dancing can make it more difficult for the resident to quiet down and focus on a meal. Sheets or cloths on the tables transform them from game areas to dining tables. Singing can be used if residents have to wait at the tables for their meals to arrive. The therapist and staff need to be ready themselves to serve the meal and to help anyone who needs feeding. The presence of the therapist helps to encourage the social aspects of eating.

Morning "coffee club" and afternoon parties and socials are successful activities for residents with dementia because they build on social skills that usually continue throughout life. Nutritional and fun snacks can be chosen by the therapist. Residents love a party and enjoy setting the tables, serving the food and drinks, and cleaning up afterward. A "fast-food day" or pizza party also are enjoyed. Eating out at restaurants is often a delightful success. You soon learn which places enjoy having your residents. A separate dining area, if available, works best. Staff, family, and volunteers are needed, with a 1 to 2 or 1 to 3 ratio of helpers to residents.

Another "eating out" option is to set up a meal in another part of the facility rather than residents' current dining area. For example, use a staff conference room, an ice cream parlor, or a rehabilitation room. Just the journey from the residents' care area to the eating place may help residents to feel that they have gone someplace special. The same food that residents would have been served in their regular dining area can be used, although the plates, silverware, and glassware should be removed from the tray before placing them in front of the residents. The "eating out" experience will be especially successful if the staff have taken the time and effort to put tablecloths, centerpieces, and fancy napkins on the table, and, if appropriate, have soft music playing. This mealtime fun will be enhanced when the staff sit down and enjoy the same meal the residents have been served.

FAMILY INVOLVEMENT AT MEALTIME

Key Considerations

- Using the family as a resource to learn food likes and dislikes
- Obtaining knowledge of former eating behaviors and habits
- Supporting family members who choose to feed their loved ones

The family is a good source of information to help you maintain the resident's nutrition. They often bring in favorite "yummies" to delight the resident. Food likes and dislikes certainly can change, as the resident forgets that he or she did not like fish, for example. Did he or she prefer hot or cold food? A big meal at noon or at night? Snacks?

Family members often want to be involved during mealtime. Usually this works out well. They need to feel welcomed, but care needs to be taken that they do not feel guilty if they do not feed their loved one on a regular or sporadic basis, or if they do not want to feed him or her at all. They may prefer to feed another resident rather than their family member, if allowed by regulation. Certainly, the family should feel assured that their loved one will be fed patiently and lovingly by staff whether they are present or not. Observation and monitoring can limit the following potential situations:

1. Poor feeding ability by the family member may demonstrate a need for in-service training on how to feed, speed of feeding, and so on.
2. The family member may be too demanding or not demanding enough of the resident to eat.
3. The family member may be too talkative and distracting for the resident to focus on eating.
4. The resident may experience increased anxiety or agitation because the family member is feeding him or her or is present in the room.
5. The resident's favorite food may be provided at an inappropriate time, may not be in keeping with specific diet orders that must be followed because of doctor's orders, or is not of the consistency that can be tolerated.
6. The family member may eat from the resident's tray.

Men, especially, like to be present during mealtime to feed their wives. Usually, this is a very satisfying experience and the couple often enjoy the meal in a room apart from other residents. The husband living alone can be encouraged to order a tray for himself so that he has a substantial meal each day. The husband often takes great pride in how well he is able to encourage his wife to eat. This also can be the feeling when other family members are present to help with meals. However, in time, the resident will eat less and less and then refuse to eat altogether. The staff should be there to explain this development to the family and to provide support so that they do not feel that they are failing in feeding techniques or do not take their loved one's diminishing appetite personally.

LATE OR TERMINAL CARE NUTRITIONAL ASSESSMENT AND CHALLENGES

Key Considerations

- Ongoing assessment to provide necessary food and food consistency changes
- Team approach for the resident receiving terminal care and offering of support for the family
- Awareness of options as preparation for end-of-life decisions

Poor nutritional intake and the possibility of malnutrition and dehydration are often experienced during the terminal stage of dementia. Vitamin, mineral, and protein deficiencies as well as the lost weight may make residents more susceptible to systemic infections and other health problems. Residents may refuse to eat for a number of reasons and sometimes exhibit behaviors that make eating unsuccessful. These may include biting down on the utensils, holding food in the mouth, refusal to open the mouth or lips, meeting the food at the front of the mouth and pushing it away with the tongue, spitting food out, pushing the caregiver's hand away, or turning the head away from the caregiver. It appears that some residents, even in the very late stages of Alzheimer's, find an inner strength to communicate their wishes for control, and they can demonstrate this by permitting or not permitting food or drink to enter their mouth.

Interventions that may help to maximize nutrition at mealtime during end-stage care include

1. Alternating warm with cool food
2. Alternating sweet with nonsweet food
3. Use of pureed foods
4. Adding unsalted beef or chicken broth to foods to make them easier to swallow
5. Adding honey to food
6. Placing pureed food in milk for the resident to drink when a spoon is not allowed in his or her mouth
7. Use of a rubber-coated baby spoon with a resident who has a tendency to clench his or her teeth or lips

Weight can be lost quickly once food intake is decreased. Choking or excessive coughing may indicate that the resident is having swallowing difficulties. Residents may eat well during the terminal-care period, but weight is still lost. Appropriate hydration is extremely important. Bringing together the interdisciplinary team can start the assessment process for developing interventions for the possible reversal of the weight loss or approaches for maintaining the resident's current weight. The team should include the physician, registered dietitian, speech therapist, occupational therapist, staff, family, and the resident if she or he is able to contribute.

The late-stage nutritional assessment should include the following:

Resident

- Eating or swallowing abilities and difficulties; any choking or excessive coughing that demonstrates a swallowing problem
- Teeth, dentures, oral hygiene
- Current medications and effects on oral cavity moisture
- Responses to current diet; assessment of calorie, protein, and fluid needs
- Positioning needs
- Physical well-being or illness that should be addressed, including assessment for malnutrition and dehydration and possible constipation
- Level of cognitive decline
- Responses to facilitation interventions, cueing, and assistance
- Sensory responses (i.e., visual, auditory, gustatory, tactile, olfactory)
- Mood and emotional needs
- Weight loss pattern and history

Foods

- Calories, protein, and fluid count
- Foods and drink enjoyed
- Foods and drink rejected
- Favored consistency and tolerance, temperature, color

Meals

- Frequency and timing
- Size
- Utensils (i.e., size, type, rubber-coated or metal)
- Appropriate feeding time allotted
- Staff (i.e., attitude, sensitivity, and feeding techniques)

Hydration

- Measuring fluid intake and urination output

Environment

- Presence of overstimulation or understimulation
- Noise
- Light and temperature
- Presence of other residents that is helpful or distracting

Family

- Response to family members being present or not present

Fortified foods and drinks rich in nutrients can help prevent or curb weight loss. Foods, such as oatmeal, pudding, soup, and mashed potatoes, can be prepared with cream, half-and-half, dried fruits, nuts, honey, sugar, jam, butter, sour cream, bacon, avocado, or cheese to add calories. Protein can be added by adding peanut butter, cheese, hard-cooked eggs or egg substitute, dry milk powder, or chopped meat, when appropriate, to foods. Rich drinks, such as oral liquid supplements, instant breakfast powders, nectars, fruit or vegetable juice, cocoa, and pasteurized eggnog, can be substituted for tea and coffee. Offering the resident "regular" food for as long as possible is suggested before turning to liquid supplements. A registered dietitian is the best resource for these recipes. See Appendix 6-3 for examples of recipes of fortified and nutrient-dense foods.

As the late stage of dementia advances, residents will usually slowly stop eating. Focus remarks of praise on what the resident has eaten, not on the food that remains on the plate. Encourage the resident to take "just" a bite of the food. Then encourage the resident to take another bite. Feeding the resident becomes an activity consuming a great deal of time. The emphasis continues to be on providing adequate calories and protein as well as fluid. Every bite counts.

Family members are called on to make choices about end-of-life decisions (see Chapter 13). The decline in the resident's ability to eat is, in time, part of the progression of the dementia. Hospice can become involved at this time if the family chooses. Comfort measures are then used as the caregiving team surrounds the resident and the family with support and presence.

HEALTH CARE PROVIDER AND STAFF ISSUES

Successful eating and mealtime activity require a team approach throughout a health care facility. Issues ranging from the size of the plates to the quality of the food, staff that are appropriately trained, and a dietary department that supports the ever changing needs of residents with dementia requires support from ownership and management.

Weight loss can happen all too quickly for residents with dementia. Support for the residents' overall cognitive, physical, and psychosocial wellness does not happen without assessment, problem solving, commitment, and follow-through.

Creative interventions may require specific policies and procedures that support the unique needs of residents with dementia. For example, pouring honey on food may be necessary because the resident is only willing to eat sweet foods, or someone who is monitoring the meal may need to be seated during mealtime because of the resident's anxiety that he or she is not eating (see Appendix 6-1).

> An Alzheimer's special-care unit of 16 residents was eating lunch when two state regulators arrived to survey the mealtime. A third person was present with them for the observation. The three visitors stood watching the residents eat

Alzheimer's Disease: Activity-Focused Care

while marking down their observations on clipboards. The residents became concerned that the visitors were not eating. The agitation increased as the staff became nervous about the residents not eating. The end result was not a total "food fight" but very close to one. No one ate. This care unit now has a policy and procedure that safeguards the residents, especially at mealtimes. It requests that no one stand during the meal except for the serving of food, the helping of residents, or the changing of seats. Training for surveyors on this requirement that everyone is to be seated has led to their responding with thanks. The surveyors stated that they did not realize the discomfort they were causing the residents and are, therefore, more than willing to accommodate the policy to be seated.

Staff are required to cooperate with the emphasis on eating as an activity. Meals are not dished out and then taken away without first assessing if the food should be adapted, perhaps into a sandwich, for the resident to be able to eat. Or, perhaps some residents take up to 1½ hours to eat and even though the kitchen is clamoring for the dirty dishes, the caregiving staff hang on to them while the resident slowly eats.

Staff are also deeply affected when all their very best efforts to feed a resident are met with clenched lips or teeth and a refusal to eat. Staff may feel helpless and let down that the resident appears to have made a choice not to eat and is therefore seen as uncooperative. Near the time of a resident's death, staff may also struggle with their personal convictions when family members do not want any artificial means of feeding or nutrition, or both, and are content with allowing the resident to gradually slip away into death. Hopefully, social services and other caring staff are there to comfort the hands-on staff as well as facilitate the use of a hospice bereavement counselor when appropriate.

The industry surrounding the development of specialized foods and recipes for medically compromised persons is quickly evolving and growing. A resident's nutrition and hydration can be supported for an extended period as the dementia progresses. The bottom line, no matter how sophisticated the foods are, comes down to the nature of the staff. A dedicated staff support residents with dementia when they generously offer them and their families kindness, patience, and respect.

SUMMARY

Ensuring and supporting the food intake of residents with dementia takes a team approach and commitment to quality care. The emphasis must be on the resident and his or her unique needs. Caregivers are called to be sensitive to the resident's needs, including the resident's feelings of humiliation when he or she forgets how to eat or needs to be fed. Eating is not only a complex activity but also the most significant activity of each day because of the many consequences and the effects on the resident when nutritional intake is minimized. Activity-focused care calls for creativity and flexibility as well as facilitation interventions that should be a basic component of all mealtimes. Residents' often erratic responses to food, environment, staff, family, and others present a challenge in the fulfillment of residents' nutritional needs and well-being.

SUGGESTED READING

Griffin RL. Factors contributing to minimizing weight loss in patients with dementia. Am J Alzheimer's Dis 1995;10:33–36.

Hellen CR. Eating: an Alzheimer's activity. Am J Alzheimer's Care Rel Dis Res 1990;5:5–9.

Kovach CR. Late-Stage Dementia Care: A Basic Guide. Washington, DC: Taylor and Francis, 1997.

McCann RM, Hall WJ, Groth-Juncker A. Comfort care for terminally ill patients. The appropriate use of nutrition and hydration. JAMA 1994;272:1263–1266.

Volicer L, Seltzer B, Rheaume Y, et al. Eating difficulties in patients with probable dementia of the Alzheimer type. J Geriatr Psychiatry Neurol 1989;2:188–195.

Watson R. Measuring feeding difficulty in patients with dementia: developing a scale. J Adv Nurs 1994;19:257–263.

Zahler L, Keiser A, Gates G, Holdt C. Staff attitudes towards the provision of nutritional care to Alzheimer's patients. Am J Alzheimer's Care Rel Dis Res 1994;9:31–37.

A6-1

Sample Policy and Procedures: Supporting Optimal Nutrition for Residents with Dementia

It is the policy of this care center that residents with dementia will receive adapted methods of food presentation, dining area environmental modifications, food items supporting specific need, and acceptance of self-feeding methods needed to support their optimum nutrition.

Discussion
Dementia may affect eating and drinking processes in the following ways:

- Chewing or swallowing skills, or both, are forgotten or diminished, which is often a cause of choking or food refusal.
- Food may be not eaten because of
  - decreased attention span, inability to attend to the activity of eating
  - food not being recognized as something to eat
  - inability to motor plan or remember how to move the food to the mouth
  - environmental distractions
- Food is kept in the mouth, chewed endlessly.
- Food is eaten too fast, gulped down.
- Food is played with; may be eaten from another resident's tray.
- Utensils are not used appropriately or not used at all; food is eaten with the fingers.
- Nonedibles are eaten (e.g., paper napkins, sugar packets, garnishes).

Procedures
Residents will receive ongoing observation or assessment to determine specific needs for modification of presentation, environment, specific food item adaptations, and methods enabling self-feeding.

Food Presentation Considerations

- Garnishes will not be used when residents cannot respond by knowing if they are edible or nonedible.
- Packets (e.g., salt, sugar, sweetener, jelly) will not be placed on the tables when residents do not understand appropriate usage, but will be available for the staff to offer or use.
- Finger foods are encouraged, including sandwiches made from any mealtime food item.
- Food items can be presented one at a time if necessary to reduce confusion and anxiety.
- Sweet food items (e.g., honey, pudding, sugar) may be placed on top or within food not being eaten (e.g., sprinkling sugar on top of mashed potatoes, honey on top of eggs) if medically appropriate.
- A single utensil (e.g., spoon, fork) can be used when necessary to reduce confusion and encourage independence.
- Food can be eaten by the resident in nontraditional places if that is the only place the resident is willing to eat (e.g., the bedroom, hall, or while walking or pacing).

Environmental Considerations

- Plastic utensils will not be used by residents at regular mealtimes unless there is a kitchen emergency or if the resident exhibits behavioral challenges such as stabbing or throwing.
- Plastic utensils used for snacks will be closely monitored for misuse.
- Distractions, including excess noise, visitors, etc., will be minimized during mealtimes (e.g., prohibiting group tours, limiting specific persons found to be upsetting to the residents).
- All persons in the dining area will be asked to be seated during mealtimes unless they are residents or actively involved with residents or involved in the serving of food.
- Staff will be seated while assisting residents at mealtime.

Specific Food Item Modifications

- Broth or liquid (e.g., soup, milk, coffee, tea, water, of appropriate temperature) may be used to decrease the dryness, stiffness, or food mass of foods (e.g., mashed potatoes, cake).
- Pureed foods not accepted with a spoon may be placed in liquids (e.g., milk, coffee, tea) in a cup for the resident to drink.
- Foods can be mixed together on the plate if they are not accepted individually.

Enabling Self-Eating

- All responses to self-feeding will be permitted, including eating with the fingers.
- "Messy" eaters will be permitted to continue feeding themselves, as there is dignity in feeding oneself.
- Residents unable to sit down during mealtime may be allowed to walk and eat if attempts to eat or be fed at the table have not been successful.
- The resident's meal may remain available when eating is extremely slow or the resident starts and stops eating.
- Attention will be placed on seating arrangements to diminish negative responses to tablemates (e.g., a resident preferring to eat alone may be seated away from other residents by using an individual-sized table).

A6-2
Finger Food Suggestions

When eating utensils escalate anxiety, increase confusion, or lead to the meal not being eaten, utensils can be totally disregarded and eating with fingers can commence. The important concern should not center on good manners versus bad manners. If eating with the fingers allows the person with dementia to retain independence during mealtimes, therefore promoting the resident's ability to be in control and have a positive self-image, then the emphasis shifts to finding foods that are nutritionally supportive and can be easily grasped, held, and delivered to the mouth. The following lists are some suggestions. It is hoped that the lists will encourage caregivers to be innovative, leading to the development of their own finger food creations.

FINGER FOOD IDEAS FOR BREAKFAST

- Cereals: small or large shredded wheat, sturdy flakes or shaped cereals
- Eggs: hard-boiled, scrambled in chunks (not broken up), scrambled or fried egg sandwiches, deviled eggs
- "Take-along" biscuit sandwiches with sausage, egg, and cheese
- French toast, raisin toast, cinnamon toast
- Pancakes
- Waffles
- Coffee cake, donuts
- Peanut butter and jelly sandwiches
- Grilled cheese sandwiches
- Fruits: all that can be handheld, both dried and fresh

FINGER FOOD IDEAS FOR LUNCH AND SNACKS

- Sandwiches: all kinds that can be successfully held without falling apart
    Use different kinds of breads, rolls, pocket breads, hot dog buns (e.g., roll-up sandwiches using a flour tortilla)
    Heating sandwiches, so ingredients become sticky, helps to keep them together
- Hamburgers, hot dogs
- Fruit plates with cheese cubes, vegetable sticks
- Pizza

- Salads: all kinds that have pieces big enough to pick up (e.g., Cobb, pasta roll-up salads using a large lettuce leaf to wrap around ingredients)
- Fruits: all that can be handheld, both dried and fresh

FINGER FOOD IDEAS FOR DESSERTS

- Fruit
- Cookies, bars, cake, cupcakes
- Fruit gelatin cubes
- Ice cream bars, cones, Popsicles
- Applesauce cubes made with gelatin
- Candy bars
- Cream puffs

FINGER FOOD IDEAS FOR DINNER

- Meats, poultry, fish, seafood: if soft and safe to make into bite-sized pieces, nuggets, or rolled; placed in sandwiches or cooked into balls, loafs, or pies
- Dinner sandwiches: use mashed potatoes to hold in meat and vegetables (toasting bread helps to keep sandwich from falling apart)
- Dinner roll-up: use large cooked cabbage leaf to wrap around meat, vegetables, and rice or potatoes
- Quiche pieces: vegetables, meat, seafood
- Pasta (use ones that can be filled with meat or cheese) with or without an extremely thick sauce, or pasta shells, rotini, or elbow macaroni
- Vegetable pieces: carrots, zucchini, cucumbers, tomatoes, brussels sprouts, celery, beets, beans, corn, green peppers
- Potatoes: baked, roasted, french fried, hash browned, oven baked, small boiled
- Rolls, biscuits, breads, bread sticks
- Cubed cranberry sauce (heat first and then add gelatin to increase firmness), pickles, olives
- Desserts: see Finger Food Ideas for Desserts

Alzheimer's Disease: Activity-Focused Care

A6-3
Nutrient-Dense Recipes

Super Pudding*

2 cups whole milk
¾ cup dry milk powder
2 tablespoons vegetable oil
1 package (4½ oz) instant pudding (resident's favorite flavor)

Stir together milk, milk powder and oil. Add instant pudding and mix well. Pour
into dishes and refrigerate.
Yield: Three 1-cup servings
Nutrient analysis per 1-cup serving: 495 calories, 14 g protein
Tips:
- Serve with cream, heavy cream, whipping cream, vanilla ice cream, or vanilla
  frozen yogurt.
- Substitute cream, heavy cream, or evaporated milk for the whole milk.
- For more calories, use dry milk powder made from whole milk.

Super Cereal†

2½ cups dry oatmeal
⅔ cup 2% milk
3½ cups water
1 cup nonfat dry milk
¼ lb margarine
½ cup brown sugar
½ cup granulated sugar

Mix water, dry milk, and ⅓ cup of 2% milk. Bring to a boil. Pour in oatmeal (or
other hot cereal) and cook over low heat until done, approximately 5 minutes.
Add margarine, sugars, and remaining ⅓ cup milk. Cook an additional 5 minutes.
Yield: 4 servings
Nutrient analysis per 8-oz serving: 564 calories, 13 g protein, 24 g fat, 74 g car-
bohydrate

---

*Courtesy of Carol Johnson, D.T.R., Lutheran Home, Arlington Heights, Illinois.
†Courtesy of The Wealshire, Lincolnshire, Illinois.

Breakfast Take Alongs*

⅔ cup butter or margarine
⅔ cup sugar
1 egg
1 teaspoon vanilla
¾ cup all-purpose flour
½ teaspoon baking soda
½ teaspoon salt
1½ cups oats (quick or old fashioned, uncooked)
1 cup (4 oz) shredded cheddar cheese
½ cup wheat germ
6 crisply cooked bacon slices, crumbled

Beat together butter, sugar, egg, and vanilla until well blended. Add combined flour, baking soda, and salt; mix well. Stir in oats, cheese, wheat germ, and bacon. Drop by rounded tablespoonfuls onto greased cookie sheet. Bake in preheated oven (350°F) 12–14 minutes or until edges are golden brown. Cool 1 minute on cookie sheet; remove to wire cooling rack. Store in loosely covered container in refrigerator or at room temperature.
Yield: Three dozen cookies
Nutrient analysis per two cookies: 160 calories, 6 g protein (three of these breakfast cookies provide approximately 11% of the U.S. Recommended Daily Allowance of protein)

High-Calorie Oatmeal*

4 cups cooked oatmeal
3¼ cups heavy whipping cream
15 oz frozen eggs
4 tablespoons margarine
15 tablespoons instant nonfat dried milk
15 tablespoons brown sugar (packed)

Prepare oatmeal according to package directions. Add remaining ingredients. Mix well.
Yield: Ten 6-oz servings
Nutrient analysis per 6-oz serving: 502 calories, 11.6 g protein, 38.4 g fat, 287 mg cholesterol, 2.06 g fiber, 177 mg sodium

High-Protein Mashed Potatoes*

4 cups whole milk
1 cup egg substitute
2 teaspoons margarine
1 teaspoon salt
1⅔ cups potato flakes

---

*Courtesy of Carol Johnson, D.T.R., Lutheran Home, Arlington Heights, Illinois.

Combine milk and egg substitute. Cover and steam until 160°F. Whisk until smooth. Add remaining ingredients. Cover and hold at 180°F until service.

Yield: Five 6-oz servings

Nutrient analysis per 6-oz serving: 226 calories, 13.4 g protein, 10 g fat, 27 mg cholesterol, 1 g fiber, 214 mg sodium

7

Physical Wellness: Mobility and Exercise

What is physical wellness? Wellness is more that just not being sick—it is a positive state of health. Wellness reflects a holistic sense involving the body, mind, and spirit with feelings of being in control of physical outcomes, including dignity and purpose.

Residents with dementia who are able to move and walk independently are usually capable of maintaining a positive outlook and quality of life as near normal as possible. As cognitive control of their lives decreases, the ability to walk encourages confidence and the sense of retaining control of themselves and their environment.

The aging process directly affects mobility. Body rhythms, the speed at which the resident moves and performs daily tasks, slow down. The body needs to move to maintain use of muscles and joints while promoting overall physical fitness, including the functional skeletal, cardiovascular, respiratory, digestive, excretory, and epidermal body systems. Problems, such as dizziness, swelling of the ankles or feet, arthritis, Parkinson's disease, osteoporosis, strokes, and a decrease in endurance, are but a few of the contributors to limited or compromised mobility. Safety becomes an issue. The elderly often become fearful of falling and many experience an increasing possibility of falls.

Caregiving stress can be eased when the resident is able to reduce anxiety by walking and being mobile. Walking also sustains a more normal day-night activity pattern because the resident experiences a healthy fatigue. When the resident is capable of participating or helping the caregiver, less physical strength is required for transfers or repositioning. Certainly, there are mobile residents who can cause or increase caregiver stress because of their constant safe or unsafe pacing and wandering. Considering ambulation as a resident's activity addresses mobility's positive and negative aspects and their influence on the relationship between the resident, caregiver, and environment.

As the process of dementia progresses, affecting the overall physical abilities of residents, the emphasis on physical well-being does not diminish but becomes increasingly the responsibility of the caregiver. Interventions calling forth the caregiver's flexibility and creativity can continue to facilitate residents' sense of wholeness and connectedness with their own bodies, as well as the continued relationship with other persons and their environment.

DEMENTIA FACTORS AFFECTING MOBILITY

Mobility is the culmination of not only physical wellness but also the integration of awareness of self and one's surroundings with the desire to ambulate. Dementia can pull apart or annul the coming together of all the necessary components for success. At times, it might appear that the resident is truly not a candidate for independent mobility but then he or she is up and going. Identifying how mobility is affected by the resident's cognitive, physical, and psychosocial responses enables staff to offer creative interventions for promoting independent or assisted ambulation. Examples of factors affecting mobility are listed in the following sections.

Cognitive Factors

- Limited attention span and orientation to surroundings
- Inability to follow directions or to understand communications or clues that enable safety
- Decreased ability to judge necessary aspects of safety or environmental hazards, or both (e.g., staying off of wet floors, putting shoes on the wrong feet, not pulling pants up adequately, or finding someone or something in the way and not knowing how to cope or adjust to the situation)
- Inability to interpret or report pain, possibly caused by sore feet, ill-fitting shoes, or skeletal or arthritic problems
- Inability to understand or respond appropriately to tiredness or inability to remember how to sit down, leading to the increased occurrence of falls
- Being grabbed by another resident intent on walking and being pulled along, not knowing how to get loose and away from the resident
- Decreased ability to remember how to initiate the activity of movement and ambulation
- Slowness or lack of response to being off balance and the inability to make the necessary adjustments to avoid a fall
- Intermittent ability to walk or walk safely due to limited body awareness and understanding of the environment
- Spatial or perceptual problems or inability to interpret or judge the environment, including

    Visual clifting, or the inability to understand or perceive depth or to interpret changes in the appearance of the floor, or both, so that the resident catches his or her feet on a rug or steps too high when walking from one floor surface to another (e.g., a rug to another surface such as a vinyl kitchen floor)

    > Irving could not judge the relationship between the floor and the wall even with a black, 10-in. contrast stripe at the base of the wall. One day, he walked into a corner and kept stepping from one foot to the other because he was not able to remember how to turn around to maneuver out of the corner.

    Tripping over obstacles such as chair legs or extended footrest on a geriatric chair

Walking into janitorial "wet floor" signs

Falling up or down stairs

Thinking that the floor is wet because of the shine or glare

Walking into walls or bumping into door frames

Interpreting patterns on the floor cover or rug as items to be picked up or thinking that dark areas are holes to be jumped across or walked around

> Sophie is very frail but can manage walking short distances independently. She becomes at risk for falls when she walks into the family room and attempts to bend over and pick up the design embedded in the linoleum floor.

Inability to judge distance (e.g., walking into furniture or people and not understanding how to walk around someone or something)

Physical Factors

- Experiencing apraxia, the inability to purposefully move the body or to interpret the body's relationship to space because of the brain's difficulty putting together the necessary information

> Margaret walks slanted to the right from the waist up. At times, she appears almost ready to fall to the right. When reminded or given physical clues to stand up straight, she does not respond because she is unaware of her body's position or how to make the needed change. At other times, she walks with a normal posture. To help prevent a possible fall, the staff attached the strap of a heavy shoulder purse to her left shoulder. The weight of the purse helped to straighten her posture.

- Poor balance due to decreased postural and righting reflexes
- Walking with feet close together in a narrow-based or a foot-crossing gait
- Walking with the body tilted to one side; forward or backward leaning
- Reaching out and grabbing when passing by an object or person, throwing the body off balance
- Tremor or rigidity of the trunk due to Parkinson's disease-like symptoms or the effects of medications
- Difficulty with narrow doorways or small spaces, leading to "freezing," which prohibits the resident from lifting his or her feet
- Sudden jerking movements of arms or legs that compromise balance

> Susan could walk easily, but when she changed direction her feet would turn quickly, while her trunk, shoulders, and arms were still facing forward. This pulled her body off balance and led to constant falls. She was not able to respond to reminders or instructions asking her to take small steps around a half circle when she wanted to walk in the reverse direction.

- Festination: Walking faster and faster and not being able to initiate the movement to slow down, possibly leading to the resident's running
- Exhaustion due to excessive walking or pacing
- Decreased abilities often precipitated by the effects of dehydration because the resident does not remember to drink
- Compromised mobility due to lack of or refusal to wear glasses, an incorrect prescription that distorts the visual environment, or the resident wearing someone else's glasses

Psychosocial Factors

- Reduced or rejected desire to ambulate due to a real or perceived fear of falling
- Reduced or limited mobility due to depression, mood changes, or visual or auditory hallucinations
- Becoming fearful and grabbing persons, doorways, bed rails, or other items, causing the walking or movement to stop suddenly
- Positive or negative responses to persons walking with resident
- Safe or unsafe responses to stress
- Disliking people in the way, shoving them, and being thrown off balance
- Feelings of paranoia or a need to search or look for someone or something
- Possible falls due to anger or feelings of having personal space or territory invaded, leading to the resident pushing, kicking, or hitting

PROMOTING MOBILITY AND INDEPENDENT AMBULATION

The resident's past and present mobility patterns and habits become necessary components for facilitating mobility. Caregivers should look at and understand the positive and negative aspects of mobility and assess their effects on the resident's abilities and inabilities. The questions to be answered are

- How does the activity of mobility affect the resident's quality of life?
- What are the risks involved and how do they lead to falls or possible injuries?
- Is mobility a priority in spite of the risks?
- What are reasonable expectations and goals?
- Is the decision to foster mobility, although the resident is at high risk for falling, supported by all persons responsible for the resident, including the attending physician and the family members responsible for care?

Assessment and Monitoring Components

A functional assessment of the resident's physical well-being can be made easily by observing the basic activities of daily living. Difficulties with any of the tasks reflects the possible need for a corrective program. These daily life functional tasks include

- Bed mobility
- Balance (sitting and standing)

Alzheimer's Disease: Activity-Focused Care

- Transfer skills (to and from the bed, chair, toilet)
- Walking skills (e.g., balance, turning, bending down, reaching up, overall endurance, effective use of an assistive device if used)
- Dressing (e.g., reaching, pulling up clothing, buttoning, zipping, over-head dressing, step-in dressing)
- General range of motion
- Lack of or minimal effect of disability due to other factors such as sight, hearing, pain

Other assessment and monitoring components are

- Considering all physical aspects of the resident's health, past and present.
- Determining what medications are being used and their side effects.
- Testing for joint range of motion, muscle strength, balance, and endurance.
- Monitoring foot care and acting on possible problems; selecting safe, sturdy, and well-fitting shoes.
- Assessing safety, especially as it pertains to standing from a sitting position.
- Assessing the bed for proper height so when the resident sits on the bed his or her feet touch the floor and knees are bent at a comfortable angle of approximately 90 degrees.
- Determining if adapted equipment is being used correctly (generally, adapted equipment is not used successfully if introduced after the onset of the dementia).
- Assessing if enough calories are being consumed to maintain proper weight and nutrition, especially when pacing or wandering is excessive.
- Checking vision and hearing, making necessary changes and improvements if possible; residents often forget to wear glasses or they will wear someone else's; hearing aids are sometimes placed in the trash or refused.
- Realizing that the ability to move and walk can remain the same, change very gradually, or experience a rapid decline, with the cause not always known or understood. A fall sometimes can cause a resident to cease walking even though he or she did not experience physical damage or pain. The same effect can result from the resident sustaining an illness or hospitalization.
- Constantly monitoring for safety or change.

> Bob had been limping for 2 days. He had not fallen and no
> bruises were observed on his body. A sock pushed down
> into the toe of his shoe was found to be the source of his
> limp. When it was removed, Bob resumed his normal gait.

Approaches

- "Listen" to the resident's verbal and nonverbal communication.
- Use clueing, verbal and nonverbal, breaking down the task of walking or transfers into simple steps.
- Be aware of timing and the resident's mood or level of agitation.
- A familiar staffperson may improve the resident's responses.
- Understand and, if possible, accept the resident's pacing and wandering as his or her activity.

- When resident does not want to walk, try singing or use food as a motivation or a distraction technique.
- Use a consistent type of approach but be flexible and make changes when necessary.

Maintaining Mobility

Residents with dementia who have been restrained or bedfast for a period may not have the ability to resume mobility. Even 3–4 days of inactivity can affect residents' ability to remember how to walk.

Mobility must be allowed and encouraged if ambulation is to continue. Exercising or movement of body parts, or both, on a daily basis helps to decrease the possibility of immobility (see Appendix 7-1). Normalization tasks, such as sweeping the floor, reaching and washing windows, and dancing, help to maintain strength, coordination, range of motion, and balance. Consider mobility as the resident's activity (see Chapter 9).

Have a workout club with charts to record achievements, and wear special T-shirts. You also might set up a physical fitness trail (see Appendix 7-2) with exercises and equipment that will strengthen both the upper and lower extremities. The trail could be outside, in a room, or in a hallway. It might include over-the-door pulleys; finger ladders; stretchy, wide rubber bands attached to a railing; knobs or wheels to turn; and exercises described and depicted in pictures and words.

A walking club can be effective all year long if inside space is available when needed. In a health care facility, staff from throughout the home can conduct a walking club for selected residents. Staff could include secretaries, dietary staff, housekeeping staff, and non–hands-on staff, including administration.

Use the following suggestions to adapt and modify exercise according to residents' abilities, body positions, and attention spans.

- Scarves, plastic golf tubes, dowels, weights, dumbbells, or objects held in the hands help to increase concentration and give clueing for following exercises.
- Try different kinds of music (e.g., loud, soft, and with or without a beat or rhythm). Observe residents' responses and make changes as necessary.
- Encourage residents to count or clap, setting a rhythm as a method to encourage participation and reduce rigidity.
- Use simple, clear directions with visual and verbal clueing (e.g., "Reach your arms up to the sky. Move your arms [side to side] like treetops in the breeze.").
- Place your hands over the resident's hands to facilitate movement, if necessary.
- Use routine and familiar exercises.
- Start exercises from the head and neck down and proceed toward the feet
- Use exercises calling for bilateral arm motions.
- If the resident has weakness of one extremity, place the stronger hand over the weak one for grasping an exercise wand.
- Exercise at the same time each day if possible. Mornings are usually the best. If possible, conduct exercise groups two or more times daily.

Environmental Safety

- Use chairs with arms and legs that do not splay out in the back.
- Pick a chair with a seat color or tone in contrast to the color of the flooring to provide perceptual clueing.
- Use a chair with a solid, firm seat rather than a soft, saggy seat. The same is true for wheelchair seats.
- Avoid low coffee tables or couches.
- Eliminate floor clutter and keep furniture in a familiar arrangement.
- Avoid wet floor surfaces or spilled food on the floor.
- Do not use carpets with thick or high pile or scatter rugs.
- Use grab bars and handrails, especially in the bathroom.
- Be willing to modify the environment as needed to promote maximum safety.
- Maintain a defined walking path area throughout the environment.

ASSISTING MOBILITY

Assisting the resident to ambulate starts with a relationship of trust and comfort between the resident and the caregiver. It is up to the caregiver to be aware of the resident's mood and willingness to be cooperative. The reality of assisted mobility is that sometimes the resident is able to achieve success but there will be times when the resident is not able to attend to the task of walking.

- Use a safety belt around the resident when providing assistance.
- Assess whether assistance from the side, back, or front is safest or facilitates the best response.

> Helen was feeling shy and insecure and would not dance with the staffperson when they were standing face to face. She seemed more secure and increased her participation when she was held from the back against the staffperson's chest.

- Assess the resident's safety for using a rolling walker. If the back two legs catch on the flooring or rug, punch holes in tennis balls and insert one on each leg so the walker will slide along.
- Use a bar, railing, or the back of a wheelchair to aid the resident's ease in walking and to reduce his or her fear of falling.
- The resident's focus and attention span can be improved if he or she holds on to something while ambulating.
- Hold the resident with his or her back against your chest and use your foot to move his or her feet one at a time.
- If possible and safe, ask the resident to take your arm rather than your holding the resident's arm. When the caregiver takes hold of the resident's upper arm to assist with mobility, the resident may experience an increase in muscle tone leading to rigidity of the trunk and extremities, complicating the ability to move.
- Use singing or counting of the number of steps taken. This is especially effective when parkinsonian-like rigidity or "freezing" is affecting a smooth gait and

the ability to walk through doorways. For example, say to the resident, "Let's count your steps from here to the hall. Ready? Count with me—one, two, three."

- Simplify and adapt a mobility task (e.g., getting into a car) using the same counting system for setting a rhythm (see Appendix 7-3).
- If the resident has stopped walking and seems unable to progress forward as though his or her feet are stuck on the floor, ask the resident to lift up his or her toes inside his or her shoes or take one step backward and then go forward.
- Set up a walking list to remind staff to assist the resident two or three times each day.
- Encourage walking to the bathroom or to activities or back to the resident's room after meals.
- Transfer resident, if at all possible, from the wheelchair to a regular chair for all meals.
- Use staffpersons as needed to assist with the resident's mobility (e.g., male staff employed in non–hands-on caregiving positions can assist the caregiving staff, especially when the resident fears falling and the helper appears as a strong person).

> Marvin had fallen and broken his hip. His recovery was slowed due to his overwhelming fear of falling. When the therapist tried to work with him on the parallel bars, Marvin could not tolerate the confining space. He would become very parkinsonian, his body would become rigid and his feet just could not move. It was as though his feet were nailed to the floor. The therapist wanted Marvin to hang on to the parallel bars because his physical size and poor balance made therapy difficult and, at times, unsafe. Marvin's fears continued, along with his limited progress, until Steve, the director of housekeeping, came to the rescue. Steve helped to support Marvin on one side while the therapist took his other side. The three practiced walking in a wide, open hallway. Marvin felt confident with Steve by his side and was able to strengthen his physical well-being and mobility skills. With his fear of falling diminished, Marvin slowly resumed his walking independence.

CAREGIVING FOR IMMOBILE RESIDENTS

Residents who cannot move independently need total assistance from caregivers for positioning and overall physical wellbeing. This requires a comprehensive plan of care for responding to the resident's needs for comfort and skin integrity. Suggestions for assisting the resident include the following:

- Assess abilities and inabilities and set realistic goals, realizing that mobility skills can change and vary.
- Understand that immobility is the usual outcome of dementia's progressive course but may occur just before the resident's death.

Alzheimer's Disease: Activity-Focused Care

- Use wrap-around walkers and rehabilitation techniques if independent ambulation has stopped or has become extremely unsafe due to recurrent falls or having a resident that sits down on the floor suddenly and without any warning. Residents should be assessed for ability to use these devices safely. Tall or very short residents require a wrap-around walker of an appropriate size.
- Become skilled in giving the resident passive range of motion (PROM) therapy at least once daily. PROM therapy can be demonstrated by a nurse, rehabilitation staffperson, or physical or occupational therapist.
- Position and reposition the resident every 2 hours, wherever he or she is: bed, chair or geriatric chair, or wheelchair.
- If the resident is seated, use a lap board to help the resident's arms rest on the board, thereby enabling his or her trunk to be supported.
- Use a wedge-shaped seat cushion that is higher in the front and slants to the back of the seat for helping the resident sit straight or to prevent the resident from sliding out of the chair.
- A soft piece of the plastic type of non-skid material placed under a rug to keep it from sliding can be placed under the buttocks of a dressed resident to prevent sliding.
- A rolled towel or pillow under the seat cushion on one side can help to straighten the resident who is leaning to one side. Place the roll on the side the resident is leaning toward.
- Continue good hygiene care and monitor the skin constantly to avoid reddened areas that lead to skin breakdown. Use specialized seat cushions and bed mattresses to reduce pressure sores. Seek medical help as needed.

ASSESSING FOR FALLS

Fisher and colleagues (1988) stated that one-third to two-thirds of individuals older than the age of 65 years sustain one or more falls per year and that falls are the sixth leading cause of death overall after the age of 65.

Residents with dementia are at high risk for falling. Awareness of the resident's cognitive, physical, and psychosocial abilities, strengths, challenges, and risks should be used as a basis for monitoring mobility components, determining risks for falls, and thereby possibly preventing falls.

A fall assessment (see Appendix 7-4) includes the following considerations:

1. Facility admission within the past month
2. History of recent falls
3. Age, especially if the resident is older than 85 years
4. Sensory assessment (e.g., vision, hearing, color discrimination, acuity)
5. Decreased trunk stability, slower righting reflexes
6. Spatial-perceptual dysfunction
7. Proprioceptive input (i.e., ability to integrate and interpret stimuli originating in muscles, joints, and other internal tissues to provide information about the position of one body part in relationship to another)
8. Cognitive awareness, mental status, distractibility, and depression
9. Judgment

10. Hostility, anger, and mood changes
11. Hallucinations
12. Sleep disturbances
13. General physical well-being and limitations, including cardiovascular conditions
14. Mobility, gait stability, stride, joint stability, postural sway and postural control, changes in posture and body alignment that cause the resident's center of gravity to change
15. Use of adapted equipment, often carried along and not used correctly
16. Reduced ability or reflex to reestablish equilibrium when off balance
17. Balance, dizziness, and orthostatic hypotension
18. Endurance and muscle tone
19. Urinary problems (e.g., incontinence, frequency, and urgency)
20. Ability to communicate or understand communications
21. Improper footwear or podiatry problems
22. Improper clothing (e.g., someone else's shoes, robe too long, pants not pulled up)
23. Medications: side effects
24. Environment (e.g., flooring, clutter, lighting, glare, uneven floor surface, rug nap, slippery flooring, unstable furniture, lack of or unstable grab bars, electrical cords, bedspreads that splay out and onto the floor surface, inaccessible items that the resident might try to reach, noise, intercom that may lead the resident to think that he or she is being called and therefore hurry off to find the source of the call)
25. Other medical situations that compromise mobility (e.g., Parkinson's disease, degenerative joint complications, compromised breath control, osteoporosis)

If a resident's hip breaks because of a fall, the possibility of successful rehabilitation may vary from resident to resident. All attempts should be made to help the resident walk again if at all possible. An experienced therapist, able to communicate and use distraction techniques with the resident, is needed. It may be impossible to judge the outcome of therapy even when there are no additional difficulties other than the dementia and the broken hip. The resident's alertness, good nutrition, and determination, combined with the caregiver's caring, consistent approach are needed for reestablishing mobility.

Other precipitating fall risk factors are the general effects on posture due to aging. Men tend to walk with a more flexed posture and a wide-based, short-stepped gait. Women take a smaller step but have a narrow-based, waddling gait. Many older persons furniture-grab, hanging on to one piece of furniture after another as they walk from area to area. Grabbing also includes reaching out to hold a faucet, for example, to steady oneself while stepping into the bathtub or shower.

Falls should be assessed, recorded in detail, and reported to the physician and family. Necessary adaptations for the resident, others, and environment may need to be made to prevent another fall. An interesting possible deterrent to falls might be when residents bring in their bed from home. They "know" this bed, and it is usually a bit wider than the typical facility bed. The residents know just how far to roll over and how to position their bottom so they can sit down without missing the edge. It seems to give them a better sense and understanding of the room size in relationship to other objects such as the closet or the toilet. Regulations may require that the mattress be cleaned before using.

Medications often are implicated as precipitating factors to a fall, especially when tranquilizers or sleeping pills are used. Encourage the attending physician to monitor medications, decreasing and discontinuing their use, if appropriate. However, falls can happen under the best conditions, even when the resident's mobility is observed and monitored closely.

FUNCTIONAL MAINTENANCE AND REHABILITATION PROGRAMS

Supporting physical wellness throughout the dementia disease process requires a multidisciplinary approach focusing on the resident's remaining abilities (see Appendixes 7-1 and 7-2). However, a fall resulting in a broken hip can result in wheelchair dependence. Residents with dementia can have difficulty accessing or receiving Medicare treatment because of the strict guidelines requiring residents' ongoing improvement. Consistent improvement is often difficult to demonstrate due to residents' cognitive dysfunctions. When residents recovering from a hip fracture are placed in a rehabilitation program that progresses at their speed of recovery and ability to cognitively follow through, reaching treatment goals is more likely. The resident may need to have a rehabilitation period of care followed by rehabilitation inactivity and then the rehabilitation continued again, perhaps after a month or so.

Before discontinuation of active therapy, treatment plans are made by the therapist for setting up a functional maintenance program. This program helps the resident to access residual skills, assuring that he or she is functioning at his or her highest possible level of ability. The resident's strengths are focused on improving function. Functional maintenance programs are designed by a skilled professional who performs an evaluation and uses the findings to design and implement an individualized plan for the resident. All programs are with physician's orders. The therapist then teaches and supervises the facility staff to continue the program. The desired outcome of a functional maintenance program is not to make more work for the staff, but to help the resident be able to do more for herself or himself. The emphasis is on activity-focused care, in which the daily living tasks become the resident's activity with the staff not doing "to" or "for" the resident, but working "with" him or her.

The basic requirement of a physical maintenance or rehabilitation program is that the therapist be willing to enter into the resident's world and go along with what the resident wants to do. It is that simple. The therapist must be creative and then adapt the treatment modalities to fit the resident's responses. Tying in the selected movement or preferred physical response to a normal life activity will be most successful (e.g., assisting the resident to shampoo his or her hair when the therapy goal calls for increased shoulder motion and reaching to head height). Asking the resident to carry a bunch of flowers down the hall to give to his or her favorite friend will elicit more cooperation than saying, "I want you to walk 75 feet."

Suggestions for promoting optimum rehabilitation results include the following:

I. Follow communication basics.
   A. Use short, simple sentences.
   B. Avoid lengthy explanations.

C. Use touch, avoiding a manipulative touch.

D. Relate to resident at his or her eye level.

E. Frame your requests (e.g., "Please help me with . . ." "I really need your assistance with . . .").

F. Offer choices of only two items.

G. Try to stop asking questions.

H. Assure the resident that he or she is safe and that you will be with him or her.

II. Consider attention span and follow-through issues.

A. Address possible excess disability needs (e.g., glasses, illness).

B. Accept the resident's difficulty in initiating activity.

C. Use objects for the resident to hold in his or her hand (e.g., golf tubes, wands, therapy balls, fabrics).

D. Evaluate distraction factors (e.g., face the resident toward the wall or away from a door; do not position yourself between the resident and the window because the light behind your face will darken your features).

E. Assess the environmental distractions such as television, other residents in the area, noise.

F. If possible, avoid having the resident wait for therapy; have objects for the resident if he or she has to wait (e.g., busy box, scrapbooks, a familiar item brought in by the family such as a stuffed animal, family picture).

G. Use multisensory cueing.

H. Be aware of timing of therapy and adjust if possible; mornings are generally the best.

I. Try to facilitate the therapy in an environment familiar to the resident.

J. Switch therapists if the resident shows excess combativeness or dislike.

III. Understand the resident's behaviors as his or her method of communication, and track antecedents of the behaviors to evaluate what the behavior is "saying."

IV. Use distraction techniques (e.g., singing, food, "You have a phone call") for bringing back a wandering resident.

V. Incorporate an activity into the therapy procedures and goals (e.g., walking to retrieve a ball, placing a book on a table, hanging clothes on a hook, washing hair in the shower).

VI. Know the resident's life story and incorporate aspects of familiar information and tasks into the therapy (see Chapter 3).

VII. Understand task breakdown and simplification.

VIII. Be willing to shift therapeutic strategies if something is not working (e.g., the resident may have a limited response if the program takes place in a confined area).

IX. Use family members or favorite staff to assist as needed.

X. Use various interventions to enable response (e.g., hand over hand; starting a motion so the resident can take over [chaining]; counting, clapping, or singing to set a rhythm; mirroring the task for the resident so he or she can watch you).

XI. Limit use of adapted equipment, use only if necessary.

XII. Use the following suggestions for walking residents requiring one foot to be nonweightbearing:

A. One shoe on, one off. Assess to see which foot should wear the shoe (i.e., the resident may have a decreased tendency to step on a foot without a shoe or step on a foot when both the sock and shoe are off).

Alzheimer's Disease: Activity-Focused Care

B. Place a colored yarn tassel on the shoes, red for, "Do not step down on this foot," and green for, "OK to step down on this foot."

C. Place a sock filled with marbles or large sponges on the nonweightbearing foot so it looks or feels strange, especially when it touches the floor.

XIII. Provide staff training and monitoring to ensure follow-through with all program goals and implementation.

XIV. Engage family members to participate in the rehabilitation's follow-through.

PHYSICAL RESTRAINTS: DEFINITION, ISSUES, AND EFFICACY

The focus on limiting the use of restraints and emphasis on a "restraint-free environment" developed from the Omnibus Budget Reconciliation Act of 1987 (OBRA, Public Law 100-203). This act includes strict controls on the use of restraints in nursing facilities and makes a positive statement supporting the rights of nursing home residents to be free from restraints. The Nursing Home Reform Act, which was included in OBRA 1987, was implemented in October 1990. According to Section 1819 of the Social Security Act, restraints may only be imposed to "ensure the physical safety of the resident or other residents and only upon written order of a physician." This order must be specific as to duration and circumstances of the restraint use. Enforcement regulations and interpretative guidelines have been expanded to help address the definition of a restraint plus the context for using or not using.

Restraints are used for varying needs. In the past, for the sake of the staff's convenience, residents have been restrained. However, staff are now better educated in restraint alternatives and understanding of the negative aspects of restraint use.

Sometimes, certain items are called restraints that a caregiver might not consider as such. For example, bed rails in the up position are considered a restraint. A one-piece outfit, such as a jump suit that zips up the back, could be considered a restraint if the resident cannot open the zipper independently or on command.

Resident-related needs or possible indications for the use of restraints include difficulties with ambulation, balance, positioning, unsafe behavioral responses, and when the safety of life support mechanisms is jeopardized.

There are two basic types of restraints.

1. *Chemical*: drugs prescribed to control mood, behavior, mental status
2. *Physical*: any method, device, material, or equipment that cannot be removed by the resident that restricts freedom of movement or normal access to one's body

Whether to use restraints or reduce the current application of restraints, therefore, requires study, problem solving, and response to the following issues:

- Resident rights, care, and safety
- Legal issues for misuse, including resident abuse
- Liability and financial issues
- Risk management
- Family issues
- Staff: education, facilitation, and program support

Since OBRA went into effect in 1990, the courts have ruled in favor of restraint-free care. Such care for residents with dementia calls for a creative and careful response within the context of informed dementia care awareness. It also calls for complete facility staff cooperation and education.

DEMENTIA FACTORS AFFECTING THE USE OF RESTRAINTS

The decision to use a restraining device for a person with mid- to late-stage dementia is determined by assessing and incorporating information. OBRA considerations and guidelines become part of the decision. Cognitive, physical, psychosocial, and environmental factors that affect residents with dementia include the following.

Cognitive Factors

- Limited memory, cognitive ability, awareness, or attention
- Visual or spatial dysfunction
- Poor judgment
- Impaired ability to act or react in a safe manner (e.g., oral intake of nonedibles, walking on wet floors, trying to walk independently when unable, inappropriate use of adapted equipment)
- Inability to interpret sensory input
- Disorientation due to limited awareness
- Confusion: constant or sporadic episodes
- Limited ability to understand or communicate with others
- Response to hallucinations or delusions or both

Physical Factors

- Gait, motor planning dysfunction
- Limited range of motion
- Poor balance: sitting, walking, or standing
- Fenestration (walking too fast or running)
- Constant wandering or pacing, not sitting down to rest
- Poor trunk stability or inability to maintain body alignment
- Decreased strength and endurance, exhaustion
- Physical inabilities due to medication
- Inability to maintain seated position
- Seizures
- Poor vision
- Dizziness
- Pushing, hitting, or shoving others
- Inability to tolerate life-sustaining equipment (e.g., tube feeding or hydration intravenous support)

Psychosocial Factors

- Aggressive or combative behaviors
- Excessive anxiousness or frustration, feeling of loss of control, or agitated response to feeling manipulated
- Decreased self-image
- Inability to be flexible or adaptive to change
- Abusive to self or others: verbally or physically or both
- Fearful of others
- Fear of falling; presence of other fears, either real or imagined
- Depression
- Stripping, removing clothing at inappropriate times or places

Environmental Factors

- Floor glare, window reflection
- Food on floor or wet floor areas
- Excessive noise or disturbed response to the intercom
- Excessive use of color or decorations (e.g., too many holiday decorations and constant playing of music)
- Excessive clutter

NEGATIVE EFFECTS OF RESTRAINTS

The consequences of immobilizing the resident with the application of restraints must be considered seriously. The resident is the most affected, but family members and staff are often distressed when observing and responding to a resident being restrained. At times, restraints appear to break the human spirit of a resident. This great loss of personal integrity may be due to the resident's intuitive insight involving the depletion of freedom and compromised holistic wellness.

Cognitive and Psychosocial Effects: Reduced Personhood

Examples of the negative cognitive and psychosocial effects of restraints include

- Decline in positive mood (e.g., depression, passivity, sadness, anger, withdrawal, feelings of isolation, fear, panic, embarrassment, humiliation, decreased self-esteem, feeling caged, dehumanized)
- "Checking out": decreased interest to initiate or respond cognitively
- Decreased interest in or participation in communications
- Resistance to care
- Reduced opportunities for social contact
- Broken human spirit

Physical Effects: Compromised Functional Well-being

Examples of the negative physical effects of restraints include

- Increased agitation (e.g., hitting, spitting, scratching, kicking, yelling, calling out, screaming)
- Decreased functional and physical wellness and body performance (e.g., loss of body control, decreased range of motion, decreased overall strength and endurance, constipation, incontinence, reduced nutritional intake, compromised skin integrity, infection, reduced ambulation, dehydration, orthostatic hypotension, contracture, bone demineralization, lowered metabolic rate, blood volume changes, edema, loss of muscle mass and possibility of developing orthostatic hypertension, increased risk for pressure sores, respiratory difficulties or pneumonia or both, disturbed sleep pattern, possible risk of death due to suffocation or strangulation)
- Increased risk that falls may be more serious when the resident is allowed to move freely

ALTERNATIVES TO RESTRAINTS

Restraint-free care should be individually designed for each resident and part of the plan of care. The questions of "Why is this difficult behavior occurring?" and "What would be an appropriate intervention that continues to support the abilities of the resident while refocusing or adjusting for the individual's difficulties?" should be answered first. Another important question for staff to ask about a challenging resident is, "Who has the problem?" (see Appendix 8-3). There are many restraint-free options to choose from, ranging from verbal distraction techniques to environmental modifications.

Another consideration is whether the least restrictive alternative has been used. Working with a multidisciplinary team to provide information for assessment and interviewing the resident (if possible), family, and staff should be part of the assessment. The assessment also should include information about what has happened when the resident has been removed from restraint, and whether the resident's total time in restraints has been reduced. Staff must develop an individualized care plan that includes the resident's abilities and strengths as well as deficits or difficulties (see Appendix 1-2 and the Glossary at the end of this book). As the resident changes, the care plan must reflect the changes with appropriate approaches.

Alternatives to the use of restraints include physically based alternatives, cognitive and psychosocial distraction techniques, meaningful activities as interventions, and environmental adaptations.

Physically Based Alternatives

Provide companionship and supervision, and try the following:

- Offer favorite foods, drink, exercise.
- Cut out all caffeine.
- Provide for daily rest period or nap.
- Use warm bath or whirlpool.

- Have resident walk outside whenever possible.
- Have resident use wrap-around walker with seat.
- Use hand mitts or hand splint to prevent pinch grasp or use an air splint to prevent the resident's hand from reaching his or her mouth or nose area when a tube is being used or a life support system is being jeopardized.
- Consult physician and change treatment to discontinue intravenous tubes or have treatment occur during hours of sleep, rather than during wakefulness, if possible.
- Have a functional maintenance or restorative program available to use when appropriate.

Cognitive and Psychosocial Distraction Techniques

Examples of cognitive and psychosocial distraction techniques include the following:

- Respond and validate mood, then use an activity or an "I really need your help"–type distraction.
- Relate approach to positive aspects of the resident's life history (e.g., "Professor, please help me lead this class," or, "Professor, it is time for the staff meeting, come with me this way").
- Have trained staff that can "rescue" the agitated resident and take him or her to a safe, quiet area. The rescue staff may be management staff that the hands-on staff know they can call when the resident needs a different face or they need relief (see Chapter 8).
- Set up a "patrol" system (see Chapter 8).
- Do not use restraints when staff are monitoring, such as during mealtime and activities.
- Engage a companion for one-to-one attention, active listening.
- Telephone a family member.
- Have staff take the resident to sit in their office or follow them around as they work.
- Give the resident a sweater or favorite clothing item belonging to a loved one and reassure the resident that his or her loved one will return.
- Use therapeutic fibs, if appropriate (e.g., "Maria, the children are in school").
- Increase the use of touch, reassurances, and reminders such as, "You are safe, I will be here with you." Talk softly with the resident.
- Recognize the resident's nonverbal language expressing need and respond immediately to initiate distraction or refocusing techniques (e.g., use the resident's LifeStory Book [see Chapter 3]).

Meaningful Activities as Interventions

Examples of meaningful activities as interventions include the following:

- Refocus behavior using familiar normalization activities and active exercise opportunities.
- Supply safe areas for walking and wandering that can be accessed independently.

- Use calming music (try a tape player placed in a fanny pack with large earphones), relaxation techniques, guided mediations.
- Use activities that reduce agitated behaviors (see Chapter 9).
- Use regularly scheduled exercise and walking programs, structured routines.
- Provide interesting props to carry or use a fanny pack with items.
- Try to give the resident chewing gum to help reduce anxiety, combativeness, or verbal outbursts.
- Have a baby doll available to be picked up and cuddled.
- Take resident on trips into the community.
- Use a high-touch approach to care (e.g., massage).

Environmental Adaptations and Suggestions

Examples of environmental adaptations and suggestions include the following:

- Chairs: with slanted back or deep seats, heavy chairs that are difficult to move, recliners, rockers, gliders, beanbag chairs, Adirondack-style chairs, use of wedge cushions, wrap-around walkers
- Beds: place near wall, lower bed and use a soft mat, mattress on the floor, use half-length bedrails or one bed-side rail only
- Signs: "stop" or "keep out," "Jim, turn around," "Jim, do not touch this door," directional and way-finding signs
- Monitoring system: television monitoring, enclosed areas, exit alarms, nursery intercom, sensitive pads for under the mattress or in a chair that set off an alarm when the resident rises from the seat or mattress
- Hiding: covering intravenous (IV) poles with a hook and loop closure sewn along the seam of long pillowcase-type covering that is made from washable fabric and is colored to "fade into" the environment and not call attention to the IV stand, covering door knobs if allowable, placing fabric strips (1 yd wide) across doorways
- Personalizing the environment with familiar "stuff" from the resident's past
- Use of a nonskid, plastic-like material under the resident so that the chance of sliding out of the chair is decreased
- Reducing environmental noise that stresses residents (e.g., intercom, paging systems, television)
- Use of firm wheelchair seats

RESTRAINT USE CONSIDERATIONS: CAN THERE BE POSITIVE OUTCOMES?

Little is written about the positive use of restraints as an accountable therapeutic intervention for persons with dementia. The OBRA guidelines, which demand that nursing home staff introduce restraint alternatives, serve to highlight circumstances when restraints should not be considered. Restraints, therefore, should only be used if they enable or support the resident's needs. The resident with dementia has the same basic needs as all humans.

Restraint use considerations include

- Involvement of the resident's physician
- Assessment of needs, circumstances, and desired outcome
- Have restraint alternatives and less restrictive solutions been tried?
- Does the use of the restraint fulfill the need or escalate conflict and deny fulfillment?
- What is the shortest possible duration of time for using the restraint?
- Is an assessment and monitoring system in place that makes sure that the restraint is the correct size and in good repair before using?
- Are necessary policies and procedures on restraint use and application being used?
- Are staff trained in the correct use and application of the restraint?

Maslow's (1954) "hierarchy of motives" states that humans are motivated by basic needs that are related to each other in a hierarchical and developmental way. Maslow found that a person moves from one level to a higher level only if his or her needs are met at the lower level first. Level one and level two must be met before advancing up the hierarchy pyramid. An interesting question, therefore, asks, "Does the use of restraints enable the resident to have his or her needs met at the lower levels as described by Maslow?"

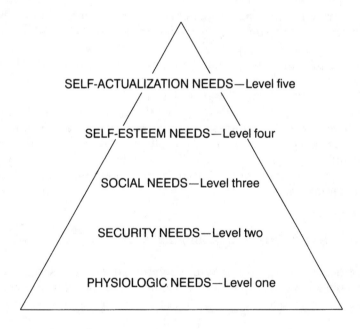

Level One Needs: Physiologic

Body system functions for sustaining life include circulation, respiration, nutrition, fluids, bowel and bladder function, sleep, rest, activity, exercise, muscle-skeletal ability, mobility, and sensory stimulation.

A resident who is not able to eat while walking or who is too restless to sit at the table may need restraints during mealtime to enable maximum caloric intake. An example would be the use of a geriatric chair with a lap table just for mealtimes. A resident may not interpret inner signals of fatigue from constant pacing or may be unable to remember how to sit down, and therefore may benefit from a therapeutic rest while confined to a geriatric chair. Similarly, an exhausted resident climbing in and out of bed all night due to fearfulness may feel safe and "held in a nurturing embrace" when a restraining vest is used to prohibit leaving the bed and as an aid to encourage rest or sleep.

Level Two Needs: Safety and Security

Level two needs include a therapeutic environment to reduce anxiety and potentially harmful situations, interventions to reduce risk of falls, methods to promote safe mobility, assured walking and sitting balance, and reduction of fears that lead to combativeness with other residents or staff.

A resident with dementia may experience a sporadic inability to safely ambulate and may need a restraining device due to lack of awareness of the dysfunction. Hallucinations or possible psychiatric dysfunctions may incite a resident's combative behavior that does not respond to distraction interventions. Restraints may decrease or eliminate injury to the resident and to others. A resident constantly pushing aside staff in a frantic desire to leave a safe environment may be diverted from exiting by using a door security system. A resident with limited body awareness who may not know when his or her compromised sitting balance will cause falling out of the chair or of the possibility of hitting his or her head on a table or other furniture pieces may need a chest vest, torso restraint, or trunk stabilizer cushions during periods of dysfunctional trunk stability.

Level Three Needs: Love and Belonging; Social Needs

Level three needs include giving and receiving affection, responding to companionship, having a relationship with the resident peer community, accepting family support and attention, welcoming and enjoying visitors, and accepting staffpersons.

Levels Four and Five Needs: Self-esteem and Self-actualization

Levels four and five needs include feeling useful and productive; a sense of a positive use of time; fullest achievement of capacity; gratification and increased self-worth from participation in activities of daily living; the ability to gain pleasure in appearance; the desire to express emotional capabilities; autonomy, or in control of self and the environment; and the ability to respond to inner spirituality and worship experiences.

Use of Restraints Discussion: Enabling Levels Three, Four, and Five

The promotion of the resident's positive self-esteem is dependent on basic needs being met. Only then can the resident have the energy and drive to function with maximum capabilities. In activity-focused caregiving dedicated to facilitating the resident's abilities and wellness, the accountable use of restraints might be the considered approach to support an affirming and safe quality of life for the resident. Examples may include wrap-around walkers, chair "buddies," or a torso restraint. The definition of a restraint is whether the resident can remove the device if desired or on command. Restraints for these levels move from the viewpoint of being a negative factor to one of becoming an "enabler." Therapeutic use of restraints for enabling levels three, four, and five would be extremely limited because the resident would probably respond favorably to psychosocial interventions.

HEALTH CARE PROVIDER AND STAFF ISSUES

Physical wellness and mobility are one of the primary focuses of resident care. Rehabilitation therapies and functional maintenance programs become the backbone of the physical wellness emphasis. Staff education and motivation for carrying out programs supporting the resident's physical functioning and mobility require commitment and dedication from everyone involved in care and management.

Falls within a facility are regarded as incidents and therefore a report is filled out and filed. When a resident's ability to ambulate becomes compromised, placing the resident at a high risk for falling, some administrators and regulators express great concern. The development of a policy supporting the resident's mobility, even when greatly impaired, may be helpful if expectations are that the resident will remain independent for as long as possible. Information about the resident's difficulties should appear on the plan of care, with input from the physician, staff, and family as to the approach and intervention selected. Family members should be in agreement about ambulation as a negotiated risk.

Why do nursing home staff use restraints? Some nursing assistants compiled the following honest answers:

- The nurse told me
- The restraint was in the room
- Safety concerns (e.g., possibility of falling, need for positioning, tendency to pull out tubes, threat to others, threat to self, eloping or leaving an area unsupervised, need for rest, threat from others)
- Life sustaining concerns (e.g., need help sitting still for meals, tendency to take food from others that is not appropriate for the resident to eat, elevating legs when needed)
- Infection control (e.g., tendency to urinate or spit on others)
- To give medications
- Staff convenience
- Family insists

Restraint-reduction programs are being addressed by health care facilities, especially long-term care centers. Literature is pointing out that most residents can be released from physical restraints and still be safe, in fact safer than being restrained. The success of such programs requires that the administrative staff be committed, knowledgeable, and involved in the emphasis on assessing resident needs and finding appropriate restraint alternatives. Restraint-reduction programs require full cooperation from the entire staff, in-servicing, ongoing and open communications, and certainly family support and input. The multidisciplinary team is the key component for a successful restraint-reduction program. A successful outcome is best achieved when team planning, training, and support from nursing assistants is assured. Models for this type of program are available in nursing and rehabilitation literature as well as from state and federal regulators.

SUMMARY

Promoting and supporting the resident with dementia to maintain physical well-being, mobility, and ambulation is an important challenge. Activity-focused care offers meaningfulness to residents' physical wellness and movement abilities by understanding how to honor and adapt, if needed, each component of these all-important resident activities. The cognitive, physical, and psychosocial benefits almost always outweigh the possible difficulties. Certainly, as the dementia progresses the possibilities for continued independence decrease and assistance is needed. The caregiver needs encouragement and support to continue trying all possible interventions and methods of assisting the resident's physical wellness and mobility for as long as realistically possible.

All alternatives to restraint usage need to be attempted before any consideration to use a restraint is entertained. Therefore, the informed decision in determining the therapeutic and accountable use of a restraint should be guided by this definitive judgment: At this time, in this place, in these circumstances, what is the ultimate best course for the resident's well-being?

Physical wellness, supported and maintained throughout the resident's dementia experience, takes caregiver teamwork and commitment. The outcome of wellness is that the resident and the caregiver are able to share the challenges of daily living with mutual respect.

REFERENCES

Fisher AG, Bonder BR, Falconnier L. Falls in older persons: a multifactorial study. Gerontologist 1988;28:2081.

Maslow AH. Motivation and Personality. New York: Harper & Row, 1954.

SUGGESTED READING

Blakeslee JA, Goldman BD, Papougenis D, Torell CA. Making the transition to restraint free care. J Gerontol Nurs 1991;17:4–8.

Brady R, Chester FR, Pierce LL, et al. Geriatric falls: prevention strategies for the staff. J Gerontol Nurs 1993;19:26–32.

Cohen C, Neufeld R, Dunbar J, et al. Alternatives to physical restraints. J Gerontol Nurs 1996;22:23–29.

Ebel S. A new approach for physical therapists in long term care of Alzheimer's patients. Am J Alzheimer's Care Rel Dis Res 1992;7:12–18.

Gehlsen GM, Whaley MH. Falls in the elderly. II. Balance, strength and flexibility. Arch Phys Med Rehabil 1990;71:739–741.

Hulsebus T, Aitken M. Alternatives to restraints. Gerontology 1997;20:1–2.

The Kendal Corporation. Untie the Elderly: Resource Manual. Kennett Square, PA: The Kendal Corporation, 1994.

Levine J, Marchello V, Totolos E. Progress toward a restraint-free environment in a large academic nursing facility. J Am Geriatr Soc 1995;43:914–918.

Lohman H, Padilla RL, Byers-Connon S. Occupational Therapy with Elders. St. Louis: Mosby–Year Book, 1998.

Newman LA. Maintaining Function in Older Adults. Boston: Butterworth, 1995.

Rader J. Modifying the environment to decrease the use of restraints. J Gerontol Nurs 1991;17:9–13.

Werner P, Koroknay V, Braun J, Cohen-Mansfield J. Individualized care alternatives used in the process of removing physical restraints in the nursing home. J Am Geriat Soc 1994;42:321–325.

A7-1
Exercises, Balance, and Strengthening

Exercise is physical activity that provides a planned, structured, and repetitive bodily movement for the purpose of maintaining or improving physical well-being. Working closely with occupational and physical therapy will enhance exercise program planning and facilitation. If possible, exercise programs should be conducted at least two times a day for maximum effectiveness. A warm-up, work, and cooldown period of exercise helps to maintain residents' abilities to participate and safeguards against possible muscle and joint damage.

Participation in an exercise program requires a physician's endorsement or prescription. Factors that may limit a resident's participation in an exercise program may include

- Joint movement limitations or weakness
- Overall muscle and physical well-being limitations, including muscle tone, balance, and pulmonary function
- Fear of falling, overexertion, loss of breath
- Limited cognitive awareness to follow directions or respond to the program
- Sensory losses and perceptual problems
- Foot problems
- Coexisting medical problems
- Pain after exercising beyond expected discomfort

Possible warning signs to watch for and respond appropriately to during exercise include

- Shortness of breath or irregular heart rate
- Pain in the chest, arm, or jaw
- Cool or clammy skin
- Increased confusion
- Complaints of dizziness, headache, or nausea
- Decrease in overall balance ability

Exercises, as with all activity based on the resident's abilities, should meet the following criteria:

- Safe
- Adaptable
- Simple

- Repetitious
- Dignified
- Fun

In addition to the exercise suggestions discussed in Chapter 7, Maintaining Mobility, the following exercises will encourage a resident's overall coordination, balance, and strengthening and will enhance and maintain physical well-being:

1. Dancing: fast, slow, large or small steps, dancing alone, as a couple, or in a circle with others
2. Mini knee bends holding onto a chair
3. Push-ups while seated in a chair
4. Weight shifting, side to side, while sitting in a chair
5. Haunch walking while seated (i.e., moving from right to left buttock)
6. Arm motion exercises that require crossing through the midline of his or her body
7. Using a small ball to pass around his or her body while standing
8. While seated, picking up a soft, large ball using both feet, making a circle with the ball, and then placing the ball on the floor
9. Walking a marked path down a hallway, then walking it again, with a small, soft pillow on his or her head for improving posture and balance
10. Ankle dorsiflexion repetitions
11. Reaching activity (e.g., dusting, washing windows)
12. Tug of war using a fabric "rope"
13. Kicking objects (e.g., balls of various sizes and weight) seated or, if appropriate, standing, perhaps through a goal or wicket, or at other objects such as bowling pins
14. Walking, stepping over or around objects (monitor for safety)
15. Aggression-reducing exercises (see Chapter 9, Movement Activities: Encouraging Physical Participation Activities for Therapeutically Reducing the Prevalence, Onset, or Intensity or Aggressive or Combative Behaviors, and Appendix 9-9)
16. Any throwing exercises (e.g., beanbags into a basket or at a target)
17. Standing on one foot
18. Stepping forward and backward or grapevine walking
19. Pulling objects of various weights on a clothesline (e.g., a basket of books, a chair)
20. Hitting a ball with a paddle for eye-hand coordination
21. Parachute activities (e.g., lifting, lowering, rotating)
22. Postural exercises, including
    - Scapular exercises: ask the resident to pinch his or her shoulder blades together toward his or her spine, then back; ask the resident to lift his or her shoulders, pull them backward, then down and forward, as though there was an eraser on the resident's shoulder and he or she was erasing a chalkboard in a circular motion; ask the resident to lace his or her fingers together behind his or her neck and push his or her elbows back
    - Ask the resident to walk with a pillow on his or her head without a planned path and then walk around chairs

- Ask the resident to touch his or her body parts, while seated or standing, requiring crossing the midline of his or her body to the other side
- Ask the resident to perform hamstring stretches from a sitting position with his or her foot on a stool, knee in extension, reaching forward as far as possible to touch his or her foot
- Side bending and trunk rotating
- Bouncing or dribbling a ball while standing or seated

23. Exercises to increase pulmonary function include
    - Blowing a pinwheel, whistle, or bubbles
    - Blowing into a straw placed in water to make bubbles or move a floating object about
    - Blowing out candles

Other exercise ideas incorporate a story line that can be acted out by residents as they follow through with movements that reflect the tale. Examples are

1. Cycling to a specific place such as the zoo, botanical garden, and so forth
2. Swimming contest that includes all the strokes
3. Visiting the zoo and imitating all the animals
4. Competing in the Olympics and doing all the events
5. Movements depicting all leisure sports such as fishing, golf, and tennis
6. Going to a department store and trying on clothing, shoes, and hats
7. Going for a hike, including putting on boots, marching, skipping, tiptoeing, applying insect repellent, jumping across a stream on rocks, looking up in the treetops for birds, and bending over to pick flowers
8. Helping Santa in his workshop preparing toys (e.g., winding up a mechanical dog, testing out a new bike, turning a jack-in-the-box handle and springing up, moving arms on a toy clock to different times)

A7-2
Fitness Trail

A physical wellness–focused fitness trail can be developed for either outside or inside a care center. Placement is often along a hallway that allows for stations to remain set up. This allows for families to also use the trail with their loved one during visits.

The trail stations can be described in words, pictures, stick-person drawings, or diagrams. Bright-colored pictures, large printing that is easy to read, and creative decorating of the trail stations can help to attract the resident and facilitate active participation. The trail can be developed for either the standing or seated resident, or can have stations able to be accessed in either position. Include directions to lock the wheelchair brakes before engaging in the exercise, if appropriate.

EXAMPLES OF EXERCISES FOR FITNESS TRAIL

A. Shoulder exercises: designate number of repetitions; include drawing of stick person
  1. Shrugging shoulders
  2. Raising arm straight out in front of the body and down
  3. Raising arm to the side of the body, up toward the head, and down
  4. Raising both arms up and over the head
  5. Moving hands together in chopping motion from one shoulder down, across the body
B. Elbow exercises: designate number of repetitions; include drawing of stick person
  1. Bending elbows and touching fingers to the shoulders
  2. Straightening elbows to the side
C. Trunk twisting exercises: designate number of repetitions; include drawing of stick person
  1. With arms folded on chest, twisting trunk to the left
  2. With arms folded on chest, twisting trunk to the right
D. Pulley exercises: use a rehabilitation pulley over the door or wall-mounted pulley with two handles; give instructions for use and number of repetitions
E. Stretch pull cords or rubberized exercise sheets: tie to a grab bar or door knob and designate number of pulls and the placement of the cord in the hand, or against the wrist or in the space made by a bent elbow
F. Hand exercises: designate number of repetitions
  1. Opening and closing the hand
  2. Fingers spreading and then moving back together so they touch

G. Pulls toward the handrail: designate number of repetitions
    1. Face the handrail, lock wheelchair brakes
    2. Place hands on the handrail
    3. Pull and lean forward as far as possible, bending the elbows
    4. Push back as far as possible
H. Leg exercises: designate number of repetitions
    1. Seated, place one side against the wall
    2. Lock wheelchair brakes
    3. Kick left leg out to front
    4. Straighten knee as much as possible
    5. Bring leg down, bending knee
    6. Repeat with the right leg
I. Other fitness trail suggestions:
    1. Finger ladder, or tape markers on the wall to finger climb and exercise the shoulder as well as arm and elbow extension
    2. Shoulder wheel for shoulder range of motion
    3. Clothespins and clothesline for reaching up and pinning baby clothes
    4. Cut a hula hoop in half, place drapery rings on the tube, and mount in a wooden base at both ends so the resident can slide them from one side to the other
    5. Punching bag
    6. A punching bag–type, 3-ft figure (e.g., a clown) that the resident can hit and have pop back upright because the base is filled with sand
    7. Pinwheels to blow
    8. Busy board of locks, keys, latches, and other hardware to manipulate

A7-3

Activity-Focused Mobility Task Example: Getting Into a Car

Goals for the mobility task example of getting into a car are

- To minimize stress and difficulties leaving a residence and getting into a car
- To provide a purposeful use of time during the task
- To give dignity by inviting the resident into the task (i.e., doing with the resident, not to the resident)
- To provide verbal, visual, and auditory cueing, task breakdown, and a musical rhythm to facilitate body movement

The task has three components: (1) leaving the residence, (2) walking to the car, and (3) getting into the car.

Areas of Challenge	Assistance or Intervention
Leaving the house	
Overcoming fear of leaving security of the home	Set up a task to be completed using a prop (e.g., a letter to be mailed, flowers to take to a friend).
Not understanding the request	Ask for resident's help (e.g., "Let's go to the post office and mail this letter," or, "This bill is due, please help me take it to be mailed.")
Not wanting to go to the day care center or designated place	Have resident hold the prop, which helps to focus on the task and acts as a distraction to decrease anxiety about leaving.
Striking out when feeling manipulated	Use simple commands (e.g., point to the door or open door, tapping it with your hand, for increased cueing).

Areas of Challenge	Assistance or Intervention
Walking to the car	
Spatial perceptual	Sing as you escort the resident, to enable rhythmic movement, especially when changing floor surface.
	Hold resident's arm by placing yours under his or her arm from elbow to hand.
Rigidity or freezing when going through a door	Ask resident to count, with you, out loud, the number of steps to the car.
Apraxia: general body awareness and movement difficulties	Ask resident to march with you while you sing a march (e.g., "We Are Marching to Pretoria").
Getting into the car	
Freezing, trunk rigidity	Sing, and encourage resident to sing with you.
Not understanding needed body movements	Briefly describe the task in short sentences, then ask the resident to dance with you, then hum or sing a song, such as "Let Me Call You Sweetheart," as you gently turn the resident so his or her buttocks are lined up with the car seat, then say, "Thank you for the dance, let's sit down," and guide resident's buttocks onto the seat. The resident's arms have been on your shoulder and holding your hand, so he or she is less likely to grasp at the door frame as he or she is seated.
Fear of a small space	Assist with resident's legs and feet, if needed.
Difficulty being able to "back up" into the seat to sit down	Distract the resident from focusing on his or her movement difficulties by thanking him or her for holding the prop and helping you.

A7-4

*Sample Fall Assessment Form**

Fall Assessment: Predisposition for Falling

Resident name: _____ Room: ____ Evaluation date: _____

Attending physician: _____ Admit date: _____

Blood pressure: Standing: _____ Lying down: _____

Select fall risk items applicable to resident and insert the number in the parentheses on the line in front of the item. The items have a weighted score based on the severity of possible predisposition for falling. The total is compared to the scaling guide for determining further intervention.

I. Age   ☐50–70 (1)   ☐70–79 (2)   ☐80+ (3)

II. Mental status (count all that apply)
- __ impaired receptive communication (1)
- __ oriented at all times (0)
- __ confused at all times (1)
- __ intermittent confusion (2)
- __ distracted by people (1)
- __ becomes lost easily (1)
- __ distracted by environment (1)
- __ impaired expressive communication (1)
- __ aware of self-limitations (0)
- __ decreased perceptual spatial skills (2)
- __ decreased functional spatial skills (2)
- __ overall poor judgment (1)

III. General mood (count all that apply)
- __ calm (0)   __ anxious (2)   __ combative (2)

IV. History (count all that apply)
- __ seizures (1)
- __ vertigo/syncope (2)
- __ cardiac arrhythmia (1)
- __ abnormal laboratory tests (1)
- __ fluid imbalance (1)
- __ other
- __ no fall history (0)
- __ fell within past week (2)
- __ fell within past month (1)
- __ fell within past 3 months (1)
- __ history of multiple falls (2)
- __ back problems

Total score for page 1 _____

---

*Courtesy of The Wealshire, Lincolnshire, Illinois.

Page 2: Fall Assessment: Predisposition for Falling
Total score brought forward from page 1 _____

V. Coexisting conditions (count all that apply)
__ lower extremity edema (1)   __ anemia (1)
__ uncompensated visual   __ contracture, upper extremity (1)
   deficit (2)   __ contracture, lower extremity (2)
__ uncompensated hearing   __ general weakness (2)
   deficit (1)   __ hallucinations (1)
__ paralysis or cerebrovascular   __ sleep disturbances (1)
   accident (1)   __ arthritic or painful joints (1)
__ Parkinson's disease (2)   __ bifocals (1)
__ limb amputation (1)   __ diabetic (1)
__ foot problems (2)   __ other

VI. Gait and balance (count all that apply)
__ wide base of balance (0)   __ loss of standing balance if
__ poor trunk control (1)   nudged (1)
__ lurching, swaying gait (1)   __ balance problems when
__ ambulates with assistance (2)   walking (2)
__ transfers independently (1)   __ decrease in muscular coordina-
__ hypermotion, startled   tion (1)
   reaction (1)   __ transfers with assistance (1)
__ self-propels wheelchair (1)   __ abnormal posture (1)
__ jerking or instability when making turns (2)
__ use of assistive devices (e.g., cane, walker, furniture) (1)
__ gait pattern changes when walking through doorways or changing
   floor surface (1)
__ grasps furniture (1)

VII. Elimination (count all that apply)
__ independent and continent (0) __ incontinent (1)
__ catheter or ostomy or both (0) __ independent and incontinent (2)
__ elimination with assistance (1)

VIII. Medications (check all that apply)
☐antihistamine   ☐antihypertensives   ☐antiseizure/antiepileptic
☐benzodiazepines ☐cathartics ☐diuretics ☐hypoglycemic agents
☐narcotics   ☐psychotropics   ☐sedatives/hypnotics
☐other (specify) _____

Indicate below how many medications patient is currently taking or
took before admission.
__ no medications (0) __ one medication (1) __ two or more medications (2)
__ change of medication or dosage or both within the last 30 days (1)

Total score for page 2 _____

Page 3: Fall Assessment: Predisposition for Falling
Total score brought forward from page 2_____

IX. Current safety devices
__ not needed (0)
__ chair or bed alarm system (0)   __ side rails (1)
__ safety vest—bed (2)   __ waist belt—wheelchair (1)
__ safety vest—wheelchair (1)   __ self-releasing belt (1)
__ positioning pillow (1)   __ geriatric chair (1)
__ wrap-around walker (1)   __ misuses or neglects to use device (2)

X. Footwear
__ appropriate (0)   __ inappropriate (2)

XI. Admission within past 4 weeks (2)

Assessment total _____

Scaling Guide
  0–10 = Annual review
 11–20 = Biannual review
  21+ = Quarterly review
  25+ = To be reviewed for rehabilitation services: gait training, balance and
        strengthening, functional maintentance, physical or occupational
        therapy, medication review, or restraint reduction.

Signature: _____

Date: _____

8

Behaviors: Understanding, Creative Interventions, and Refocusing

"Alzheimer's behaviors." The words alone promote anxiety, fear, anger, and apprehension in most caregivers. The progression of dementia can trigger difficult and often bizarre changes in residents' responses to themselves, others, and their environment. Persons with Alzheimer's disease are often labeled as "behavior problems." Appropriate attempts to limit or circumnavigate possible antecedents of unwanted behaviors must be a part of the plan of care.

Behaviors, being a part of living, affect the person with dementia in positive and negative ways. Alzheimer's disease and related disorders might be the primary diagnostic factors. In the aging resident, however, not every symptom or problem can or should be blamed on dementia or preclude the possibility of a pre-existent illness or the onset of a new physical or mental illness.

We all have behaviors. Behaviors are demonstrations of who we are and how we communicate our response to daily living. We are willing to accept or reject our own behaviors. We are sometimes more accepting and less critical, sometimes not. Our flexibility can vary based on how comfortable we are with ourselves, others, and our surroundings.

Persons with dementia should be offered the same open-minded and flexible approach. "Behavior" typically connotes bad or uncooperative actions or reactions, when in fact the behavior is often an expressed solution for a problem or situation. The behavior, therefore, becomes a means of communicating feelings and needs. Behavior has meaning and is usually goal directed.

At times, this expression of needs, demonstrated by the behavior, becomes an activity. Rummaging through bureau drawers or wandering room to room can be viewed as the resident's activity. The criteria for a therapeutic or positive activity are the same as for other purposeful uses of time or energy: The activity should focus on the resident's abilities and self-esteem and be a safe tool to reduce or eliminate the negative or unwanted behaviors, as well as a vehicle for verbal and nonverbal communication.

Generally there is a reason for the behavior—it does not just happen. At times, if one has the insight and takes time to investigate a behavioral response, the thought or action being demonstrated may be understood. At other times, it is impossible to perceive the basis of the reaction. An example would be a combative behavioral response to a hallucination or a perceived dislike of someone, whether real or imagined.

The caregiver who is willing to look at what a behavior is "saying" and who is flexible enough to adapt or make appropriate changes rather than manipulate or force the resident to change often will be able to help the resident decrease unacceptable behaviors and promote positive responses. Negative behavior may be the resident's only or selected way to invite or force interaction with other residents, staff, or family members.

A behavior usually does not happen in an instant. There is a buildup of the feelings that the resident is trying to express. Caregivers skilled in observing nonverbal behavior can very often pick up on the situation and assess the unspoken need. The important challenge to caregivers is to react to the very first signs of the resident's concern or demonstrated response. If the situation or behavior is refocused during the initial stage, rather than waiting until the response is out of hand and the resident is overwhelmed, the resident is safeguarded from perhaps an embarrassing or unsafe experience.

Caregivers are challenged to rethink and reevaluate their selected criteria or limitations of "good" and "bad" behavioral responses. Rarely are the negative behaviors enacted on purpose or to manipulate the caregiver, but rather are a result of the disease process. The behaviors can be a problem to others but not to the resident, who is oblivious to the resultant aggravation or concern. At times, the need or value of the chosen behavioral outcome is weighed against the ease or stress involved in soliciting the desired response. This is like "picking your fights," deciding which issues to focus on changing or decreasing and which issues to just let go.

BEHAVIORS AS EXPRESSIONS OF ABILITIES AND INABILITIES

Behavior can express the resident's abilities or demonstrate inabilities or challenges to the resident. Certainly, a behavior can have both positive and negative components. Stress is reduced when the positive aspects of behaviors are supported and the resident care is focused on abilities.

Behaviors: Demonstrating Resident Abilities

With the progression of memory loss; decrease in orientation to persons, places, things, and themselves; and diminishing language skills, the resident "acts out" or demonstrates feelings, concerns, and needs. Behaviors provide the stage for allowing the resident to be "heard." Behaviors are used as the residents search to feel accepted, have a positive self-image, and attempt to foster self-wellness. The caregiver should watch and listen, gathering this behavior-related information for the basis of accountable resident care and support. Examples are provided in the following sections.

Behaviors: Providing Cognitive Support of Abilities
Wandering provides environmental changes and contact with others that stimulate verbal and problem-solving responses. Rummaging, sorting, and rearranging books, file cards, and bureau drawer items promote "being-at-work" patterns and increase attention span.

Behaviors: Providing Physical Support of Abilities
Pacing decreases stress and restlessness, increases well-being and appetite, and helps to produce healthy fatigue. Hyperactivity often demonstrates needs such as hunger, use of the toilet, or onset of an illness.

Behaviors: Providing Psychosocial Support of Abilities
Taking clothes from the closet to the bed and back to the closet provides a perceived purposeful use of time. Or, the resident may feel secure by carrying items in his or her arms such as towels, magazines, and papers. His or her desire to feel in control may be exhibited by rearranging or taking apart items such as a phonograph or draperies. Fear or anxiety may be demonstrated by increased agitation or combativeness.

Behaviors: Precipitating Challenges, Risks, or Inabilities

Negative or unwanted behaviors do occur. Residents and others can be affected emotionally and physically. A resident's behavior can seesaw back and forth, ranging from enabling a positive outcome to creating a fully developed negative response. For example, rummaging can promote feelings of being in charge and making a positive use of time, or it can increase frustration and anger as a hunted-for item, such as a purse, cannot be found. The person with dementia, experiencing inabilities being escalated or challenged, responds. Increased anxiety, frustration, outbursts, and combativeness can communicate a real or perceived need. Examples are provided in the following sections.

Behaviors: Precipitating Cognitive Challenges, Risks, or Inabilities
Wandering and becoming lost may precipitate increased disorientation. The resident may not understand a task or what is expected of him or her, which may initiate combativeness or a catastrophic reaction.

Behaviors: Precipitating Physical Challenges, Risks, or Inabilities
Unwanted weight loss or exhaustion may be caused by constant pacing. Safety may be compromised by wandering on wet floors, high traffic areas, or uneven ground surfaces. The resident may attempt to eat or drink a toxic cleaning solution, non-food item, or spoiled food.

Behaviors: Precipitating Psychosocial Challenges, Risks, or Inabilities
The resident may exhibit paranoid tendencies, accusing others and becoming combative. He or she may also experience depression or withdrawal due to negative feedback from others.

RISK FACTORS PRECIPITATING BEHAVIORAL MANIFESTATIONS

Almost every behavior is a demonstration of a purpose or reflection of a reason. The list of possible factors precipitating unwanted behaviors is endless. There are many variables, such as time of day, people present, what has just happened, and all the considerations listed under Implementing a Behavioral Profile: Why Is the Behavior Happening?

Other risk factors precipitating behavioral manifestations that should be considered are

1. Undiagnosed fractures: especially in residents with high risk for osteoporosis
2. Chronic pain: residents who cannot report pain should have prescribed medications administered on a consistent basis, not waiting until they grimace or show signs of agitation
3. Fatigue: impaired sleep cycle, exhaustion
4. Current pain: assess for possibilities such as a toothache, earache, ingrown toenail; do not rely on the resident to self-report pain or discomfort
5. Possible urinary or bowel retention, anemia, hypoglycemia
6. Dehydration: a possible causative situation leading to late-day agitation
7. Nightmares: inability to move from the dream sleep state into the awake reality
8. Other physical causes for the physician to assess: hypoglycemia, seizures, anemia, discomfort from possible causes such as prostate problems, prolapsed bladder, uterus or bowel complications
9. Depression: mood-influenced behavior, usually difficult for the resident to express
10. Misidentification of persons in their environment or what is happening to or about them, or both
11. Relocation stress: the homeostasis or comfort of the past location is responded to with distress or disequilibrium because of a move or change
12. Disconnection-connection: not being called forth or validated as a person of worth during the day to be involved in a meaningful way, often seen when the staff does too much for the resident and does not engage the resident in activity or activities of daily living (ADLs) (therefore, a response to learned helplessness); not having decision-making opportunities; having too much done "to" rather than "with" the resident
13. Feelings of abuse or being invaded: residents interpret ADLs as abuse (e.g., having teeth brushed, tightening a small waistband, rubbing wet hair dry); response to tactile defensiveness
14. Caregiver response: negative reaction to caregiver's size, age, gender, race, foreign accent or foreign language being spoken, approach; response to too many caregivers present or involved at one time

GUIDELINES FOR UNDERSTANDING AND REFOCUSING BEHAVIORS

It is almost impossible to account for the multiple variables that affect residents' behaviors and the variety of possible responses to them by caregivers. It is equally impossible to describe "the" single answer or solution when assistance or intervention is needed. What works at one time or place may work or not work in the next similar circumstance. Therefore, guidelines or problem-solving tools are needed for outlining or diagramming the behavior's components. Guidelines bring together the best possible information for enabling the insight and understanding needed to select a change or response. The challenge is to discern the positive and negative aspects of the behavioral activity and then to identify the assistance needed either to promote the behavior's continuation or to take the needed action to distract the resident from or end the unwanted response.

Prevent: Be Prepared

- Start with the resident's LifeStory Book (see Chapter 3) and bring out positive aspects of his or her life history throughout the day.
- Be aware of the resident's past coping skills or problems when handling stressful situations, change, or overt fear.
- Be willing to be a detective and size up situations and prevent negative situations before they happen. Deal with any excess disabilities that escalate the resident's unease.
- Realize that fear is usually the number one emotion felt by persons with dementia. Constant reminders of, "You are safe with me, I will be here with you today," help to dispel or lesson a negative behavior arising from fear.
- Recognize "triggers" or antecedents of possible difficult behaviors. Prevention of an unwanted behavior is always preferable to allowing the resident to go through a possible frightening experience. For example, basic care, such as drying the resident's hair or fastening a tight pair of trousers, could be misconstrued by the resident and become a trigger for acting-out behavior.
- Act immediately; do not wait. As soon as the caregiver perceives that the resident is beginning to be concerned or is exhibiting agitation, the caregiver should act right then and there. Waiting allows situations that can easily be changed or stopped to develop into major confrontations or overwhelming feelings of being out of control.
- Prevention can also occur when the caregiver is willing to step back, take a deep breath, and "go with the flow." This means relaxing expectations, letting go of the need to always be right, and giving oneself permission to change and enter the resident's "world" and not try to force-fit the resident into the caregiver's "world."

Interpret: Message and Meaning

- Ask what the behavior is "saying." Behaviors are usually the resident's method of communication when words are inaccessible or the feelings are inexpressible in any other way.
- Be a detective: look at the clues, put the pieces together to find the meaning. Be especially sensitive to the resident's mood, facial expression, voice tone, and body stance.
- Review the resident's LifeStory for cues (see Chapter 3).

- Remember that the resident's behaviors are rarely on purpose: the resident does not plan or try to be difficult, although it may seem that he or she is being stubbornly difficult.
- Look at all aspects of possible difficulty: cognitive need or misunderstandings; physical need such as illness; psychosocial need such as fear or anger; environmental factors (e.g., too much noise or a frightening television show).

Analyze: What Is the Problem?

A resident can display a difficult behavior that presents a problem for caregivers (e.g., excessive pacing or leaving an area of safety unsupervised). At the same time, from a resident's point of view, it may not be a problem at all. The resultant behavior activity might represent a need to act out anxiety or boredom. Be able to separate your needs as a caregiver from the needs of the resident. Be willing to let go, not always needing to be right.

Problem solving requires looking at the behavior's symptoms and possible triggers or antecedents, and then analyzing an appropriate response. A behavior profile (see Appendix 8-1), behavior observation form (see Appendix 8-2), behavior analysis form (see Appendix 8-3), and sensory profile (see Appendix 5-2) can supply information for assisting the analysis and help to develop a refocusing intervention. Focus on feelings and expressed emotions.

Respond: Reframe and Refocus

Reframing a difficult behavior occurs when the caregiver has analyzed the implied communication, determined who has the problem as reflected by the behavior, and then applied creativity and an open mind to reframe or reconsider the entire situation. Perhaps the behavior can be ignored without any unpleasant outcome. Perhaps a small change (e.g., the removal of a mirror when the resident becomes angered because he or she thinks that someone is watching him or her) can be instituted and the difficulty avoided.

Refocusing occurs just before or during a difficult behavior. The resident's attention or focus is channeled into a less threatening or difficult outcome. The resident's concern or feeling behind the behavior is acknowledged first and then the behavioral refocusing technique is used as part of the problem-solving procedure. The negativeness of an incident can then be turned into a positive outcome.

How can the resident's self-esteem, dignity, and remaining abilities and strengths be part of the behavior problem solving? Caregivers aware of the resident's strengths and well-being, as well as his or her challenges, can incorporate the resident's abilities into an appropriate response for refocusing difficult behaviors. Residents long for validation as persons of worth.

IMPLEMENTING A BEHAVIOR PROFILE

The resident *with* dementia *with* a challenging behavior deserves caregivers willing to take the time to ask the right questions. The process of using a behavior profile (see Appendix 8-1) allows not only meaningful information to be gathered but also facilitates effective interventions to be created and put into action.

The questions to ask are: What? Why? Who? Where? When? What now?

What Is Happening?

Identify and assess exactly what the exhibited behavior is. Does the behavior have physical or emotional manifestations? Can the actual response be described?

Physical Focus

- Pacing
- Wandering: purposefully, aimlessly
- Rummaging
- Hitting or striking
- Stripping off clothing
- Wringing hands
- Packing
- Picking skin, hair, clothing, or other items
- Repetitive motions, tapping, wiping
- Sexual manipulations

Emotional Focus

- Anxiousness
- Fearfulness
- Paranoia or suspiciousness
- Response to hallucinations
- Depression or withdrawal
- Screaming, yelling, or shouting
- Stubbornness
- Crying
- Mood changes
- Verbal abuse
- Catastrophic reaction

Why Is the Behavior Happening?

Because a behavior is a form of communication or a solution to a problem, the "why" must be answered, if possible. Is the action or reaction really a problem and, if so, to whom? Pacing or moving furniture from place to place may be annoying to the caregiver but not to the resident. Rarely is the resident with dementia capable of a negative or manipulative behavior just to irritate the caregiver. Is there an excess disability? An excess disability is when a problem or situation affecting the resident compounds or exasperates the difficulties already experienced by the person because of his or her dementia. Examples of excess disabilities are illness, environmental overstimulation or understimulation, sensory deficits that could be corrected, or other situations listed under Cognitive, Physical, Psychosocial, and Environmental Focus. Inability to understand or interpret the cause or antecedent of the resident's behavior can become the source of caregiver anger, frustration, guilt, and depression.

Cognitive Focus

- Limited awareness or ability to interpret others or environmental, physical, or emotional stimuli
- Task is too complicated or unfamiliar; unclear instructions
- Being asked to respond to too many questions; feeling like he or she is being tested
- Responding to arguments between others; thinking that he or she is part of the confrontation
- Decreased understanding or ability to communicate
- Not enough time given to respond
- Violence, trauma, or emotional situations on television
- Limited attention span
- Lifelong personality pattern and past experience or history of responding or coping with stress
- Memory deficit
- Being scolded or criticized or being told, "No" or "Don't"
- Limited ability to make choices or changes in a schedule or routine
- Spatial or perceptual dysfunctions that lead to misinterpretation of people, space, objects, or tasks
- Mistaken identity of persons or places
- Decreased or lack of familiar routine or structure to the day
- Activities that are insulting or too childlike
- Staff's not speaking English or the common language spoken by the resident

Physical Focus

- Inability to manipulate or move the body due to decreased motor planning or body awareness
- Physical responses due to sensory deficit misinterpretation, especially hearing and vision
- Being touched from the back or being grabbed without eye contact
- Dehydration
- Fatigue or disruption of sleep patterns
- Harmful or negative responses due to medications, side effects
- Use of restraints
- Hallucinations: auditory or visual
- Onset of an illness, discomfort, or hunger
- Surprised by unexpected physical contact

Psychosocial Focus

- Paranoia, suspiciousness, or depression

- Lack of personal or positive validation as a person of worth or both
- Familiar person out of sight
- Fear, anxiety, or frustration
- Searching or feeling lost
- Unrealistic demands from others; not having preferences respected
- Feeling contradicted, scolded, or manipulated
- Disliking a person, place, or thing or inability to find a friend
- Change in routine
- Unrealistic expectations
- Overstimulation from holidays or special events
- Relocation stress

Environmental Focus

- Unfamiliar surroundings
- Sensory overload (e.g., noise, overdecorating)
- Sensory "underload": nothing going on
- Sudden movements; startling or unexpected noises
- Lack of cues or information needed for orientation
- Loud sounds; constant or disliked noises
- Darkness or poor lighting
- Glare; reflections
- Clutter or crowded areas
- Barriers: real or perceived
- Going from varying areas of light (e.g., from a well-lit area to one of dimness or darkness)
- Twinkling decorations or decorations hanging from the ceiling that turn with air currents
- Sudden weather changes that affect the lighting and sounds in the environment

Who Is Involved?

Is the behavior involving just the resident? Other residents? Staff? Family? Visitors? For example, if the behavior is a response to a specific person, it can tell you something about that relationship. Is the response consistent? Are difficult behaviors due to gender, race, culture, age, size?

> Isabel would display agitation and refuse to continue eating if her husband arrived to visit during mealtime. He would stand over her, arms folded, and stare at his wife. She almost seemed to "feel" his arrival, even before she saw him. Isabel resented his disapproving scowl and lack of a caring response. Her nervous tremors increased and she often acted out her discomfort by pushing the food tray to the floor. These behaviors ceased when her husband was requested to visit after meals.

Where Is the Behavior Exhibited?

The environment greatly affects the residents' behavior. The actual room of the house or facility, hall, or area can often supply the cues needed to understand the behavioral response. Is being outside or inside a factor? Does an unfamiliar environment precipitate a desired or unwanted behavior or can the same response be noted in familiar surroundings? Is the response consistent?

> Arlene was agitated easily and would yell verbal abuses
> when the family room became too crowded or noisy. She
> was not able to tolerate the pacing of other residents. The
> yelling was reduced when Arlene sat with quiet residents in
> a small group or when she was busy alone in her bedroom.

When Does the Behavior Usually Occur?

The resident experiences "good and bad days" as well as "ups and downs" throughout the day that affect mood and responses. For example, late afternoon and the time before and after supper often affect residents' behavior in what is referred to as "sundown syndrome." Increased anxiety, restlessness, or combativeness may be exhibited. Observing the specific time of behavior may give the caregiver insight into the cause and needed intervention. Is the response consistent?

> Samuel was always hungry first thing in the morning. The
> staff did not know that his wife always gave him a sand-
> wich as soon as he awoke while he was dressing. He hit and
> shoved a staffperson across the room before information
> that helped to solve the morning behavioral response was
> understood and an early morning snack was supplied.

What Now? Assistance

The what, why, who, and when form the basis of responses to the demonstrated behavior. If time permits, the actual listing of these components helps to enable an accountable action plan. Does the behavior follow a repeated pattern of response to certain circumstances? The accumulated information then is held up against the criteria defining the behavior as one that supports the resident's abilities or exacerbates the resident's inabilities. The focus then is shifted to the "why" of the behavior. This is often where the needed changes must start. Understanding of the cognitive, physical, psychosocial, and environmental aspects that have precipitated possible instigation of the "why" becomes the fundamental reasoning behind adapting, modifying, or making complete changes. Knowledge and skills in communication, breaking down and simplifying tasks, distraction techniques, and supporting positive activities are the tools to carry out the required changes and provide needed assistance.

TRACKING BEHAVIORAL PATTERNS: A BEHAVIOR OBSERVATION FORM

Discovering a pattern related to the onset or display of a difficult behavior is usually helpful. Most behavior challenges have identifiable triggers or antecedents. At times, the behavior might appear to have a random onset. By using a behavior observation form (see Appendix 8-2) everyone involved with the resident's care can assist in trying to identify the triggers and help in making necessary changes. Hopefully, a pattern is identified with appropriate refocusing interventions. The form also allows a history of the behavior to be documented. Included on the form are the following areas:

1. *Date and time of day*: This is especially important if the behavior incidents cluster around a certain time.
2. *Observed activity and behavior*: Documenting exactly what happens during the behavior is imperative; it can be an emotional time for all involved and sometimes the resident's acting out or responses are not evaluated clearly.
3. *Trigger*: What started it all? Can the possible cause be identified and changed?
4. *Intervention*: What stopped the behavior from proceeding? Does the same intervention happen on a consistent basis? Why not?
5. *Time elapsed*: How much time was needed to stop the behavior? When the behavior was stopped or refocused, how long before it happened again?
6. *Observer*: Include names of caregivers who were involved and may need to be consulted when more information is needed or for team problem solving.

PROBLEM SOLVING: A BEHAVIOR ANALYSIS FORM

Putting together the puzzle pieces to be able to solve or refocus a difficult behavior requires analyzing information about the behavior, the resident, and general tolerance for the occurrence. The focus becomes studying the resident as a "person with a behavior," not a behavior that defines the resident.

Components of a behavior analysis form (see Appendix 8-3) are as follows:

1. *Behaviors exhibited*: What exactly is going on?
2. *Emotions expressed*: What is the resident trying to say or express as manifested in the behavior?
3. *Whose problem*? Is it totally a resident-owned problem? A safety issue? Affecting other residents? A family request? Are staff tolerance or administration or regulatory factors involved? Can the environment handle the behavior?
4. *Excess disabilities*: What else is going on with the resident? Illness? Sensory factors? Cognitive or communication challenges? Emotional? Environmental? Family or caregiver related?
5. *Resident abilities*: Listing the resident's strengths enables appropriate interventions that uphold dignity and well-being.

6. *Refocusing interventions*: Listing ways to refocus the behavior that incorporates the resident's cognitive, physical, social, and spiritual well-being as well as support drawn from the environment and caregivers' skills.

SAFETY IN THE COMMUNITY: ELOPEMENT AND A POLICE DISPATCH FORM

Unless a lock and key are used, most safety measures for resident security can be violated. Most doors are also fire exits, and even with sophisticated alarm systems, the resident can still elope.

> Dick, a tall and athletic man, defied the security system of a nursing home. He was strong enough to hurdle the 6-ft fence before heading out to the highway. One night, armed with crisp bills from the Monopoly game, Dick went out his window, over the fence, through six lanes of traffic, to the local tavern. After enjoying the beer and burger he had ordered, Dick proudly reached into his pocket to pull out his "money." He peeled a $20 bill off the stack of bills and handed it to the bartender. Laughter ensued while Dick continued to try to pay with the game money. He became embarrassed, leading to agitation, when his money was unacceptable. After all, he thought it was good money. A staffperson's spouse was in the tavern that evening, realized the situation before it got out of hand, and intervened. The local police were called and because of their training in dementia and refocusing behaviors, Dick was escorted back to the facility without further confrontation.

Ideally, a care facility or program caring for persons with dementia has taken the time and effort to reach out to gain a supportive partnership with the local police and fire departments. Civic and community professionals are usually anxious to learn about the impact of Alzheimer's disease and related dementias on the people residing within their community (see Appendix 8-4).

The Alzheimer's Association also has excellent programs to offer these professionals. The Safe Return program is especially effective. The program provides a bracelet for the resident to wear and registers the resident on a national listing available 24 hours a day. This network enables family members, staff, and other health care professionals to seek help when a resident has eloped or when a person with dementia has been found and is unable to provide pertinent information. The Association also has helpful hints on how to encourage the person with dementia to wear the bracelet. One of the most effective ideas is to have the bracelet given to the resident by his or her grandchild. Reinforcement can be offered by admiring the bracelet on the resident and remarking what a wonderful gift the grandchild has given to him or her. The Safe Return bracelets come in a silver tone. If this presents a problem to the resident who "only wears gold," spray paint the bracelet a gold tone.

The Wealshire, of Lincolnshire, Illinois, working with the Lincolnshire Police, developed a form that is used if a resident elopes from the facility (see Appendix 8-5).

The form includes information that the police need to identify the resident. Also included is a listing of helpful information the police can obtain from the care center that will help officers when they make contact with the resident. This dispatch form can be kept on the charts of residents that are high-risk elopers. At the stressful time of seeking assistance for a missing resident, it is helpful to have a copy of the form that the police will be using so the staff have the answers ready before making the 911 call. Local police departments can help a care center with the development of an elopement policy and procedure and provide suggestions for searching a building. In return, offer police, fire, and other civic workers inservices about dementia and how it affects residents they may come in contact with. Law enforcement departments are a great resource for assistance. Working together benefits everyone.

BEHAVIOR ANALYSIS EXAMPLES

An example of a problem-solving tool for understanding the resident's communication spoken through the medium of a behavior is the use of an analysis system. This tool analyzes the resident's abilities, challenges or inabilities, and suggestions for assistance. Two examples follow: wandering and pacing and "redistribution of stuff"—rummaging.

Behavior Analysis Example: Wandering and Pacing

Wandering and pacing are activities that involve movement, either walking or in a wheelchair, with or without a sense of purpose or goal.

Demonstrating Resident Abilities
PROVIDING COGNITIVE SUPPORT OF ABILITIES.   Wandering and pacing behavior

- Provides environmental changes and sensory stimulation
- Brings contact with others and increases orientation and familiarity with surroundings
- Leads to decision making through choice of where to go
- Expresses sensory overload

PROVIDING PHYSICAL SUPPORT OF ABILITIES. Wandering and pacing behavior

- Decreases stress and restlessness
- Increases physical well-being and gross motor skills
- Maintains activeness; positive use of energy
- Increases appetite and healthy fatigue
- Expresses needs (e.g., hunger, urination, exercise)
- Expresses medication reaction; decreases weight
- Indicates possible onset of physical problems, illness, or uncomfortable clothing

PROVIDING PSYCHOSOCIAL SUPPORT OF ABILITIES.   Wandering and pacing behavior

- Provides sense of purposeful way to spend time; gives dignity
- Avoids boredom: resident receives greetings, responses from others

- Promotes former role pattern (e.g., going to the health club, doing housework)
- Allows resident to feel "in control"; decreases feelings of anxiety
- Provides a way to express needs (e.g., fear, anxiousness, loneliness)

Precipitating Challenges, Risks, or Inabilities

PRECIPITATING COGNITIVE CHALLENGES, RISKS, OR INABILITIES.   Wandering and pacing behavior

- Can cause resident to look for something he or she cannot name or describe to himself or herself or others
- Adds to confusion, disorientation, not knowing where he or she is
- May cause resident not to know or recognize signs of fatigue or how to stop and sit down; not realizing when he or she has become lost
- May cause resident to respond because of not knowing or understanding what is expected of him or her

PRECIPITATING PHYSICAL CHALLENGES, RISKS, OR INABILITIES.   Wandering and pacing behavior

- Can lead to increased fatigue; unwanted weight loss
- Can compromise safety and increase chance of falls or contact injuries
- Can increase difficulty experienced in accomplishing ADLs

PRECIPITATING PSYCHOSOCIAL CHALLENGES, RISKS, OR INABILITIES.   Wandering and pacing behavior

- Can cause feelings of being lost, searching
- Can increase stress and anxiety
- Can cause negative feedback to be received from others (e.g., when in the wrong room)
- Can cause feelings of insecurity, tension, being manipulated
- Can cause increased negative feedback from others when invading their space

Assistance Suggestions

COGNITIVE ASSISTANCE SUGGESTIONS

- Assess what the wandering is "telling" you. Does the resident have an agenda and, if so, how can you offer the resident reassurance that his or her concerns will be met? Is the wandering purposeful? Self-stimulating? Caused by fear of abandonment?
- Use calm approach, eye contact, arms at the side.
- Use signs for clueing (e.g., the resident's name on the bedroom or bathroom, familiar objects from the past, arrow to activity room, signs on walls or the floor).
- Use stop sign on door or large "NO."
- Color or decorate a door you do not wish used so it blends in with walls and does not look like a door, or put up a full-length mirror where the resident will see "someone watching them," if appropriate and accepted by the resident.
- Use distraction techniques to break up the pacing pattern (e.g., offer to sit with the resident, have a drink of juice, look at pictures or the view from the window).
- Simplify tasks and requests to reduce communication difficulties.

- Try a strong voice and words such as, "You're going in the wrong direction."
- Say, "You've got a phone call," to direct the person back to a safe place.
- Assess whether leaving the unit or a trip out of the house-facility precipitates, on return, the escalation of problem wandering. Coats may need to be hidden to decrease the reminder of going outside.

PHYSICAL ASSISTANCE SUGGESTIONS

- Assess physical health for problems and needs (e.g., illness, seizures, response to medication).
- Use good evening lighting, avoiding shadows, and a night-light to help when needed to separate dreams from reality.
- Assess for sensory deficits, especially vision and hearing.
- Walk with the resident, converse, and build trust, then redirect; do not force the resident. Single staffperson intervention is preferable.
- Avoid use of rugs with nap and scatter rugs, which may lead to falls. Provide safe, uncluttered area to pace.
- Check that all toxic or harmful items are locked away or removed.
- Monitor fatigue and if the resident will not sit down to rest, use a geriatric chair with a tray or restrain the resident for 15–30 minutes if resident has physician orders for restraints.
- Maintain fluid and food intake, and monitor weight weekly.
- Monitor the resident's feet and watch for blisters, calluses, and so on.
- Offer stimulating activities (e.g., dancing, exercises).
- Make door frames a contrasting color from the wall and chair seats a contrasting color from the floor.
- Close the door or use fabric strips across doorways.
- Acquaint staff with resident to increase safety monitoring.
- Use a medic alert bracelet or name wristband, perhaps a specific color for wanderers.
- Establish a lost-resident policy and procedure.

PSYCHOSOCIAL ASSISTANCE SUGGESTIONS

- Provide reassurance, acceptance, and attention—do not argue or confront.
- Walk with the resident, using time spent as a social activity or opportunity to do a purposeful task (e.g., delivering an item).
- Look for and eliminate persons or situations that led to the pacing. Note environmental hypo- or hyperstimulation needs.
- Set up a walking group or club. Take facility "tours."
- Train staff in distraction techniques or ways to reroute wanderers. Use familiar objects, such as chairs and bedspreads, to help increase sense of comfort.
- Use consistent, familiar, trained staff.

Behavior Analysis Example: "Redistribution of Stuff"—Rummaging

Rummaging and pillaging is the activity of searching, looking at, touching, holding, and moving items from one place to another.

Demonstrating Resident Abilities
PROVIDING COGNITIVE SUPPORT OF ABILITIES.   Rummaging behavior

- Provides a way for resident to select, gather, and "own" familiar items
- Encourages resident to make choices and decisions; increase interest in sur-roundings
- Offers a "valuable" use of time for resident; resident has attitude of being at work
- May be a method to attract attention; attempt socialization
- Is a way for resident to use items as a reminder of the past and present (e.g., who resident was, where resident is); resident may substitute gathered held items for "ungathered" thoughts
- Enables resident to take things apart to understand them (e.g., knows purse should be full but does not understand what to put in it, so "saves" napkins, spoons, sugar packets).

PROVIDING PHYSICAL SUPPORT OF ABILITIES.   Rummaging behavior

- Increases opportunities for resident to use touch as a primary sensory stimu-lant or link to reality
- Encourages resident's need to be physically active, but not knowing what to do
- Increases well-being and gross motor skills such as moving, bending, and reaching
- Uses fine-motor skills such as taking things apart
- Offers an outlet for restlessness or end result for wandering and pacing

PROVIDING PSYCHOSOCIAL SUPPORT OF ABILITIES.   Rummaging behavior

- Becomes a vehicle to act out expressions of fear and boredom
- Provides the comfort of familiar roles and tasks (e.g., housekeeping, managing)
- Provides a sense of mission, purpose, feeling useful, being a helper
- Decreases anxiety (e.g., saving food decreases worry about being hungry and not knowing where the next meal will come from)
- Provides feelings of possession, ownership, being in control
- Makes resident feel important (e.g., having items for pocket or purse)

Precipitating Challenges, Risks, or Inabilities
PRECIPITATING COGNITIVE CHALLENGES, RISKS, OR INABILITIES.   Rummaging behavior

- Can increase confusion, limiting clear thinking or planning
- Can lead to thinking about or taking items that are not the resident's

PRECIPITATING PHYSICAL CHALLENGES, RISKS, OR INABILITIES.   Rummaging behavior

- Increases safety risks, especially with toxic substances, spoiled food, sharp items, unsafe environments (e.g., kitchen, bathroom)

PRECIPITATING PSYCHOSOCIAL CHALLENGES, RISKS, OR INABILITIES.   Rummaging behavior

- May lead to accusing others of stealing
- May cause increased frustration, especially when confronted by persons wanting resident's items or negative response to the invasion
- May cause increased anxiety, not knowing what the resident is looking for

- May cause feeling lost, leading to searching
- May cause verbal, nonverbal messages from others that the resident is a thief

Assistance Suggestions

COGNITIVE ASSISTANCE SUGGESTIONS

- Provide love and a sense of security that needs will be met.
- Mark items with the resident's name.
- Use "straightening up" as an activity.
- Have "stuff" available for rummaging in the top drawer of a bureau or desk, or in kitchen.
- If you need to take an item that the resident has, give the resident something else in its place to hold.
- Learn favorite hiding places, especially tissue boxes, under the mattress, and behind drapes.
- Have sorting activities and "stuff" available that is safe (e.g., baby clothes, washcloths, playing cards).
- Have familiar items from the past that the resident can hold and carry.
- Make cloth scrapbooks, sew on straps, and attach the books to the resident's chair.

PHYSICAL ASSISTANCE SUGGESTIONS

- Keep the resident physically busy with activities.
- Check for unsafe items or surroundings.
- Train all persons and staff to understand safety monitoring.
- Set up special areas, such as drawers and closets, for rummaging.
- Shut doors or use 24-in. fabric strips across doors.

PSYCHOSOCIAL ASSISTANCE SUGGESTIONS

- Do not view rummaging as a negative activity.
- Be with the resident and make the activity fun, thereby changing it from being a fear-driven endeavor.
- Do not punish, scold, tease, or respond with anger; be gentle, speak softly.
- Find a calming environment to reduce fears.
- Use distraction (e.g., "Come with me; let's get a glass of juice") to move the resident from someone else's space or possessions.
- Give tasks to make the resident feel helpful.
- Make busy boxes with safe items to handle (e.g., ribbons, artificial flowers, balls of yarn) for acceptable rummaging.
- Ask the resident's family to bring in safe, expendable items that are familiar and work-related or associated with pleasurable activity (e.g., clipboard, order blanks, spools of thread, and balls of yarn).

SAFETY ISSUES: PHYSICALLY AGGRESSIVE, COMBATIVE, OR VIOLENT SITUATIONS

Act, do not react. A physically aggressive or combative resident is a frightened resident. Try to remain calm. Refrain from arguing. Intervention should happen long before the resident feels the need to *respond* by hitting out, pushing, shoving, kicking, hair pulling, scratching, or biting. Usually, the resident has displayed signs of the impending escalation of emotions.

The following are some specific suggestions for dealing with a physically aggressive, combative, or violent situation:

1. *Be alert.* Staff require training in all aspects of dementia caregiving. Emphasis is first on residents and their personal experience of dementia and their LifeStory. Prevention of difficult behaviors starts with communication skills and an awareness of the resident's nonverbal language as well as that of caregivers themselves. Training must also include a working knowledge of how to handle the aggressive resident, assuring the upset resident's safety, other residents' safety, and safety of the staff. Developing a relationship with the local hospital's psychiatric program may provide an instructor on techniques that can be modified for nursing home staff caring for residents with dementia. Offering such training will allow the staff to have confidence that they can handle difficult situations. Staff must be able to count on each other's assistance.

Examples of redirection interventions include

- Assuring the resident that he or she is safe.
- Opening the resident's LifeStory Book and try to gain his or her interest.
- Having tabletop "stuff" available that may catch the resident's eye, so he or she can pick it up and take off with it and thereby perhaps feel more in control.
- Using statements, such as, "Would you please help me?" or, "I need your assistance," in hopes of attracting the resident's attention and offering him or her a meaningful task, or feelings of self-worth.
- Offering something to eat or drink; cookies are usually successful. Be sure that whatever is handed to the resident will not hurt anyone if it is thrown back.

2. *Be prepared.* Have a system in place for obtaining needed assistance. Training staff to respond to, for example, "Code Wealshire" would alert staff that help was needed. Include also the place of the need: "Code Wealshire, in the shower room." Size up the situation and ask for help if there is reason to suspect a combative situation.

3. *"Know" the residents.* Identify potentially difficult residents who exhibit strong or combative responses to challenging situations. This does not mean labeling (e.g., "Jim is combative") as though Jim is always a troublemaker. Also identify potential combinations of residents that can lead to difficulty and which distraction techniques to use before a confrontation occurs. Knowing the individual resident's triggers for provoking anger or fear is also necessary. Prevention is still the best approach to reducing or eliminating violence.

Warning signs include

- Changes in physical activity, such as pacing, other movements, or becoming quiet or withdrawn; clapping hands; upper-body shaking or tremor
- Body language (e.g., threatening gestures, reddened face, fists, rapid eye movement, refusal to respond to redirection, no eye contact with person attempting to offer redirection)
- Verbal cues (e.g., raised voice, rapid speech, muttering, humming, whistling, obscene or threatening language, stuttering, calling out)

4. *Initiate "rescue" or "patrol" intervention.* If the staffperson involved with the resident is not able to help the resident to change his or her behavior, another staffperson can arrive on the scene, send the first staffperson away, and maybe effectively gain the confidence of the resident, who feels "rescued."

Suggestions for resident contact after the "rescue" are

- Take the resident for a walk away from the crisis area
- Seek a quiet area
- Reassure the resident that he or she is safe
- Offer cookies or other food.

There are certainly times when the upset resident needs one-to-one attention. However, it can be exhausting trying to redirect a resident acting out of control. Consider the following suggestions:

- Training all staff in the health care facility in "rescue" techniques. Staff not working directly in the resident care area (e.g., administrative staff) can offer their services to assist staff when the going gets tough. Staff comfortable with an upset resident, confident in their ability to offer redirection, and with relaxed and nonconfrontational body language can be available as needed. Hands-on staff should be trained to call in a manager or administrator when assistance is required or needed. At times, just taking the resident away from the area to another part of the building allows everyone to regroup as well as offers the resident a successful intervention.
- "Patrol" duty. This intervention works and also allows the rest of the staff to calm down and feel less stressed or overburdened. A resident that is upset, calling out, eloping, or escalating into a combative situation can be a candidate for "patrol."

> Pedro, a strong resident, pushed his way through the facility's front door 20–50 times a shift. Staff were constantly called to the front door to help redirect Pedro. It seemed impossible to get any work done; just when a staffperson tried, the front door alarm would go off again. The staff began to become disgusted, negative, and worn down by the need to constantly respond and chase down Pedro. Pedro would sometimes feel the staff's displeasure in his behavior and strike out in response. "Pedro patrol" was put into action. Staff members were each assigned a half hour shift when he or she would be responsible to redirect Pedro. It was a tough half hour, but the benefit far outweighed the task because for the next 2–3 hours that staffperson did not need to respond to Pedro. Only the person "on duty" was responsible unless help was needed and a code was called. Everyone was a winner, staff as well as Pedro.

"Patrol" can work in many situations in which there is a constantly reoccurring difficulty with a certain resident. Having one person assigned for a particular period helps everyone else to take a deep breath and go on with their work.

5. *Defuse confrontation and aggressive actions.* **Physical intervention should be the last resort!** Suggestions include the following:

- Immediately assess the situation for the need to call 911 due to the severity or possibilities of hurt residents, family members, or staff because the confrontation cannot be refocused or defused.
- If the resident will be safe, back away from the confrontation while continuing to monitor the situation.
- Respond immediately. Call a code if needed.
- Safety for the resident and all involved is the number one concern.
- Keep your voice calm. Try whispering in the resident's ear if deemed safe to be physically close.
- Or, try yelling (e.g., *"Let go."*).
- Try firmness (e.g., "Hilda, you are coming with me, *now."*).
- Try startle techniques (e.g., clap, sing [especially the "Star Spangled Banner" while telling the resident to stand at attention], drop something noisy, fake a sprained ankle and ask for help, talk quietly back to the yelling of a resident).
- Use simple, direct language, do not argue or try to reason, do not ask the resident questions that require use of memory.
- Be aware of your nonverbal gestures (e.g., facial responses, finger pointing, shaking your head as a negative gesture).
- Speak in positive tones with positive words. Eliminate "don't" and "no." Be nonjudgmental—this is the resident's fear speaking out.
- Acknowledge the resident's feelings (e.g., "I am sorry that you are upset," "You look frightened, you are safe with me").
- Show concern for the situation, without anger. Be aware of your nonverbal language. Keep your hands at your side, if possible. Do not stand in front of the resident, which is a confrontational position, and it could result in being kicked. Stand to the side. Do not turn your back on the resident. Be sure you have an open way out of the room.
- Let the resident have his or her space, if needed, while maintaining his or her safety.
- If the resident can be left alone and be safe, leave him or her alone, but continue to visually monitor from a distance.
- Do not make large gestures that may make the resident more apprehensive.
- If the resident needs to be held: *call a code if assistance is needed.* Staff should approach from each side of the resident, taking hold of his or her arms above the elbow and pressing the resident's arms close to his or her side. Stand close to the resident and push into his or her body. Grasping his or her arms above the wrist joint helps to reduce the resident's ability to strike out because the range of motion is limited. Use your weight, not your strength, as you press toward the resident. Another approach is for two staffpersons, one on each side of the resident, to reach around the resident's midsection to subdue his or her arms. One staffperson stands facing the resident's side, then reaches around, usually at the same time as the other staffperson. The resident will resist at first but will probably relax when feeling safe because of being held. During this time, one staffperson only will speak to the resident, offering reassurance that all will be well. If the resident is also kicking, each staffperson can take one of his or her legs and bring his or her thigh and knee over the resident's leg that is closest to him or her. This movement holds the

resident's leg from kicking. Again, the staffperson should talk with the resident, calming his or her fears. Any other noninvolved staff in the area need to stand by if assistance is needed but also be alert to the other residents witnessing this situation. If possible, move other residents out of the area or at least calm them.

- If two residents are involved in combative behavior: Identify which resident is going to be the "easiest" to redirect and attempt to move that resident away from the other. Or, use the hold technique on the resident doing the majority of the hitting out; this requires two staffpersons, one on each side. Moving swiftly but calmly is imperative. Raised voices add to the violence of the situation. If the staffperson is alone, grabbing a pillow or object to safely place between the residents is preferred to actually getting in between fighting residents. There are times, however, when the risk of getting in between the residents is taken because the two residents are hurting each other.
- Hair pulling: Cup your hand over the resident's hand and squeeze firmly while pushing your head in toward the resident. Do not attempt to pull away from the grasp.
- Grabbing: Talk calmly with the resident, saying that he or she is hurting you. Do not attempt to pull away. Stroke the resident's lower arm of the hand that is grasping. If this does not work, place your hand over the resident's hand and squeeze firmly.
- Another intervention for grabbing is to pick up one of the resident's fingers that is part of the grasp and gently pull it up until the grasp is released. Pulling your hand away, by a rapid motion, up and against the resident's thumb, often where it encircles the caregiver's hand, releases the resident's grasp because this is the weakest part of the hold.
- Biting: Do not pull away. Yelling, "Stop," might startle the resident enough that the bite is released. If possible, push the part of you being bitten (e.g., a finger) back into the resident's mouth toward the throat. This also startles the resident and may lead to feelings of choking, which will also end the biting. Placing your finger on the resident's upper lip, just below the nose, and pushing up firmly will also stop the biting behavior. Covering the nose so the mouth opens may be helpful. A last resort is to place your finger under the jawbone in the area closest and just in front of the ear and push firmly in and up. This technique can be used for biting or grabbing.
- Confrontation with a raised cane, walker, chair, or other object: "Lock up" the object being held by the resident. This means grabbing a chair, pillow, or other object that can tangle with the raised object the resident is holding, rather than being hit by the resident's object. Locking the two objects together will allow you to lower the objects to a safe position rather than one of being raised and on the attack. Do not try to reach out and grab at an object a resident is swinging around; chances are high that you will miss and be hit.

6. *"Deep breath" time.* The confrontation is over, what now? Recognize that any confrontation is difficult on everyone—not just the people involved but also others in the area. Certainly, the staffpersons and the involved resident or residents are exhausted emotionally and still feeling stressed. Time for separation is necessary. The staffperson can take a break or have an opportunity to de-escalate feelings. Other staff can use this time to affirm their colleague and talk about the situation, what was handled well, what was not handled well, what was learned, and what can be done differ-

ently the next time. The resident also needs time to regroup. The resident should also be comforted even though he or she might have instigated the entire behavioral confrontation. Staff must take the initiative and time to go to the resident, when calmness has been restored, and assure the resident that he or she will be all right and safe. Residents very often have a sense that they have caused a difficult incident based on their behavior. They may become frightened again. When they are consoled and calmed, residents will usually indicate with words or body language that they are sorry.

RESIDENT BEHAVIORAL RESPONSES

Residents with dementia are unique human beings. They each experience dementia with varying responses. It is the "listening" to the behavioral responses and what message they are attempting to relate that becomes the essential component of a compassionate caregiver.

Anxiety and Agitation

Anxiety and agitation are fear- and anger-provoked reactions to incapabilities, sensory deficits, or the environment, leading to tenseness and uncertainty, demonstrated by increased physical movement or verbal responses. Displays of anxiety and agitation can include restlessness, hand wringing, fidgeting, crying, insomnia, withdrawal, screaming, being uncooperative, rapid speech, disorganized thinking, being argumentative, delusions, paranoia, and hallucinations. The emotional instability could escalate to a catastrophic reaction.

> Jim appeared to not enjoy the daily activities in the nursing home. His wife thought that she could ease the adjustment to his admission by telephoning daily and encouraging him to participate. He was able to talk with her briefly on the telephone and seemed to be enjoying the conversation. After the call, the anxiety began. Jim would go room to room hunting for his wife, saying, "She must be here, I just talked with her." He became more and more anxious as he searched. The staff distracted Jim by first talking about his wife and then giving him some juice. In time, it became evident that Jim's wife had to be asked not to call him for the time being. If she wanted to know how he was doing, she was encouraged to call the nurses. Jim's ability to receive his wife's phone calls without becoming overly anxious would be assessed within a month's time.

Possible causes for anxiety and agitation can be the dementia and changes in the brain. Other considerations include the environment, sensory deficits, communication incapacities, dehydration and other medication side effects, and poorly timed diuretics.

Responding to the resident demonstrating the slightest elements of anxiety at the earliest time possible may refocus emotional stress by introducing a meaningful activity (see Chapter 9). Comfort the resident by constant affirmation that he or she is safe and that you will be with him or her. Another refocusing technique is to ask the resident to hold something belonging to the caregiver because it will be needed later. This allows an opportunity for the caregiver to thank the resident for helping.

If the anxiety increases, as well as the agitation, walking with the resident and going to a quiet place may help to reduce the emotional responses. One-to-one care is usually required at this time.

Catastrophic Reactions

Catastrophic reactions are overreactive responses of distress demonstrating the inability to understand, interpret, or cope with a real or imagined situation, person, environment, or self. A resident experiencing a catastrophic reaction is affected cognitively, physically, and psychosocially. Identifying the response, behavior, or activity of the reaction as well as the possible cause or antecedent will enable an appropriate intervention (see Appendix 8-6).

Displays of catastrophic reactions can include a sudden change of mood to anger or violence, often with misdirected behavior, combativeness, crying, pacing, restlessness, repetitive hand motions, such as clapping or stamping feet, or increased strength for picking up heavy objects such as televisions.

Possible causes include unrealistic demands, too difficult a task, being rushed, inability to express needs or fears, feeling manipulated, unfamiliar environment, too much noise or confusion in environment, caffeine, strangers, reflections, misunderstanding a television show, barriers, disliked persons present, inability to motor plan (mobility to perform purposeful movement), and onset of an illness.

There are several ways to provide assistance or intervention. Perceive or anticipate problems or stressors, rephrasing negatives, such as "don't" and "no," to positive statements, such as "Come with me" or "We can do it this way." Other suggestions are to distract with food or ask the resident for assistance, simplify interactions and tasks, use familiar routines, allow time to respond, reduce environmental stimuli, and allow physical movement to defuse agitation. Do not restrain the resident unless he or she is endangering himself or herself; use caring touch and verbal reassurances, and do not try to reason, argue, or confront. Use well-trained and familiar staffpersons.

> Eileen felt in a hurry to get off the bus after returning from an outing to a restaurant. She was heard stamping her feet as she anxiously waited for her turn to "get home." At other times, after large group activities, she paced the hall while shaking both fists held up at chest level. Physical combativeness was avoided by anticipating her need to leave the bus as soon as it arrived. A quiet place helped to relieve the fist shaking. Both were signs of feeling anxious about changes in familiar routines. Her participation in outings and large group activities were scheduled for a time when staff could observe and intervene if needed.

Combativeness and Aggression

Combativeness and aggression include physically striking out due to fear, anger, misinterpretations, history of past coping response, or challenges to understanding of personal survival. Unmanageable behaviors, including combativeness and aggression, are the most common reason for placement of a resident in a care facility. Caregivers must learn skills to be able to monitor and respond to residents as they start to experience an escalation of agitation that could lead to physical aggression.

Responses are similar to those demonstrated during catastrophic reactions and also can include verbal abuse. Anticipation of antecedents of the behavior and awareness of response patterns may limit or defuse the situation. Being surprised, experiencing an invasion of privacy, or feeling manipulated are often contributing stressors. Other antecedents include the physical stress and misinterpretation of ADLs, illness, side effects of medications, sensory dysfunction, and inconsistent or demeaning staff approaches. The caregiver often is mandated to change approaches or the environment.

> Leon is strong and active. He becomes fearful during daily
> care and hits the caregiver while yelling verbal abuses.
> Using chewing gum as a distraction technique occupied
> Leon's attention so that he did not strike out. He also
> appeared unable to chew gum and swear at the same time,
> which allowed him to join others and be socially appropri-
> ate. Gum chewing would not be advised for all aggressive
> residents, but it worked with Leon.

The primary cause of aggression is fear. Combativeness is fear speaking out. There are certainly times when the resident becomes extremely difficult to control physically during an aggressive incident. When this occurs, caregivers need to have the training and the confidence to be able to handle the situation. Refer to Safety Issues: Physically Aggressive, Combative, or Violent Situations. For assistance in using activities to reduce the onset of aggressive behaviors, refer to Chapter 9.

After the aggressive situation has quieted down and all involved are calm, go to the resident or residents involved in the confrontation and assure them that they will be all right, they are safe, and you will be there for them.

Sundowning

Sundowning includes combinations of increased behavioral responses, occurring in the mid- to late afternoon and evening, that reflect physical and emotional exhaustion and spatial-perceptual dysfunctions or misinterpretations. Sundowning is a response from the resident attempting to keep it together, struggling to maintain homeostasis or "stay on an even keel" despite the effects of dementia.

A partial or complete change or escalation of inabilities expressed in the resident's emotional or physical well-being, or both, can occur as the "sun goes down." These can be demonstrated by pacing, increased confusion, restlessness, combativeness, yelling, paranoia, feelings of insecurity or fearfulness, demanding, suspiciousness, disorientation and wanting to go home, impulsiveness, or other maladaptive behaviors. The resident is basically more demanding but at the same time unable to gain relief from one-to-one assistance or appropriate refocusing activity.

Possible causes include fatigue; failure to continue coping; limited tolerance of others or the environment, or both; need for simplification of requests or participation expectations; dehydration; unfavorable response to shift changes; lighting changes; programs and news on the television; brain changes due to dementia; and lack of sensory stimulation due to darkness.

There are several ways to provide assistance and intervention. Simplify approaches and environment. Use adequate lighting, allow a safe area for physical activity, and do not restrain the resident. Find the appropriate balance between activity and inactivity, quietness and comfortable auditory stimulation, privacy and time apart in balance with inaction with a small group of friends. Do not argue. Give reassurance, a caring touch, and sensitive redirection as needed. Urge the resident to drink fluids during the day. Offer normalization and familiar activities, and offer baby dolls or stuffed animals if appropriate. Limit the number of family members or other visitors at one time. This may be a time to encourage certain family members to be present if they are calm and helpful. Evening vespers, Bible reading, and a prayer circle are helpful, if appropriate.

> Susan appeared comfortable with her daily routine, which was filled with aimless wandering, rummaging in bureau drawers, or resting on a bed, not necessarily her own. As the afternoon staff arrived, Susan began to become anxious. Her wandering escalated into pacing as the supper hour approached. Her attempts to feel in charge or purposefully busy changed from moving items from one room to another to directing other residents and staff. She yelled at persons who did not obey her commands and sometimes would threaten to hit them. Part of "being in charge" included removing the restraints or geriatric chair trays of other residents, which led to accidents. Susan's pre–nursing-home activities were discussed with her family, but there was no obvious connection between the exhibition of her authority late in the day and her past. Perhaps it was triggered by thinking that she was at home and was disciplining her children as she prepared for supper. Rather than using restraints or medications, Susan was given a "job" of delivering clean bedding and towels for evening care. Pushing the cart up and down the hall kept her occupied and supported her need to feel important. The staff thanked her for the assistance she gave. She did need monitoring to maintain the other residents' safety.

If the late afternoon agitation continues and does not respond to interventions, the attending physician should be contacted. At times, rearranging the delivery of medications can help to relieve the resident's sundown response.

Inappropriate Sexual Responses: Hypersexuality and Stripping

Fondling or other sexual behaviors that upset or endanger the resident, other residents, family, or staff are inappropriate. Behaviors or demonstrations related to sexual inappropriateness are discussed in Chapter 10. Threats, scolding, or forms of behavior modification are usually ineffective in refocusing sexual acting out. Creative interventions include distraction techniques, relocation, active involvement in acceptable activities, re-establishment of masculine roles for male residents acting out, and application of a behavior profile (see Appendix 8-1), sensory profile (see Appendix 5-2), and behavior observation form (see Appendix 8-2). The resident's medications and effects should be a major consideration when assessing inappropriate sexual behaviors.

Picking or Repetitious Movements

Picking or repetitious movements can include using the hands and fingers to take apart or pull at items, hit or wipe surfaces, or make noise such as clapping. Other repetitious movements are chewing on clothing or fingers, rocking the body back and forth, arm or leg flexion and extension, and facial grimaces. Causes of repetitious movements could be medications, boredom, or a result of the disease process.

At times, one-to-one interaction will distract the resident, but he or she will resume the movement when you leave. Holding a ball or an object, such as a doll or teddy bear, may work, but the resident often pushes the object onto the floor (see Chapter 9, Daily Life Stuff: Meaningful Activities and the description of Shoestring and Wearable Activities for Residents with Short Attention Spans). Wearing earphones attached to a cassette player may refocus the sensory focus from the tactile skin fixation to the ears and auditory awareness. Resident safety and skin integrity will need monitoring if the picking causes skin or hair problems. Monitoring is also needed when repetitious movements are so constant that they lead to possible skin breakdown.

Hyperorality

Some residents may find an uncontrollable need to put everything into their mouth that will fit. This may include food stuffing during meals as well as eating nonedibles such as plant leaves, paper, and hygiene products.

Monitoring the resident is required in addition to taking all safety precautions to keep noxious liquids or items from being available. Foods that should not be eaten by the resident (e.g., staff lunches or a 3-pound box of candy) should be locked away or placed where the resident does not have access unless supervised.

Wandering and Pacing

Wandering is often without an agenda and is aimless or exploratory. Pacing is ambulation (independent or in a wheelchair), often repetitious movement, with a self-perceived agenda (see Behavior Analysis Example: Wandering and Pacing).

Alzheimer's Disease: Activity-Focused Care

"Redistribution of Stuff"—Rummaging

Rummaging includes looking at, touching, holding, and moving items from one place to another. It appears that residents seem to want to gather up all of the objects in their surroundings as a projection of wanting to gather up their remaining cognitive abilities and hold themselves together (see Behavior Analysis Example: "Redistribution of Stuff"—Rummaging).

Sleep Disturbances and Nocturnal Wandering

Sleep disturbances include irregular sleep patterns with wake cycles at inappropriate times leading to sleep deprivation.

Fatigue and exhaustion limit the ability of the resident with dementia to engage his or her cognitive, physical, and psychosocial wellness. A cycle easily begins, sometimes resulting in a totally opposite pattern from the caregiver or other residents. Sleeplessness leads to the resident's experiencing difficult behaviors that very often have negative effects on those around him or her. Assessment of the behaviors requires looking at possible causes for the sleep disturbances. These could include pain, incontinence, difficulty breathing, sensory dysfunction, seizure activity, depression, environmental over- or understimulation, and medications. The resident's physician should re-evaluate current medications and make appropriate changes, eliminating, it is hoped, some of the side effects that are instigating the problem. The physician can also evaluate the appropriateness of sleep medication. Problems occur when the resident has difficulty waking up, resulting in the possibility of being at high risk for falls.

Monitoring the resident during the day and before the usual bedtime may be helpful. Trying to keep the resident awake by providing meaningful activities at appropriate times, no caffeine, limited naps, a snack and warm milk before bedtime, and a nightly ritual of perhaps prayers or a song the resident used to sing to his or her children might be helpful. Night wandering may be refocused by using a body pillow in the bed for company, monitoring the lights so the resident does not think that the day has begun, playing soft music in the room, and having a bedtime routine that is consistent.

Sleep cycles change as a person ages and the need to rise and urinate increases, sometimes leading to difficulty falling back to sleep. Dementia compounds the resident's challenge to experience an appropriate sleep pattern.

Demonstration of Hallucinations, Aberrations, and Delusions

The resident may misinterpret perceived physical or emotional responses to visual, tactile, or auditory stimuli. He or she responds to a seemingly real experience when no other person has the same experience.

Delusions are based on false ideas attributable to invalid awareness of someone or some situation. The delusion may become an absolute focus for the resident even if presented with information to the contrary. For example, residents may think that the place they are living is their place of work and that all of the people around them are their employees, so they give orders and perhaps develop anxiety that leads to a catastrophic reaction because the workers are not doing their "job."

Hallucinations can be visual, auditory, or sensory, or a combination. They can be pleasant or extremely frightening both to the resident and to the caregiver. There should be an assessment of the possible danger to the resident and caregiver. Is there a pattern or antecedent to the hallucination? Can the resident be distracted by touch or movement from the area?

> Joseph had experience in Europe during World War II. Because of his dementia, he would sometimes think that he was surrounded by the enemy and had to fight his way to safety. This was acted out by combativeness with staffpersons. When possible, he was taken to his room, and being alone with "no one to fight" often would end the hallucination. During Operation Desert Storm when the television showed troops, tanks, etc., Joseph experienced a dramatic increase in war-related hallucinations. Turning off the television was the obvious solution to limit the war-related behavior.

> Libby carried her daughter's picture in her arms constantly. At mealtime, she would insist that her daughter "sit here" and would put the picture on the table beside her place. Libby often would converse with the picture and certainly felt reassured that her daughter was with her. Prints of the picture had to be made when Libby started to "feed" her daughter treats.

It is important to "check out" the resident's claims of seeing or experiencing things that the caregiver is not aware of. At times, there is an element of truth in the situation that can be changed, thereby reducing the resident's agitation or antecedent for hallucinating or experiencing delusions. For example:

> George came out of his room nightly at approximately 3 A.M. Each time, he appeared agitated and concerned about the "things" in his room. Each night, the experience was different (e.g., bugs on the walls, men in the closet, tigers under the bed, babies crying outside the window). Each night, the staff validated his concern, gave George a cup of tea and a slice of toast, told him that they would go and check out his room and get rid of whatever was causing his concern, escorted him back to his room, and tucked him in bed. One night, George appeared at the usual time, very anxious, saying, "There is a naked lady in my bed, a naked lady in my bed." The staff voiced their concern, went through the usual interventions, and took George back to his room, where they actually did find a naked lady in George's bed! Helene, from across the hall, had perhaps taken a "wrong turn" after using her bathroom and had wandered into George's room.

If possible, find the antecedents or causes of the hallucinations and delusions. They could be caused by medications, drug toxicity, infections, urinary or bowel retention, dehydration, pain that is acute or chronic, and environmental stressors.

Demonstration of Accusing, Demanding, and Paranoia

The resident may insist on a specific thought, whether real or perceived, expressing fears or anxiety or both about his or her self or belongings while blaming others. For example, not remembering where the resident has placed her purse, she accuses the staffperson of taking it.

Memory loss and the inability to interpret needs or surroundings can result in paranoid responses of being watched, abused, robbed, and so forth. Frustration and anxiety can precipitate combativeness or catastrophic reactions or both. Residents can feel really helpless when they cannot find what they are looking for. The paranoia, therefore, may help the confused or forgetful resident to cope with his or her losses and changes of ability.

Possible causes include not being able to remember where possessions have been left or hidden away, poor vision, hallucinations, medications, changes in familiar routine, environmental stress, blame or unrealistic demands, hearing loss, suspiciousness and increased fear that people are talking about the resident, the staff's not speaking English or the common language of residents, and the staff's whispering or talking about residents in front of them. Residents can feel really helpless when they cannot remember where they have put something. Being surrounded by caregivers or other staffpersons who do not seem familiar only makes the situation worse.

There are several ways to provide assistance and intervention: Simplify requests and expectations. Change the care and the environment as little as possible. Do not argue or disagree. Use a caring tone of voice and touch, give reassurance, and do not confront or attempt to explain. Try to build a relationship of trust with the resident; therefore, becoming a confident, trusted listener and helper in times of "trouble." Empathize with the resident and help to hunt for the missing item, use food or tasks for distraction, have duplicates or extras of commonly misplaced items, and learn favorite hiding places, such as under the mattress, in the tissue box, or behind the drapes.

> "You took my money," Annette accused the aide. The aide responded, "No, I didn't, I just came into your room. I would not take your money. I didn't even know you had money. You just lost your money because you can't remember where you put it." This response did nothing to reassure Annette or even begin to deal with her fears. In fact, explaining to Annette made her more anxious and angry. The aide could have said, "I'm sorry you cannot find your money, that must be scary for you. Let me help you look for it and we can straighten out your drawers at the same time." This would distract Annette so that she could refocus her attention to a positive activity.

Screaming, Yelling, Calling, and Asking Repetitious Questions

Screaming, yelling, calling, and asking repetitious questions are all demonstrations of the resident's fear, feeling out of control, and need for acceptance due to real or imagined perceptions or situations and enacted with or without realization of the verbalization.

At times, the meaning behind the vocal behavior is unclear to the listener but appears to be intentional and meaningful for the resident. This excess noise making may be continuous or intermittent. Assessment of the response requires studying the resident's physical, psychosocial, cognitive, and environmental needs. Noting the time and place of the vocalization may provide clues as to its intended message. Over- or understimulation from the environment may be a factor. Screaming may be intensified during ADLs, especially bathing. Other reasons may be social isolation, medications, use of physical restraints, tactile defensiveness, or just the opposite, the need for tactile stimulation. Diverting the resident with an activity or making a noise that attracts attention may be helpful. Sometimes saying, "Shush, the baby is sleeping," may work.

"Help me, help me, help me" may be a call for companionship or an automatic, repetitive speech pattern. The challenge is to figure out the need that the resident is trying to express. Listen for the message. Causes for calling out could include a response to feeling isolated or having had too much done for the resident, and therefore the calling out is the resident's way of saying, "Hey, it's me, I'm here, I'm a real person, treat me like one." Interventions can include "catching" the resident when he or she is quiet and providing positive feedback that you really appreciate it when he or she is pleasantly quiet. Therefore, the resident receives attention for a positive response rather than a negative one.

> Laura would repeat "help me" many times, over and over. At times, she could be distracted when given a simple, repetitive activity, such as folding washcloths, or when someone held her hand. The calling out was extremely stressful for other residents and for staff. Because she was seated in a wheelchair, Laura would accompany the nurse at the desk or as she did her work. Being able to see and be touched by a familiar face helped to decrease the calling out, but this approach did not always work.

Using a cassette player with large earphones and quiet music may be successful to decrease calling out, screaming, or yelling. The shoestring and wearable activities listed in Chapter 9 can be used if the resident is also throwing anything he or she is handed. Establish and maintain a comfortable and familiar routine for the resident. Chewing gum may be successful if the resident has been a gum chewer in the past. An assessment of the safety of this intervention is required. "White" noise (e.g., a hair dryer with bonnet or audiotapes of waves, birds, or other relaxing nature sounds) may be used and evaluated for effectiveness.

Repeated questions, such as, "I want to go home," or "When is the bus coming?" are common. Medical conditions, environmental stimulation or understimulation, inactivity, and the overall inability to cope related to dementia can be the possible causes or antecedents of never-ending questions. Looking behind the statement at the feelings the resident is trying to express is helpful. The need to be included, to feel safe, and to feel loved is generally at the root of the behavior. A LifeStory Book may be a helpful intervention (see Chapter 3). Various distraction techniques may only result in the question being stated all over again. Train all caregivers to answer the questions in the same way, using the same words and tone of voice. If possible, one-to-one attention is helpful. The resident can be taken for a walk, thereby providing a change in the environment. Other suggestions include keeping hats and coats out of sight and using normalization and familiar activities that are related to home and success. Work out a system with the family if the caregiver and the resident can telephone them. Another suggestion is for caregiving staff to call management for assistance. Another caring face, therefore, can intervene and offer the needed attention or bring the resident to another area, or both.

Help staff to understand screaming, yelling, calling out, and repetitious questions as a symptom of the dementia disease process. The resident is rarely displaying these behaviors on purpose with intent to aggravate caregivers.

Demonstration of Withdrawal, Apathy, and Inability to Initiate Activity

A sadness or depressed response to surroundings and people can be related to the progressive dementia, mood or emotional well-being or dysfunction, or overall sadness. Retreating from others and a flat affect (appearing depressed or emotionally nonresponsive) can result from a mood change of short or long duration. Sometimes, the cause or precipitating factor can be discovered, sometimes not. A diminished or nonexistent self-esteem and sense of worth may be precipitating the withdrawal. Fear of failure and not wanting to set off conflict may lead the resident to not initiate activity. Fear, anxiety, and paranoia may be present. Depression may or may not respond to medications.

Close monitoring of nutrition, possible physical dysfunction, and environmental stress should be considered. Build trust with the resident. Finding activities that assure success can be attempted with the resident. Asking the resident to show you or to help you with the activity may be the invitation the resident needs to risk the attempt (see Chapter 2).

HEALTH CARE PROVIDER AND STAFF ISSUES

Behaviors and their need for possible refocusing become a shared responsibility for all in contact with the resident. Appropriate care starts with staff who are sensitive to the experience of dementia and how it affects each resident individually. Training is mandatory, but unless staffpersons respond to residents with acceptance, interest, and willingness to uphold their personhood, training is of limited value. A positive attitude is contagious. Focusing on the resident's abilities enables the needed paradigm change to stop labeling residents who are having a difficult time coping with their disease and all its changes.

The onus of preventing or responding to difficult behaviors rests on staffpersons. With physical or chemical interventions a last resort, staff are challenged to be creative and have the skills to problem solve. Staff then need the support and respect of administration to use their ideas. Issues for health care providers center on resident and staff safety. Environmental safety can be easily procured, but the realization that no security system guarantees safety is imperative.

Safety for residents' positive sense of self is complicated and requires staff sensitivity. Only when the effort and commitment is initiated by the administration can residents with dementia be offered an appropriate program focusing on their wellness.

SUMMARY

Understanding behaviors of persons with dementia requires great patience and the willingness to use insight, observation, and clear thinking. The "what, why, who, where, when, and what now" behavioral guidelines form the basis of understanding and may lead to a resolution or action plan. Responses must be made to prevent or decrease the possibility of maladaptive behaviors. Giving the resident needed clueing or support to refocus behaviors enables positive expressions.

Having appropriate tools for problem solving and behavior analysis arms caregivers with information for developing appropriate interventions. The emphasis on viewing behaviors as the resident's communication tool, and the realization that most difficult behaviors are not on purpose, can assist staff to reassess their personal and caregiving agenda, giving themselves permission to enter the resident's world.

Feelings of loss and grieving, as the dementia progresses, challenge both the resident and the caregiver to pursue creative and supportive adeptness during hands-on, day-to-day care. The emotional well-being of the resident becomes the focus, not only for accountable care, but also for a quality of life that is acceptable to both the caregiver and the care receiver. It is hoped that caregivers can see the person or resident first, then the behavior. Behaviors are not a defining characteristic of the person or resident. Would it not be "normal" to react emotionally when one's wellness is compromised as it is with dementia?

SUGGESTED READING

Cleland M. Prevention and Management of Aggressive Behavior in the Elderly. Portland, OR: Good Samaritan Hospital and Medical Center, 1988.

Cohen U, Weisman GD. Holding On to Home: Designing Environments for People with Dementia. Baltimore: Johns Hopkins University Press, 1990.

Gwyther L. Care of Alzheimer's Patients: A Manual for Nursing Home Staff. Chicago: Alzheimer's Association, 1985.

Mace N (ed). Dementia Care: Patient, Family and Community. Baltimore: Johns Hopkins University Press, 1990.

Mace N, Rabins P. The 36-Hour Day: A Family Guide to Caring for Persons with Alzheimer's Disease, Related Dementing Illnesses, and Memory Loss in Later Life. Baltimore: Johns Hopkins University Press, 1981.

Robinson A, Spencer B, White L, et al. Understanding Difficult Behaviors: Caregiving Suggestions for Coping with Alzheimer's Disease and Related Illness. Ypsilanti, MI: Geriatric Education Center of Michigan/Eastern Michigan University, 1988.

Teri L, Logsdon R. Assessment and management of behavioral disturbances in Alzheimer's disease. Compr Ther 1990;16:36–42.

White M, Kaas M, Richie M. Vocally disruptive behavior. J Gerontol Nurs 1996;22:23–29.

A8-1
Behavior Profile Form

Behavior Profile

Resident: _____

Date: _____ Staffperson: _____

What?
- What is happening? Identify and assess. _____
  _____
- Resident responses? _____
- Does the behavior have physical or emotional manifestations or both?
  _____

Where?
- Where is the behavior exhibited? _____
- Environmental triggers? _____
- Is the environment familiar? _____

When?
- When does behavior happen? _____
- Specific timing? _____
- After what? Activities of daily living? Family visit? Mealtime?
  _____

Who?
- Who is involved? Other residents? Caregiver? Family? Visitor?
  _____

Why?
- What happened before? _____
- Task too complicated? _____
- Poor communications? _____
- Physical/medical problems? _____
- Really a problem? To whom? _____
- What is the behavior "saying"? _____
- Is the behavior an activity? _____
- Is the response consistent to the same trigger? _____

What Now?
- Assistance suggestions? _____
- Approaches/intervention? _____
  __ cognitive
  __ physical
  __ psychosocial
  __ environmental
- Changes needed? _____
  By whom? _____

A8-2
Behavior Observation Form[*]

*Courtesy of The Wealshire, Lincolnshire, Illinois.

Behavior Observation Form

Name: _____

| Date | Time | Observed Activity and Behavior | Behavior | | | Observer |
			Trigger (What started it?)	Intervention (What stopped it?)	Time Elapsed (before stopping, stayed stopped)	

A8-3
Behavior Analysis Form

Behavior Analysis Form

Name: _____   Date: _____   Signature: _____

Behaviors Exhibited	Emotions Expressed	Whose Problem?	Excess Disabilities	Resident Abilities	Refocusing Interventions

— combative/ aggregate... aggressive
— hitting
— kicking
— pinching
— biting
— tripping
— pushing
— throwing
— physical
— pacing
— wandering
— running
— eloping
— pounding
— picking
— rubbing
— packing
— rummaging
	— cognitive
	
	— physical
		— resident
		  well-being
		  — cognitive
		  — physical
		  — emotional
		  — social
		  safety issues
		  — personal
		  — other residents
		— family
		  — staff
		— other residents
		— family request
		— staff tolerance
		— administration/ regulatory
		— environmental tolerance
		— other
			— acute illness:
			
			— physical
			  — fatigue
			  — dehydration
			  — constipation
			  — chronic pain
			  — pain
			  — motor/ movement
			  — hungry
			  — restraints
			— medication(s):
			
			— sensory impairment
			  — hearing
			  — sight
			  — touch
				— communication/ cognitive
				
				— physical
					— cognitive
					
					— physical

Behaviors Exhibited	Emotions Expressed	Whose Problem?	Excess Disabilities	Resident Abilities	Refocusing Interventions
— consuming			— smell		— social
— sucking			— taste		
— stripping			— cognition		
— sexual			— memory		
— yelling			— awareness		
— cursing			— orientation	— social	
— hiding things			— person		
— hiding self			— place		
— searching			— communication		— spiritual
— becoming lost			— expressive		
— sleeplessness			— receptive		
— catastrophic	— psychosocial		— emotional		
reactions			— fear		
— mood/affect			— anxiety		
— fearful			— depression		
— anxious			— stressed	— distractibility	
— depressed			— feels lost	— verbal/	
— apathetic			— worried	assurance	— environ-
— demanding			— other residents	— physical	mental
— accusatory			— relocation	— touch	
— suspicious			— environmental	— hug	
— stubborn			— negative milieu	— motor	

Behaviors Exhibited	Emotions Expressed	Whose Problem?	Excess Disabilities	Resident Abilities	Refocusing Interventions
— angry	— other		— overstimulation	— food	— caregiver
— crying			— understimulation	— drink	— specific
— embarrassed			— noise(s)	— other	
— delusional			— glare	— phone call	
— paranoid			— shadows	— music/singing	
— hallucinatory			— family factors	— rescue	
— suicidal			— caregivers	— response	
— activities of daily living related			— male		
— other			— female		
			— inconsistent		
			— overcaring		
			— other		

A8-4
Community and Civic Professionals Training Outline

ACTIVITY-FOCUSED CARE TRAINING FOR COMMUNITY AND CIVIC REPRESENTATIVES AND VOLUNTEERS (4 HOURS)

The experience of dementia
  Psychosocial needs and challenges
Defining dementia
  What is normal aging?
  Dementia: a set of symptoms
Reversible dementias
  Depression
  Metabolic
  Normal-pressure hydrocephalus
  Medications
  Brain tumor
Nonreversible dementias
  Pick's disease
  Multi-infarct or vascular dementia
  Lewy body
  Huntington's disease
  Creutzfeldt-Jakob disease
  Alcohol related
  Parkinson's disease
  Alzheimer's disease
Alzheimer's disease: senile dementia, Alzheimer type
  Risk factors
  Assessment, diagnosis, pathologic findings
  Disease course: early to late stage
  Care challenges
Supporting persons with dementia
  Psychosocial needs

Focusing on abilities
Activity-focused care
Communications: understanding and being understood
Progressive changes
Awareness of verbal and nonverbal language and skills
Guidelines
Redirection and cueing skills
Safety and environmental issues related to care
Information on Safe Return program
Safeguarding the home
Refocusing behaviors
Behaviors as symbols of communication and purposeful activity
Understanding and using problem-solving techniques
Catastrophic reaction
Combativeness and aggression
Wandering and pacing
Eloping
Sundowning
Rummaging
Yelling and screaming
Inappropriate sexual behaviors
Emotional or mood-related responses
Anxiety or agitation
Paranoia
Hallucinations
Delusions
Depression, apathy, withdrawal
Resources
Local assessment centers
Alzheimer's Association chapter

A8-5

Lincolnshire Police Department Resident Checklist for The Wealshire (Lincolnshire, Illinois)*

Name: _____ Date of birth: _____

Is this the first time this person has walked away from your facility?
Yes ___ No ___

If no, where was the person located in the past? _____

Have you searched your entire facility? Yes ___ No ___

Sex: Male ___   Female ___

Race: White ___   Black ___   Hispanic ___   Asian ___

Height: _____   Weight/build: Thin ___   Medium ___   Heavy ___

Eye color: Blue ___   Green ___   Brown ___   Hazel ___

Hair color: Gray ___   Blonde ___   Brown ___   Black ___   Red ___

Hairstyle: Short ___   Medium ___   Long ___   Bald ___

Facial hair: Mustache ___   Beard ___   Goatee ___

---

*Special thanks to Anne Marie Blaz Tegard, police officer, Bonnie Hansen-Johnsen, telecommunicator, and the Lincolnshire Police Department, Lincolnshire, Illinois.

Scars/marks/tattoos ___ Description/location: _____

_____

Clothing description: _____

_____

Where and what time was the person last seen? _____

_____

Direction of travel? _____

Is the person suicidal? Yes ___ No ___

Is the person combative or has person been combative in the past with authority/police? Yes ___ No ___

If so, what happened? _____

_____

Distraction/compliance techniques (names, places, songs, etc.): _____

_____

List any diagnosed condition/illness: _____

_____

Is the person on any behavioral modification medication? Yes ___ No ___

Is the person on any other medication that could pose a threat to life if not taken? Yes ___ No ___

Do you have a recent picture available? Yes ___ No ___

Names, addresses, and phone numbers of friends/relatives that the person may try to go to/contact: _____

_____

_____

_____

Alzheimer's Disease: Activity-Focused Care

A8-6
Catastrophic Reaction Analysis

Catastrophic reaction: a response of distress demonstrating the inability to understand, interpret, or cope with a real or imagined situation, person(s), environment, or self.

	Response/Behavior/Activity	Possible Cause or Antecedent	Assistance and Intervention
Cognitive-based responses	Decreased attention span; increased word-finding problems; increased misunderstanding of what is happening to or around the resident; yelling, screaming, cursing; increased inability to follow directions; misdirected or exaggerated responses; lack of impulse control	Unrealistic situations or demands; being asked too many questions; not able to perform a once-familiar task; increased confusion or feeling overwhelmed; decreased attention span; environmental confusion; too many people present; environment too quiet; bored; asked too many questions without enough time to answer; word-finding problems; asked to do too difficult a task; thinks show on television is real; mistaking someone for a person who is disliked or a disliked person present; thinking he or she is lost, needs to catch a bus, feed the children, must go home because	Use distraction techniques: juice, cookies, "Please come help me"; validate anxiety; move to a quiet place; use routines that are familiar; simplify, one step or thing at a time; make activities failure free, clutter free; allow time for a response; do not put the resident "on the spot"; do not assume that a resident once able to perform an activity or task can do it now; have realistic expectations of capabilities; limit decisions; reduce environmental stimuli; do not use long explanations; do not argue or directly disagree with a false idea; use consistent, familiar, and trained staff

Response/ Behavior/Activity	Possible Cause or Antecedent	Assistance and Intervention
	mother wants him or her, etc.; spatial perceptual dysfunction; being surprised	
Physical-based responses	Unprovoked aggression; excessive, violent behavior; uncontrolled crying; wringing of hands; repetitive hand motions such as clapping, "picking"; increased restlessness, pacing, packing as if to leave; increased strength for picking up heavy objects; hyperactivity; stamping feet	Unable to enter a familiar place (e.g., bedroom, family room) when the floor is being cleaned; discomfort or onset of illness; medication side effects; hallucinations; fatigue; wake-sleep reversal causing sleep deprivation; impaired vision; impaired hearing; response to inability to motor plan (e.g., how to sit down in a chair); being pushed or touched by another resident; experiencing an invasion of privacy; loud noises; time of staff change; small "accidents," incontinence; dropping or spilling things	If tolerated, try soothing touch, patting, hugging, rocking; use calming voice; check for excess disability, physiologic or medical causes, glasses not on, etc.; allow safe areas for pacing; do not restrain unless resident is a danger to self or others; understand importance of timing relative to activities of daily living; do not force participation; change the environment, if possible, limit "waiting" for meals, etc.; avoid the use of an area too small for the number of people; have activities to release aggression and anxiety (e.g., punch balls, dancing, marching, exercise); have calming activities to use when appropriate (e.g., music, story telling, reading); be aware of lighting changes; use consistent, familiar, and trained staff; be aware of territorial needs (e.g., favorite chair); obtain help from other staff when needed; do not approach from behind and touch the

Alzheimer's Disease: Activity-Focused Care

Response/ Behavior/Activity	Possible Cause or Antecedent	Assistance and Intervention
		resident to provide care; make eye contact before touching the resident
Psycho-social-based responses	Increased stubbornness, suspiciousness; increased anxiety, sudden changes of mood; negative responses to other residents, name calling, telling them to "shut up"	Fear; anger; feeling threatened; need for attention; feeling lost, insecure; feeling manipulated; response to others who are upset or tense; paranoia; being scolded, made to feel incompetent or not wanted	Reinforce positive qualities of the resident; do not reinforce negative qualities (e.g., do not yell at the person for screaming); use activities and approaches that give the resident a sense of meaning and purpose; observe and monitor resident, remove from stressful situations; be aware of relationships between residents; be aware of the time of day and the resident's mood changes; remain calm, reassuring, and supportive; use trained, consistent, and familiar staff; limit number of visitors at one time if needed, have in-services for families on how to visit; model approaches, interaction for the family if needed

9

Meaningful Activities: Daily Life Stuff

"What are you going to do today?" The answer might range from "I don't know," to, "Oh, stuff, you know, stuff." Daily life is made up of "stuff." "Stuff" has many definitions but basically it is the substance of each day, the expression of one's within and without engagement with self and life. It is this engagement that evolves into meaningful activity.

The question then becomes, what are meaningful "Alzheimer's activities"? A typical response would include activities such as dancing, singing, crafts, and exercising. Actually, there is no magical answer to this question because abilities, interests, and responses vary for each individual. Anything residents do or are involved with is their activity at that moment. Therefore, scheduled activities are just part of the activity picture. Hour after hour of planned programming becomes overwhelming for most residents. It is the pauses between scheduled activities that makes the day flow in a natural rhythm. Quiet periods are needed for residents to regroup their orientation to themselves, and the world about them. It is the balance of the down or quiet time with the active time that enables residents to draw on their strengths and abilities. Using activities as a frame around all that the resident does allows a freedom for entertaining numerous possibilities. Shifting the focus from doing an activity "for" the resident to one of doing "with" the resident or allowing the resident independent involvement stimulates wellness.

Whenever possible, invite a resident to be the facilitator of the activity. The resident may need to work with the activity therapist for a period if the resident's confidence needs building. Monitor the resident carefully so that the experience is positive and successful.

Caregivers are challenged to be creative, flexible, and willing to engage residents in nontraditional styles or types of activity. Normalization activities create a purposeful use of time and are adapted from tasks residents would be doing if they did not have dementia. Meaningful daily life activity, or daily life stuff, occurs within the context of self-care, work, play, and leisure activities. Therefore, cognitive, physical, psychosocial, and spiritual activities become integral components of a meaningful, holistic existence.

DAILY LIFE STUFF: HOW DO YOU SPELL SUCCESS?

Success is not a magnificently produced product, nor an outcome that meets the needs or specifications of the caregiver. If daily life stuff is the substance and experience of each day, the success comes from connectedness. Success is calling forth the resident's best in his or her relationship to self and others. Caregivers connecting with their residents enable the following components of success. Therefore, *SUCCESS* is spelled:

S: Sensitivity

- Looking at feelings with compassion
- Defining and maintaining personhood
- Supporting wellness

U: Understanding

- Adapting and using the components of activity-focused care
- Fostering abilities and strengths
- Discerning the resident's experience of dementia

C: Creativity

- Adapting activities and daily experiences
- Understanding task simplification
- Using and calling forth ingenuity

C: Connectedness

- Enabling communication skills: being understood and understanding
- Integrating the resident's LifeStory Book with the here and now
- Identifying and confronting sensory strengths and problems

E: Enabling

- Implementing pleasure
- Enabling dignity, sense of self-worth
- Facilitating empowerment

S: Safety

- Decreasing risks
- Experiencing sanctuary—offering the experience of sanctuary

S: Satisfaction

- Providing a sense of offered, accepted, and appreciated contribution
- Eliciting joy in doing, putting the process before the product
- Enabling fulfillment and meaningfulness

OBJECTIVES OF AN ACTIVITY

The objectives or goals of an activity focus on providing the resident opportunities, through participation in a meaningful activity, to live a life of quality. Objectives include

- A focus on abilities, not limitations
- A purposeful use of time and a sense of belonging
- An opportunity to support positive behaviors
- A tool to reduce or eliminate negative or unwanted behaviors
- A vehicle for verbal and nonverbal communication

A family member of a resident wrote this letter* to the activities department of an Alzheimer's care facility:

> My Mother came to The Wealshire to feel she belonged.
>   *You made that happen!*
> Vivian needed to feel necessary—to have a "reason to be."
>   *You made that happen!*
> For over 60 years she never sang, played games, or did hand-crafts.
>   *You made that happen!*
> We are grateful this holiday to see my Mother's smile.
>   *You made that happen!*

CRITERIA FOR A SUCCESSFUL ACTIVITY

The criteria for a successful activity include therapeutic components focused on enabling the resident's abilities. These include

- *Modification*: The activity can be simplified, broken down into small tasks, and adapted for success as abilities decline. The activity should have a limited chance of failure.
- *Repetitiveness*: The activity can be routine, familiar.
- *Multisensory cueing*: The activity contains multiple sensory components (e.g., visual, auditory, touch, taste, and smell).
- *Safety*: The activity does not present a hazard to the resident, other residents, staff, or family.
- *Adaptability*: Participation can be individual, small group, large group, seated, standing, or lying down; the activity can be spontaneous or planned.
- *Dignity*: The approach and involvement ensure the resident's self-respect and sense of worth, including age appropriateness.
- *Cultural*: The activity is relevant to personal value systems and life situations.
- *Fun*: The activity enables pleasure by using past interests and skills; certainly a perfect "end product" is not the required outcome.

QUALITIES OF AN ACTIVITY: COGNITIVE, PHYSICAL, PSYCHOSOCIAL, AND SPIRITUAL

An Alzheimer's activity, which meets the preceding outlined objectives and criteria, is a basis for a positive, holistic quality of life. The cognitive, physical, psychosocial, and

---

*Used with permission from Toni Mathis.

spiritual needs of the resident are assessed individually. The environment, time of day, presence of other persons, and the resident's general well-being are a few of the factors to be taken into account. Even the weather can influence a response positively or negatively. The key is in the approach or how the activity is presented. Positive communication skills, caring touch, and appealing to the resident's long-lasting socialization abilities often assure success. Almost all activities or tasks, even crayon coloring, can be given dignity when the approach is supportive. Saying, "Will you help me with this?" or, "Let's do this for the children's hospital," often elicits participation. Placing an object in the resident's hands may provide the needed clueing and centering of his or her attention to precipitate becoming more focused on the task or activity.

Cognitive Activity Qualities

- Enhancement of memory
- Increased awareness and attention span
- Encouragement of verbalization, decreasing word-finding problems
- Increased ability to sequence thoughts
- Fostering of ability to make choices
- Promotion of spatial-perceptual skills and awareness
- Reinforced understanding of the clueing or task breakdown process

Physical Activity Qualities

- Promotion of well-being
- Improved or maintained body image awareness
- Prompting of small or large motor or movement skills
- Increased or maintained joint range of motion
- Increased or maintained cardiovascular ability
- Improved balance
- Improved or maintained mobility and overall strength
- Increased appetite or weight control
- Promotion of healthy fatigue and normal sleep patterns
- Positive or acceptable outlet for stress, anxiety, restlessness, frustrations
- May allow tranquilizers or medications to be decreased or eliminated

Psychosocial Activity Qualities

- Arena of compassionate acceptance
- Sense of belonging, part of the resident/staff/family community; having friends
- Purposeful use of time, feelings of accomplishment, being in control
- Fostering of dignity and self-respect
- Encouragement of ability to adapt to change
- Former roles used to promote self-esteem
- Invites expression of feelings that can curtail the development or escalation of unwanted behaviors

Alzheimer's Disease: Activity-Focused Care

- Method to distract or change moods
- Support for "trying something new"
- Feeling of being safe
- Tool to promote affirming family involvement

Spiritual Activity Qualities

Refer to Chapter 11 for a discussion of the qualities of spiritual activities.

ACTIVITY ANALYSIS: CAN "ANYTHING" BE A MEANINGFUL ACTIVITY?

Perhaps. When "anything" meets the scrutiny of activity objectives and criteria and contains the qualities demanded of a meaningful activity, then the "anything" is ready for an activity analysis. An activity analysis is a process by which an activity is clearly understood so it can be selected or rejected as a meaningful engagement for a resident.

There are three basic components of an activity analysis.

I. Understanding the selected activity's effects on
   A. the cognitive, physical, and psychosocial abilities of the resident
   B. the cognitive, physical, and psychosocial risks to the resident
II. Adaptation qualities of the activity to
   A. be implemented one to one with the resident
   B. be implemented in a small group (three to six) of residents
   C. be implemented in a large group (six or more) of residents
III. Modification qualities of the activity to
   A. be meaningful for residents in the early stage of dementia
   B. be meaningful for residents in the mid-stage of dementia
   C. be meaningful for residents in the late stage of dementia

Example of an Activity Analysis: Using a Piece of Fabric

A piece of fabric, 6 ft long, brightly colored, contains replicas of flags from throughout the world. Suggestions follow as to how this fabric can meet the three basic components of activity analysis:

I. Activity's effects on abilities of the resident and risks to the resident
   A. Cognitive, physical, and psychosocial abilities
      1. Cognitive abilities and benefits
         a. Reminiscing about traveling and countries of the world
         b. Asking, for example, "What could we make out of this fabric?" "Did you sew?" "Who made your clothes?"
         c. Talking about the many colors and then relating them to colors the resident is wearing

       d. Counting the different flags

       e. Finding the represented countries on a map or globe

   2. Physical abilities and benefits

       a. Describing flags and having the resident place a marker on each one

       b. Tying the fabric in a giant knot and using it for a basketball

       c. Using fabric for a tug of war or a parachute exercise tool

       d. Cutting out each flag and pasting it on a poster board

   3. Psychosocial abilities and benefits

       a. Dividing residents into teams for a "Hole in One" contest, in which they receive one shot to throw the fabric ball into a box

       b. Using the fabric as a tablecloth and setting the table together for a party

       c. Laying the fabric out on a table in front of the residents and asking them to roll it up, working together and keeping it even

       d. Asking one resident to wrap the arm or leg of another resident with the fabric

  B. Cognitive, physical, and psychosocial risks

   1. Cognitive risks

       a. Not being able to track the conversation or have the attention span needed to stay with the topic

       b. Inability to correlate the visual image with words of description

       c. Inability to follow instructions

   2. Physical risks

       a. Motor planning and execution difficulties

       b. Post-exercise tiredness, stiffness, or soreness

       c. "Playing" too hard, causing a safety hazard to self or others

   3. Psychosocial risks

       a. Feeling put on the spot when not knowing the answer to a question

       b. Embarrassment when reminiscing is hampered by severe word-finding problems

       c. Desire to control the conversation or the cloth, or both (e.g., "That is my tablecloth, give it to me.")

II. Adaptation qualities of the activity

  A. One-to-one implementation

   1. Use resident's life story as a background for cloth-related activity, questions, discussion

   2. Wrap up or drape the fabric about the resident and then have him or her do the same for the caregiver

   3. Monitor responses and timing of using the cloth as an activity by responding to the resident's verbal and nonverbal input

  B. Small group implementation

   1. Ask each resident to respond about the cloth as he or she hands it to another resident while seated in a small circle

   2. Enable residents to offer positive feedback to each other (e.g., telling another resident that he or she would look pretty in the fabric or that the resident would like to hear more, if appropriate, about the other resident's trip to a country whose flag is on the cloth)

3. Use the small group as an opportunity to bring out each resident's abilities and active participation
C. Large group implementation
1. Move within a circle of residents or about a table so that all residents can see and touch the fabric
2. Use a physical activity with the cloth so the largest number of residents can actively participate (e.g., tie the cloth into knots so it is ball shaped and toss around the group or play "hot potato" with it to music)
III. Modification qualities of the activity
A. Use with residents in the early stage of dementia
1. Facilitate cloth activity (e.g., cutting, coloring flags drawn from the fabric, looking up information about the different countries, describing travels)
B. Use with residents in the mid-stage of dementia
1. Use active response-type activities with the fabric (e.g., knotting, tossing, kicking, throwing, wrapping, tearing, pulling, parachute movements)
C. Use with residents in the late stage of dementia
1. Use more sensory-centered fabric activities (e.g., wrapping, stroking, being stroked, cradling an arm and softly swinging it back and forth, scrunching with the fingers, untying simple knots, smoothing out wrinkles)

For another example of an activity analysis, see Appendix 9-1.

IDENTIFYING THE THERAPEUTIC VALUE OF AN ACTIVITY

Part of the activity analysis process is identifying the activity's therapeutic value. For example, if this specific activity is used for this specific resident, what value will it be to the resident? In other words, what outcome is hoped for by inviting the resident to participate in a certain activity? The therapeutic value of an activity is flexible and changeable because it also depends on how much or how little the resident actually participates and how the activity has been adapted. Therefore, the activity analysis and the activity's therapeutic value unite as the main criteria for activity selection for each resident.

Therapeutic Value Equals Desired Outcome

Two examples of activities and their therapeutic values are

- *Intergenerational activity*: sense of nurturing, reminiscing, being needed, being able to give and offer wisdom, being able to give and receive affection
- *Men's group*: friendship, companionship, sense of belonging, reminiscing, pride from past accomplishments, esteem from past life roles and positions, safe arena to joke and tell "men's" stories, opportunity to discuss subjects of interest such as sports, stocks, military, etc.

Examples of other activities and their therapeutic values are found in Appendix 9-10. The Activity Therapy Care Conference Report Form (Appendix 9-9) is an example of how the therapeutic value information is incorporated in a reporting format.

ACTIVITY ASSESSMENT AND GROUPING RESIDENTS FOR EFFECTIVE ACTIVITIES

A resident's activity assessment is a compilation of past and present interests, abilities, dislikes, inabilities, and life story. Information can be gathered by talking with family members, caregivers, and the resident. Some of the most useful information is composed of observations related to actual activity participation or nonparticipation. Insight into the resident's responses to daily life activities can include using the following functional assessment sources:

- *Eating a meal*: fine and gross motor muscle movement, attention span, problem solving, sequencing, figure-ground (foreground-background) perceptual ability, visual acuity, socialization skills
- *Folding a shirt*: motor skills, perceptual abilities, attention span, problem solving, following directions
- *Using an assessment box*: familiar objects to identify and use; playing cards to be put into sequence; stacking objects; sensory items to report on; tasks requiring one-step, two-step, or three-step directions; simple paragraph to read and relate main idea; yarn to wind; testing for attention span, problem solving, bilateral coordination, visual and auditory ability, fine motor skills, eye-hand coordination, cognitive awareness

The components of an activity assessment include all everyday skills: cognitive, physical, psychosocial, and spiritual. The resident's life story becomes the mirror in which the resident's abilities are reflected. Activity assessment items include

1. *Life story*: personal history, demographic information, educational history, interests, hobbies, military history, community involvement, leisure activities, travel, crafts, sports, and so on (see Chapter 3)
2. *Physical health*: well-being, coordination, disabilities, any medical information that would affect activities (such as food allergies, no sugar), endurance, ambulation and mobility, dominant hand, eyesight, hearing, fine motor skills, personal care needs that would affect activities, adapted equipment needs and ability to use
3. *Emotional health*: moods, sense of self, behavior refocusing needs
4. *Cognitive awareness*: coping, abilities, difficulties, attention span, short-term memory, long-term memory, ability to read, ability to follow directions, ability to write, initiating conversation, interacting with peers, interacting with staff, responding when someone approaches, making new friends easily, whether a registered voter, evaluation of motivation, specific talents
5. *Normalization activity interests*: home, outside the home
6. *Sensory profile findings*: see Appendix 5-2
7. *Communication skills*: understanding and being understood, languages spoken
8. *Environmental awareness*: distractibility, responses
9. *Spirituality*: Religious, Spiritual, and Sacred Center Assessment (see Appendix 11-1)
10. *Family*: relationships, support, involvement, difficulties
11. *Specific activities:* checklist showing past and current interests

Music, worship, sing-alongs, and exercise groups can often serve residents with varying levels of cognitive, physical, and psychosocial abilities. Many activities offer maximum participation, meaning, and positive outcomes when residents with similar abilities, needs, and interests are brought together. This peer community of shared comfort enables activities to be carefully selected and implemented, focusing on their therapeutic values. Grouping or clustering residents requires patience and flexibility because the experience will probably result in a group of some of the residents slated to participate, while others refuse to join. At the same time, unless there is a room with a closed door with someone standing guard, there will probably be a few residents wandering in and out of the activity that are not part of the listed attendees. That is okay; caregivers should carry out their program with these other residents present.

Identifying participants with similar interests and abilities for a specific group requires input from the multidisciplinary team. Suggestions for groups can be based on

- Gender-related activity
- Cognitive awareness and attention span
- Physical well-being
- Psychosocial abilities and needs
- Behavioral refocusing needs
- Interests, hobbies
- Previous life work experiences
- Shared religious beliefs
- Community outreach interest and ability
- Service project interest and ability

WHO DOES DAILY LIFE STUFF? CONNECTING MULTIFACETED CREATIVE THERAPIES

Doing the stuff of daily life is everyone's opportunity. Activity-focused care relates that all of life is an activity of being and doing. All caregivers, family members, and residents themselves are involved, therefore, throughout the day. Everyone becomes an activity therapist, activity giver, and activity receiver.

The best of circumstances occurs when residents with dementia have the opportunity to experience and be engaged with health care professionals representing varying areas of expertise. Therapies working together, sharing similar objectives related to upholding residents' personhood, enhance the possibilities of surrounding residents with a life of quality. Each professional therapist brings insight, skills, approaches, interventions, and his or her own therapeutic self to the caregiving milieu. Professionals sharing their knowledge and adapted aspects of their therapy with residents, volunteers, staff, and family members can enable Alzheimer's care centers to augment their activity programs.

Professional therapists offering meaningful and multifaceted activity include

1. *Activity therapists*: Using daily life activities and scheduled or programmed activities, the activity therapist creates, offers, and involves residents with dementia within their level of ability to experience a life of quality. All activities have the possibility of becoming a therapeutic medium for residents to enjoy, enter into,

and find meaning through. Therapists' wisdom, knowledge, experience, and compassion unite with carefully selected, developed, and implemented activities. These activities are then adapted for the individual needs and abilities of each resident. Success is then defined and achieved.

2. *Music therapists*: Music therapy is described as an allied health service using music therapeutically to enable abilities and well-being. A music therapist uses music to promote relaxation, decrease physical or emotional stress, reduce isolation, stimulate motivation and increased social interaction, and facilitate communication and expression of feelings. The type of music and its presentation is carefully selected with a therapeutic goal in mind. Listening, performing, music games, sing-alongs, song writing, reminiscing, drumming circles, rhythm activities, and educational opportunities are the basis of the milieu of music therapy. See Appendix 9-7 for a unique music therapy collaboration between two health care facilities.

3. *Dance and movement therapists*: Dance and movement therapy uses rhythmic movement as a means of communication and self-expression. Creative therapists offer one-to-one, small-group, and occasionally large-group activity based on participants' needs, responses, and planned objectives. Body movement and integration with awareness and sense of self unite residents in this therapy of active expression.

4. *Horticultural therapists*: Using flowers, herbs, vegetables, and other growing plants, horticultural therapy offers residents a meaningful activity, an opportunity to reminisce, and, most important, the awareness of being needed. It provides a nonthreatening way for the resident to nurture and care for a living plant, enabling an opportunity for enhanced self-esteem. Other goals include physical well-being and opportunities for creativity and self-expression.

5. *Art therapists*: Art therapy uses traditional art media as a therapeutic modality enabling communication and relationship. In turn, residents have the opportunity for private or shared expressions of themselves and their world view. Art therapy opportunities involve various media, including paper, clay, watercolors, oil paints, markers, crayons, crepe paper, sand, brushes, and sponges. The art therapist offers support, guidance, and direction as needed or required for the resident to have a positive therapeutic experience.

6. *Drama therapists*: Drama therapy uses creative drama with a therapeutic goal focused on supportive well-being. Creative visualizations, guided imagery, and familiar or created drama combined with the use of props, costumes, and scripts offer residents a connection to themselves, present and past, as well as a bridge to their peers.

7. *Pet therapists*: Being needed, receiving unconditional love, having a meaningful task, and companionship are but a few of the benefits of pet therapy. Dogs, cats, and birds are some of the animals included in pet therapy. As with any form of therapy, an assessment of the resident's past, likes, and dislikes is an integral component of the therapy. Residents who are fearful, disliked certain animals, or thought that all animals belong outside and not in the house should have their specific responses honored. Using a pet as an intervention or as a therapeutic goal for

Alzheimer's Disease: Activity-Focused Care

a resident's problem or need enables pet therapy to be an important element in a resident's plan of care.

8. *Massage therapists*: A massage therapist is trained to work with the elderly using therapeutic touch for enhancing emotional and physical well-being. Being touched by warm, caring hands offers residents feelings of being nurtured.

9. *Aroma therapists*: Aromatherapy uses various aromas to provide sensory stimulation, memory enhancement, reminiscence, and mood stabilization.

MAKING IT HAPPEN

Making it happen requires that the resident will show up at the activity and respond within his or her ability level. The most important thing to remember about making an activity happen is to create an opportunity of connection. Residents with dementia usually do not initiate an activity on their own. Connecting occurs when the resident is called forth to join with another resident, with family, or with staff.

Some suggestions to make it all happen include the following:

- Asking, "Mildred, do you want to play word games?" leaves the door wide open for the resident to say, "No." When the invitation is, "Mildred, it's time for word games and I really need your help with this activity," chances are the response will be, "Yes." Making the resident feel needed is imperative.
- Have all the materials ready for the activity, plus a backup activity to use if needed.
- Involve residents in the implementation of the activity whenever possible. It becomes too easy for staff to forget this vital fact and take over the leadership entirely. Finding meaning in an activity is usually a direct reflection of the resident's feelings of being needed and involved.
- Wear a name tag with your first name only and ask residents if they would each like one also.
- Welcome residents at the start by a handshake, calling each by name, and offering them a compliment.
- Watch residents for cues. Be ready to slow down or speed up the activity, or discard it altogether and start something new.
- Acknowledge all participation, finding something positive about each resident.
- Close by again shaking hands, thanking each resident for coming, and, again, making a personal, positive remark to each one.

BASIC STUFF NEEDED

Having basic stuff on hand is required not only when setting up an activity program but also to have available throughout the day for use by residents in unscheduled activity. There will always be residents wandering through activities and around the edges of activities. Having stuff to look at, pick up, and become involved with creates the feeling that they are involved and part of the community. If the environment is too neat with stuff all picked up and put away, residents may feel as though they are living in a hotel and therefore at loose ends.

Basic supplies suggestions include

I. Basic stuff for thinking activities
   A. Scrapbooks of pictures, greeting cards, etc., with a large printed phrase under each one
   B. Picture files by categories, pasted on stiff card stock
   C. Flash cards for mathematics: addition, multiplication, subtraction, and division
   D. Trivia books and games, other word games
   E. Reading books (e.g., poetry, Bible, fables, magazines)
   F. Games (e.g., dice, checkers, cards, simple board games)
   G. Reminiscing kits (see Appendix 9-2)
   H. Newspaper for reading alone or together (e.g., news, comics, crossword puzzle, horoscope, food sales)
   I. Crayons with adult-related pictures for adding color
   J. Car brochures and other catalogues to browse and make out wish lists
   K. Wallpaper books, drapery books to stimulate reminiscing or daydreaming
   L. Paint boxes
   M. Puzzles: simple jigsaw and puzzles of two to eight pieces made from familiar box fronts (e.g., tea bags, corn flakes)
II. Basic stuff for movement and physical activities
   A. Balls (e.g., beach, small, large, firm, soft, foam)
   B. Balloons (e.g., large, some filled with rice or small bells)
   C. Plastic flying disks (e.g., foam, small, soft)
   D. Exercise related (e.g., scarves, streamers, wands, plastic tubes used to hold golf clubs, dumb bells)
   E. Beanbags of various sizes and shapes and assorted games to use
   F. Laundry basket for ball tossing
   G. Music tapes for singing, dancing, marching, exercising
   H. Rhythm instruments
   I. Fabric squares for rubbing, sorting, discerning textures
   J. Bowling (e.g., tabletop, large floor game)
   K. Pinwheels for breathing and lung expansion exercises
   L. Fabrics that can be knotted into a circle or used as a parachute
   M. Sensory stimulation activity materials
   N. Punch clown with sand in its bottom that rights itself when hit
   O. Busy boxes made up of safe stuff to hold, move about, touch, take
   P. Yarns to wind
III. Basic stuff for psychosocial activities
   A. Toaster, small oven, fry pan, waffle maker
   B. Tea set with donated cups and saucers
   C. Pretty hats and men's caps
   D. Resident name tags, made by residents if possible, placed on a family tree–shaped wall banner when not in use
   E. Service projects (e.g., envelopes to be stuffed, coupons to be clipped)

F. Normalization activity supplies (e.g., sponges, broom, duster, clothing to be folded, stamps to be cut from envelopes, socks to be sorted)

G. Grooming supplies for men and women

IV. Basic materials and equipment suggestions

A. White board on wheels

B. Cassette or compact disk player

C. Appropriate videotapes (e.g., musicals, comedy, travel, nature)

D. Felt pens, markers, tape, various types of glue, scissors

E. Poster board for displaying residents' work or a large sheet of acrylic plastic mounted to the wall for taping on projects, drawings, poetry, and other things

F. Cooking equipment

G. Supply and storage area that can be locked

H. Pegged racks for caps, ties, aprons, purses, handheld cleaning tools

I. Local library card

J. Local newspaper for possible special events in the community or possibly activities within the facility

THINKING ACTIVITIES: ENCOURAGING COGNITIVE PARTICIPATION

Activities using past experiences and abilities, rote learning, and memories can enable the resident to engage in a meaningful response. Long-term memory is accessed through reminiscing, games, and visual clues. The cognitive stimulation of reciting previously memorized poems, prayers, or sayings and singing of past favorites or "oldies" stimulates verbal responses and often decreases word-finding problems. Do not be afraid to challenge residents with Alzheimer's disease, as they are often more capable cognitively than thought. Just be conscious of your approach and never put a specific resident on the spot; instead, ask the group for a response. For example, rather than asking Della to name the capital of Illinois, direct your question to the group of residents.

Using a white board, large enough for the gathered residents to see, and writing key words or topics that are being discussed, helps residents to stay focused and self-cue if they forget what the subject is. For example, when reminiscing about holiday food favorites for Thanksgiving, the word Thanksgiving and a listing of the foods discussed can be written on the board during the discussion so residents can keep track of what has been said.

Presenting the activity in a game-like mode is generally well accepted and increases participation. Clueing is used to encourage success (e.g., color coding, finding similarities in shape or color, and placing the word or saying you want to elicit at the end of a sentence rather than at the beginning). Clapping hands during counting by fives to 50 and backward from 20 by ones, or saying the alphabet, sets a rhythm that facilitates response. Putting together various shapes, sizes, textures, and figure-ground (foreground-background) relationships may limit the decline of spatial-perceptual incompetence. Repetition, such as singing the same song five to seven times in a row, stimulates increased participation and satisfaction. Singing also can be used to validate residents' ability to use words and can encourage increased use of speech.

Dementia Challenges Affecting Cognitive Activities

- Memory dysfunction: recent or past, or both
- Limited, short, or lack of attention span
- Disorientation as to time, place, or person, or a combination
- Easily distracted by movement or people, television, or noise in the immediate area as well as away from the group
- Limited ability or inability to follow simple directions
- Word problems in expression or reception, or understanding, or inability to sequence thoughts
- Perceptual dysfunction, poor body-motor planning or decreased sensory comprehension, or both, that prohibit manipulation of program materials or equipment
- Limited judgment that restricts use of potentially hazardous materials or equipment

Examples of Cognitive and Thinking Activities

(Reminder: Use the white board, when appropriate, for assisting residents to focus.)

1. *Adapted bingo*: Use pictures, Bible verses, shapes, colors, pictures of foods, flowers, simple numbers, or other images. Vary the number of items that have to be "covered" so that the game can be simplified (e.g., use a card having just four items).
2. *Who's who*: Use pictures or parts of speeches, for instance, to trigger old memories and identity of a famous person.
3. *Going shopping*: Bring in items or use catalogs, pictures, advertisements, etc., and guess the cost of the item. Vary the game by using an old catalog from 50 years ago and guess how much money items would cost today.
4. *Games with letters*: Use cutout letters, letters on different size cards, Scrabble (Milton Bradley Company, Springfield, MA) letters, and magnetic letters of all shapes and sizes to form words either by working alone or in small groups; cut out letters from sheets of sandpaper for increased clueing using sensory input; match all the letters that are the same; pick out the letter that the word or object starts with.
5. *Word games*: Use opposites, rhyming, fill in the blanks, end a familiar saying, name items in a category, crossword puzzles, word search, trivia games, and so on.
6. *Games with numbers*: Same as games with letters, make different sizes of individual numbers; make addition, subtraction, multiplication, and division flash cards by using a wide black marker and large file cards: use three-, four-, or five-digit numbers, and have the resident read the number; present a group of numbers and have residents put them in the right sequence. Remember that if residents are holding an item, such as a letter or number in their hands, they are more apt to focus their attention and respond.
7. *Spelling games, geography games*: Vary the difficulty of the questions, ask the whole group, and be sensitive to residents who cannot respond.
8. *Memory games*: Match cards, colors, or other images. Game can be made simple or complex depending on the number of items or steps to play.

9. *Adapting table games*: Games, such as checkers, Scrabble, Yahtzee (Milton Bradley Company, Springfield, MA), dominoes, and dice, can be simplified by using fewer pieces or adapting the rules.

10. *Sensory games*: Use various smells that would be familiar, touch games with items such as seashells, pine cones, smooth rocks; listen to tapes of sounds and try to identify them. "Smells" from jars can be out of context and too puzzling for residents.

11. *Reminiscing*: To connect the resident with the past, reminisce with pictures, music, old clothes, current events, a timeline, cooking, or items pertaining to certain topics such as travel posters, an angel food cake pan, or a box of office supplies. Introduce the topic and encourage participation through sharing memories. Holding an item stimulates a response, verbal or nonverbal.

12. *Reminiscing kits*: Boxes or kits of objects focused on a specific theme can help to facilitate memories. See Appendix 9-2 for examples of kits and objects to include in them. Other theme suggestions are: gardening, general or specific holidays, school days, baby care, cars, specific careers, fabrics, beach, seasons, stamps and world map, greeting cards, postal cards, weddings, and vacations.

13. *Fabric memories*: Use pieces of various fabrics such as burlap, satin, and flannel with plain colors or patterns. Ask what the fabric could have been used for, did the resident ever have an item of fabric like this, what would be best made of this, and so forth.

14. *Simple crafts*: Suggestions include collages using pictures or torn paper, coloring, sanding, lacing pictures, stamping using a potato stamp, stuffing pillows, and paper decorations. The craft has to be very basic, with one to three steps, or worked on in several sessions.

15. *Sorting activities*: Use items such as poker chips, buttons, contact paper–covered poker chips in different patterns, office supplies, and washcloths. Safety is an issue if the resident puts small items in his or her mouth.

16. *Poetry*: Use rhyming words or an object to elicit a response from the residents, write it down on a board or paper where residents can see it, and put it together as a free verse poem. Recite familiar poems learned years ago such as "The Village Smithy" or "The Night Before Christmas."

17. *Creative writing*: Ask residents to supply the idea for a theme, writing down on a white board or on newsprint paper ideas for characters, events, names, and overall story line. The thoughts can then be arranged in the order residents wish the story to flow.

18. *Teaching and learning moments*: Using the resident's LifeStory Book (see Chapter 3) as a reference, ask a resident to teach the others about a familiar aspect of his or her life, such as a class on U.S. geography. This activity would take planning and support from the activity therapist.

19. *Music*: Use music as a basic key to evoke responses. Suggestions include singing, rhythm bands, listening, clapping, and using music as a background for reminiscing. Music has universal appeal, can change or set a mood, and often encourages even the most withdrawn or inactive resident to respond.

> Margaret had little verbal speech other than an occasional word, and she had poor body awareness and limited upper extremity initiated movement. When "Let Me Call You Sweetheart" was

sung, her eyes brightened and her foot started to tap. Two or three times through the song her head rose and she mouthed a few words. As the song was repeated five or six times in a row, Margaret was able to sing more than half of the words.

20. *Art, drawing, coloring, painting, and related activities*

MOVEMENT ACTIVITIES: ENCOURAGING PHYSICAL PARTICIPATION

Residents with dementia are often physically well but need activities for maintaining their abilities. Being inactive soon leads to decreased function, strength, and well-being. For example, an active resident with Alzheimer's disease who is hospitalized or kept in bed for more than 3 days can decrease or terminate his or her ability to walk (see Chapter 7).

The following basic developmental principles incorporated into physical activities may increase the resident's level of functioning:

1. Begin with head-to-tail direction such as head-neck control and movement, eye tracking, mouth movements, neck bending, and turning.
2. Go from the midline or center of the resident's body to the sides. Focus on the long muscles of his or her back and sides that support his or her spine and help to maintain erect positioning. Examples are twisting the resident's trunk side to side, passing an object to the person beside or slightly behind him or her, bending forward or sideward and elevating shoulders and relaxing.
3. Use bilateral movement before unilateral activity. Exercise both arms together or both legs together and then one at a time. Use scarves, plastic tubes used to hold golf clubs, or other items, to encourage simultaneous movement.

Dementia Challenges Affecting Physical Activities

- Motor planning (apraxic) problems or inabilities in using fine and gross motor movements; standing or sitting balance
- Rigidity, especially of neck and trunk
- Spatial-perceptual problems affecting understanding of depth, figure-ground, body image, space, and so on
- Inability to follow directions
- Limited attention span
- Limited awareness of safety issues such as overfatigue, sore muscles or joints, foot blisters, or incorrect use of equipment

Examples of Movement and Physical Activities

1. *Balls, balloons, tossing items*: Foam or plastic flying disks, plastic horseshoes, beanbags, and rope rings can be tossed to and from the resident, into a box or

Alzheimer's Disease: Activity-Focused Care

laundry basket, over nets, kicked, punched, or hit with a racket. This offers a good way to release anxiety and anger.

2. *Parachute*: Use a sheet or several sheets sewn together with a beach ball or smaller balls in the center. Residents sit in a circle, holding the edges, and raise and lower the parachute, keeping the balls from falling to the floor. Another option is to cut a hole in the middle of the sheets, large enough for the ball to just get through. A dark line is drawn down the center of the sheet. The residents are put into teams and the score is kept when the ball goes through the hole.

3. *Tying large fabric pieces into a circle*: Tie fabric pieces of different colors and textures into a circle that is large enough for all residents to hold, and use the fabric circle like a parachute with up and down motions. This physical activity is especially appropriate for residents with limited abilities, because if they stop playing and stay in the circle, the activity can continue.

4. *Dancing*: Using music to encourage a mood, swing arms or move trunk of the seated resident with your arms. Dancing can be done alone, with a partner, or with a group. Circle dancing allows residents to watch and imitate each other. Marching music gives rhythm and cueing for moving feet and clapping.

5. *Punch clown or other figure*: Blown-up plastic figures with a sand or weighted bottom pop upright after being punched or hit.

6. *Busy boxes*: These can be used for tactile and movement responses. Objects must be large enough and nonbreakable to be safe and could include wood or plastic blocks, artificial flowers that do not pull apart, seashells, pine cones, fabric pieces, greeting cards, neckties, scarves, ribbons, and balls of yarn.

7. *Busy boards*: Various fixtures, such as zippers, faucets, light switches, or other items that can be safely manipulated, can be affixed to a board and offered to the seated resident, always with careful monitoring.

8. *Basic exercise program*: (See Appendixes 7-1 and 7-2.) Standard exercise equipment, such as stationary bikes and exercise videotapes, can be used with supervision. Use simple weights and balls to focus attention. A fitness trail can be set up with simple tasks and directions such as over-the-door pulleys, rubber stretch materials, and climbing finger wall ladders. Calling exercise a workout or health club may help to increase participation. When possible, walking inside and outside is still the best physical activity. Take residents "on tour" of the facility. Often, they are greeted warmly by office staff. Encourage them to respond with a song, such as a Christmas carol in December or "Take Me Out to the Ball Game" in the spring.

> Walter's day is spent in a wheelchair. He hesitates to use his hands because of the tremors that often lead to dropping his fork or spilling his milk. When a plastic 3-ft tube or dowel is placed in his hands, the tremor decreases as he grabs on tightly. With his arms working together, up and down over his head, or around in a circle toward or away from him, Walter can participate successfully in the "men's athletic club."

PSYCHOSOCIAL ACTIVITIES: ENCOURAGING PARTICIPATION

Focusing activities on psychosocial skills enables participation and peer group building. This sense of community and the need to be socially acceptable can be nurtured by presenting activities in the context of a party. Make a party for any occasion, such as opening day of baseball, first day of the week, and of course all of the traditional holidays and birthdays.

Group activities are an excellent medium to invite family members into program partnership. For example: an English tea party where a daughter brings in Mom's silver service to be polished by residents and used; a waffle party where family members bring in their waffle irons and the residents join them in small groups to stir the batter, prepare the fruit toppings, and bake the waffles. Residents also love sharing their cooking "yummies" with staff.

Dementia Challenges Affecting Psychosocial Activities

- Limited tolerance or understanding of others
- Wanting attention
- Wanting what the other person has and not realizing that it is not his or hers
- Tendency to have catastrophic reactions, paranoia, hallucinations, delusions, depression, anxiety, aggression, feelings of being lost, or fixation on a specific thing or person

Examples of Psychosocial Activities

1. *Parties*: Include the resident in all of the preparation, serving, and cleaning up. Staff guests and families give a special feeling of importance to the resident. Parties can be done simply, and food or snacks do not have to be served but are a favorite for all.
2. *Special days*: Lead up to a special day with decorations, foods, name tags, hats, and other items. Special times may include holiday parties, picnics, intergenerational day, "Farmer Jones" day, a slumber party, school days, ethnic days, "here comes the bride," senior prom, lemonade stand, white elephant sale, and a bake sale. "Clown day" can be a disaster, because when a staffperson is dressed as a clown, the familiar person has seemed to disappear, and the residents may have apprehension and feel lost.
3. *Working together*: Small group activities can be shared, such as putting up or taking down bulletin board decorations, making scrapbooks, and cleaning up the activity area.
4. *Service projects*: "Doing for others" is an often understood and familiar activity and will elicit a response. The list of opportunities is endless, with projects, pictures, and scrapbooks for children receiving the best participation (see Community Partnership and Service for Others Activities).
5. *Name tag day*: Each resident has a large name tag with his or her first name. Residents usually can read familiar names and will say them out loud. The

"named" residents forget that they are wearing a tag and are pleased that their name is known.

6. *Grooming*: This can include doing nails, styling hair, shaving, applying lotion, and so on. Costume jewelry, hats, flowers, neckties, and scarves make them feel special.

7. *Caring for pets*: Appropriate animals for residents to hug, brush, and feed are a great source of giving and receiving love and acceptance. If the nursing home cannot have a pet live in, staff can bring in "the pet of the day."

8. *Movies*: Using favorites, such as "The Sound of Music," give out tickets and serve refreshments.

9. *Bus trips*: Trips into the community have to be thought out carefully. The staff or family member ratio to residents should be 1 to 3. Be sure the place selected is appropriate. Picnic areas and restaurants are the most successful trip destinations. Many restaurants will set aside a special place or separate room if they know you are coming. The actual bus travel time should not be longer than half an hour. Remember that loading and unloading a bus of persons with dementia is time consuming, and watchful eyes for wandering residents are a must. "Wanderers" should be the first to board the bus and the last to be unloaded. Tuck a facility business card in the pocket of all residents, especially wanderers, in case they become lost. The selection of residents must be made the day of the trip, with the understanding that at the last minute a resident might not be able to go because of anxiety or illness. Ordering food should be limited to no more than three choices to prevent frustration or catastrophic reactions. It is wise always to have a nurse present in case of choking. A staff-person's car driven to the restaurant also allows flexibility if a resident loses the ability to tolerate the change of environment and needs to return "home."

> Mrs. Jones usually eats about half of the food on her tray. She tries to stuff the food into her mouth as quickly as possible and therefore eats most of her meals with her fingers. It was decided to take her on a bus trip to a local restaurant in spite of her "poor manners." In preparation for the outing, the activity therapist manicured her nails with polish, which pleased Mrs. Jones. On the morning of the trip, the staff encouraged her to select her favorite outfit and care was taken with her makeup and hair. Costume jewelry added splendor to the overall effect. At the restaurant, Mrs. Jones was seated with residents who were her "friends." The staff were not surprised when Mrs. Jones ate her entire meal with the appropriate silverware and responded to others with graciousness and enjoyment. Eating out had indeed been a successful activity.

SPIRITUAL ACTIVITIES: COMPASSIONATE CONNECTEDNESS

For information on spiritual activities, see Chapter 11.

LIFE WORK AND NORMALIZATION ACTIVITIES

"Work" is a source of a meaningful quality of life. Residents with dementia were all viable, active citizens in their homes, jobs, and community. The challenge is to take the tasks that they at one time were engaged in easily and successfully and adapt or modify them for a continued sense of purposeful participation. The activity then resembles the familiar "work" that is based on examples of what residents would be doing if dementia had not occurred. Thus, these are "normalization activities," or those tasks or activities that residents would be doing if they were "normal." The focus is now on residents' current abilities, and the tasks must assure success.

Equally important and part of the normalization focus is the "role" of the resident. The former office manager, mother, church leader, helper, etc., may still believe that he or she is active in that position. The selected activity must allow for continuation of the "role" to promote dignity and self-worth (see Appendix 9-4).

> Robert thinks the nursing home unit is his factory and all the staff and other residents are employees. He feels confident and successful when he is dressed in a suit and tie, walking around with a clipboard and pen, carrying items to distribute. He no longer gives out machine parts but now places clean linens in the rooms. He feels good about his "job" and has to be convinced that all workers need a break for lunchtime. The staff thank him for his help and give compliments about his good work.

> Martha's home was always spotless. Now she feels needed and supported when she is asked to help straighten out bureau drawers, given a cloth to wipe tables, or asked to dust the bookshelves. She takes pride in "keeping her house neat."

Normalization tasks combine all the qualities of cognitive, physical, and psychosocial activities. Symptoms or the effects of dementia can affect participation. The challenge is to find or develop appropriate tasks for residents and achieve a desired and realistic outcome. Selecting normalization tasks while meeting the objectives and criteria for a therapeutic experience is only limited by our creativity (see Appendix 9-5).

The following are examples of life work and normalization activities:

- Folding washcloths, rags, laundry, baby clothing, ties
- Buttoning shirts and folding them
- Separating types or colors of socks
- Untying knots put in socks (enjoyed by low-functioning residents)
- Hanging up clean clothing, gathering soiled clothing
- Hand washing socks and stockings and hanging them up on a clothesline
- Sorting items (e.g., poker chips, coupons, various sizes of envelopes, cards, military insignia, plastic silverware into a kitchen drawer, costume jewelry)
- Tearing paper for a kennel

- Working at a plywood busy board with hardware fixtures
- Shining silver, shoes, brass; for veterans, lacing and polishing combat boots
- Washing floors, sinks, or windows
- Untying knots and winding clothesline into a hank
- Winding twine onto a wooden bobbin (fishing)
- Winding yarn from the skein into a ball, then onto a tube, and back into a ball
- Hanging hats or aprons on a wall pegboard
- Folding or hanging up neckties
- Rolling clothing into a footlocker drawer
- Putting slides into slotted boxes or a carousel
- Putting together plastic lids and containers
- Putting silverware into kitchen utensil box
- Rolling pennies
- Stuffing envelopes
- Sweeping, mopping, dusting, wiping tabletops
- Cooking, preparing for parties, setting the table
- Gardening, caring for plants, arranging flowers
- Caring for pets
- Party planning, implementation, and follow-through
- "Shopping" (e.g., using a laundry rack, hang up clothing from a garage sale, using plastic size signs and grouping clothing appropriately, add a "Sale Today Only" sign for assuring successful shopping by catching residents' attention)

Another form of a normalization activity is to have a menu selection program.

> Bertha had been in the dementia unit for almost 2 years. She was selected to be in the first group in the unit to try menu selection. This involved choosing between two entrees for the main meal of the day. The choices were listed on a piece of paper with a place to check or circle the selection and sign her name. The activity therapist met with each resident and helped each to read the menu. At first, just making a choice was difficult, as Bertha had not been asked if she wanted "turkey or beef" for a long time. She needed encouragement. In time she could choose, circle the selection, and sign her initials. She still hesitates to sign her name, perhaps remembering feeling coerced into signing checks. She appears to feel she took part in the meals being served and tells everyone how she chose what they are eating. Surely, she is remembering the years when she selected foods to serve her family.

COMMUNITY PARTNERSHIP AND SERVICE FOR OTHERS ACTIVITIES

How about this idea? Take the local yellow pages in the phone book, start with the letter "A" and ask, "What can they do for me?" In other words, look at the nearby community as a source of supplies, donations, activities, active involvement, assistance, volunteers, or places to visit. Residents with dementia should have the opportunity to go into the community or have the community brought in to them. In return, the facility can offer the community group educational programs on Alzheimer's disease or other programs related to aging and opportunities for volunteering.

Developing partnerships with local groups can enrich both the residents and the groups themselves (see Appendixes 9-6 and 9-7).

Other examples of resident activities involving community partnership and service for others are

- Cutting coupons and soup labels for school label drives.
- Recycling cans or paper, taking them to a recycling center that offers payment, selecting and donating the money to a worthy charity.
- Cutting and soaking off postage stamps for collectors.
- Making simple toys for challenged children.
- Hosting scouts at the facility and offering to help with badge work activity. Another suggestion is to approach the local scouts office and offer the facility as a site for an Explorer Post specializing in health care. Staff from several disciplines would be involved in such a post that has young men and women ages 16–21. Scouting groups are also sources for volunteers, as the scouts work on different health-related programs.
- Baking treats for local civic groups (e.g., fire, police, public works).
- Preparing lunches and cold drinks and taking them to volunteers working at building sites for Habitat for Humanity.
- Helping to sort donations for Habitat for Humanity or other clothing distribution sites.
- Stuffing envelopes and doing mailings for nonprofit groups or the local village office.
- Volunteering (e.g., patrolling for litter around public grounds, weeding at the botanical garden, performing town hall tasks, dusting books at the library, being trail walkers at the forest preserve).
- Planting gardens of flowers, vegetables, or theme gardens and sharing the harvest with others. Examples of themes are
    Salad garden (e.g., cucumbers, tomatoes, radishes, lettuce, onions, peppers, dill and other herbs)
    Pasta sauce garden (e.g., tomatoes, peppers, zucchini, herbs, onions)
    Picnic garden (e.g., corn, carrots, melons, tomatoes, potatoes)
- Supporting a charity by having walk-, wheel-, or roll-a-thons within the facility.
- Making tray favors, scrapbooks, decorations, etc., for children in the hospital.
- Writing letters to persons in the service.

INTERGENERATIONAL ACTIVITIES: FUN FOR ALL

Bringing together persons of different ages for opportunities to interact and enjoy each other's gifts of self creates a priceless treasure to be shared by all. Intergenerational activities require planning and great sensitivity for all involved. The children and the elders should feel connected to the shared activity to feel the benefits of the relationship to each other.

The children's ages and socialization skills become the basis for planning. Children can be prepared by having stories about grandparents read to them by their teachers or parents. Residents' social skills and abilities to interact with youngsters are also part of the equation for success. Selecting residents with similar abilities can be helpful. Activities are needed that promote one-to-one, small-group, and large-group interaction. Shared events should be structured, but flexible at the same time. The time of day of the intergenerational activity and the length of time spent together should be considered. Music and treats can be the glue that holds the activity together. Sharing of wisdom, fun, games, dancing, stories, preparing and eating treats, creative arts, crafts, treasures, and a warm lap ensure a happy time for all.

ACTIVITIES FOR ENGAGING MALE PARTICIPATION, ENJOYMENT, AND SATISFACTION

The answer to, "What is a good activity for men?" is the same as to the question about what is a good Alzheimer's activity—anything that meets therapeutic objects and criteria.

Selecting activities for men to enjoy starts with their life story (see Chapter 3). Consideration then includes the men's cognitive, physical, and psychosocial well-being. Just bringing a group of men together "does not a good activity make."

Typical men's activities include sharing the newspaper, talking about sports, seeing an action-packed video, having a pizza and nonalcoholic beer, and sanding birdhouses. These activities may meet the men's interests and needs for awhile, but caregivers are encouraged to use their creativity to develop and facilitate activities that provide men with a meaningful experience in which they can feel needed and actively involved.

Start by asking the men. Using their life stories as a basis, reflect on their past interests, life work, hobbies, and cultural background. Help them to feel ownership of their group and its decisions. If at all possible, have a retired, volunteer man run the group. If not available, perhaps a male staffperson within the facility would be willing to be a leader.

Suggestions for men's activities include

- Service-related projects (see Community Partnership and Service for Others Activities).
- Community outreach and visits.
    scouts
    car dealer
    police station
    firehouse
    local schools, especially for their sports events
    park districts
- Invited community guest program: Ask retired community men to speak with the men's club about their field of experience and interest.
- "Back-of-the-house" experts program: Walk the men through the facility's working areas (e.g., kitchen, boiler room, central supply, laundry) and talk about what it takes to run a home.

- Men's club environmental consultants: Go through the public areas of the facility plus all the resident areas checking for lighting needs, furniture repairs, paint touchups needed, broken screens, ceiling leaks, and so forth.
- Past military experience–related activities.
- Flag raising and lowering for the facility.
- Monthly newsletter featuring biographical sketches of famous men or men who have been residents' role models.
- Hosts for a special event (e.g., pancake breakfast, pizza party, cocktail party, dance).
- Videotapes of special interest (e.g., sports, biography, military, specific jobs such as construction, trains)

SHOESTRING AND WEARABLE ACTIVITIES FOR RESIDENTS WITH SHORT ATTENTION SPANS

Residents who are unable to sit down and attend an activity or those with limited ability to focus on an activity for more than a minute or two pose a challenge for the caregiver. Very often, these residents will not grasp an object or, if they do, they will hold it for a moment and then drop the object or push it away.

The objective of "shoestring" and "wearable" activities is to provide an activity that can be safely worn by residents so it travels or stays with them for an extended period. If there is a concern about the safety of having any form of string or objects around the resident's neck, items can be worn over one shoulder and under the other like a mail carrier's pouch. The shoestring and wearable activities can also be affixed near the seated resident on a stable piece of furniture or to a safe part of the environment such as a doorknob or banister.

Shoestring and wearable activities can be creative and variable. A guideline is that they are accessible to use when appropriate and that they promote aspects and interests from the resident's life story. Objects should be lightweight and non-breakable. Items that have a hole in them or can be tied onto the string are preferred. If not, a hole might have to be punched into the item. If preferred, the items can be knotted into place on the string so they do not all slide to one area. The strings can be hung on a wall peg rack, draped over a chair, or laid out on a flat surface. It is hoped that residents will be intrigued and pick up the string as they wander by; if not, the caregiver can select one for them.

Actual shoestrings of soft cotton weave can be used when the objects used need the hard tip for threading onto the string. Depending on the length of the shoestring, two or three items may have to be knotted together. If the objects to be used are easy to thread and do not require a small threading tip, a washable cording or macramé string can be used. Be sure that the cording is wide or thick enough that it does not knot itself easily. A cording that has a satin-like finish is best. Shoestrings will not knot on themselves, but they can be expensive if you need to tie quite a few together. The end product should be able to hang loosely to the resident's waist when worn.

What do you put on the shoestring? Ideas are endless. Suggestions for items to use as shoestring activities are

- Kitchen-related items (e.g., measuring spoons and cups, cooking spoons, spatulas, plastic cookie cutters)

- Neckties knotted onto the string
- Curlers or hair rollers of different colors and shapes along with combs and brushes
- Service badges from the military
- Puzzle pieces of different shapes and sizes with holes punched in them
- Tennis balls of different colors or other sized balls
- Keys
- Playing cards with varying pictures and colors
- Scarves
- Milk carton lids of different colors plus plastic lids from other containers
- Thread spools with the end of the thread glued down
- Baby-related items (e.g., rattles, spoons, clothing, bootie or shoe)
- Costume jewelry that can be safety knotted onto the string
- Mittens, socks, caps
- Bells of different sizes and sounds
- Laminated pictures that relate a theme (e.g., flowers, children, cars, kitchens)
- Family-related wearable activity (e.g., families can put together shoestrings using pictures or remembrances)

ONE-TO-ONE ACTIVITIES: PERSONALIZED ACTIVITIES

What can you offer the resident who will not participate in groups, large or small? This resident may or may not walk around the edges of an activity. There will always be residents who do not go near an activity for a number of reasons, including being bedridden or "chair-bound" and needing nursing monitoring, constant pacing, inability to track voice or movement, fearful, shy, depressed, or just not interested. Developing a personalized program for these residents requires creativity and a sincere commitment to a quality one-to-one activity program.

Suggestions and guidelines for program development include

1. Firmly commit to the program and its implementation.

2. Develop a one-to-one resource library. A library of "stuff" that can be taken off the shelf and brought with the therapist or person carrying out the one-to-one program can include many different kinds of items (e.g., to stimulate cognitive abilities, promote physical wellness, provide psychosocial opportunities, and provide spiritual opportunities). Persons with dementia respond with the fullest attention when they are not "talked at" but have an item of some sort to hold in their hand or to look at. Refer to Making It Happen, Basic Stuff Needed, and Sensory Stimulation and Activities for Late-Stage Dementia Care, as well as the basic activity descriptions for encouraging cognitive, physical, and psychosocial participation. Remember that there is no "magical activity" in general and the same is true for finding an appropriate activity for a one-to-one program.

3. Make a one-to-one resource listing. This can be in a notebook or a file box. It is a handy reference of what is available for the program and helpful for staff with limited ideas of their own. The headings for the resource listing could be cognitive, physical, psychosocial, and spiritual, and then these could be broken down according to the various levels of abilities required for successful implementation.

4. The success of a one-to-one program rests on the personality and wisdom of the activity therapist or whoever is carrying out the engagement with the resident. Asking the resident for assistance or to show how to do something can be helpful. Facilitation techniques, such as hand over hand, chaining, or bridging, also help the contact to be successful (see the glossary at the end of the book).

5. Train all involved staffpersons, family members, and volunteers involved in the one-to-one program. Encourage non–hands-on staff to participate. Perhaps they have a resident they are fond of or they may be open to assist any resident assigned to them.

6. Staff involved in the program should have a scheduled time for implementing a one-to-one program. Otherwise, it is too easy to put off. Most of the involved residents do not call attention to themselves, which is why they are in the program to begin with.

7. Keep a one-to-one resident informational file on residents who are part of the program. Include interesting information from the resident's LifeStory Book (see Chapter 3) and a list of one-to-one activities that have worked as well as ones that did not work and perhaps should not be tried again. Also include the resident's best time of day for responding to the one-to-one program.

8. Create a one-to-one program cart, box, or apron. It is helpful, for example, when a staffperson doing a one-to-one with a resident wears an apron or smock that lets everyone know what is going on. This helps to limit the distractions that often occur when other staff think that the resident and the staffperson are "just talking." It also allows the staffperson to be prepared in case the "game plan" has to change quickly to another subject or activity. The apron or smock can have big pockets for bringing along what is needed for the program's implementation.

9. Start the actual program by knowing the resident's life story (see Chapter 3).

10. Begin by building up an acquaintance or trust with the resident by spending a few minutes two or three times a day with him or her. Observe nonverbal responses to assess successful connections with the resident. If all goes well and the guidelines have been followed, the one-to-one program is well on its way to success.

SENSORY STIMULATION AND ACTIVITIES FOR LATE-STAGE DEMENTIA CARE

Residents who are frail, have limited ability to respond to group activities, and have difficulty relating to the world around them usually require individualized activities. Adapted activities for residents' interests and abilities can be comforting and supportive and decrease their sense of isolation. The general pace of activities is slowed by including time to linger with the basic hands-on caregiving tasks that reflect self-worth through nurturing touch. Residents in the late stage of dementia tire easily and often have small naps throughout the day. Mealtimes become an activity in and of themselves because of the extended time that is usually needed for the resident to eat. Activities providing socialization and physical, spiritual, and cognitive responses are offered with the necessary adaptations and simplification to ensure a positive response from the resident.

Placing the activities in attractive baskets that can be kept out and accessible is helpful. Residents in late-stage dementia may also be able to respond to shoestring activities.

Activities that provide sensory stimulation can be engaged in with little expended energy. The goal is to have a balance between sensory-stimulating and sensory-calming activities. Whenever possible, the "real" item should be used for the sensory stimulation rather than, for example, smells out of a kit or bottle. These activities include

1. *Sight*: pictures from magazines, calendars, cards, coffee table books, colors, watching bubbles in the air, mobiles, wind socks, flags, mirrors, slides, videotapes, watching birds at a feeder, wind up toys to walk across the table, mirror
2. *Sound*: nature, music, music box, birds, musical instruments, reading aloud (e.g., poetry, rhymes, Bible), old radio programs, jingle bells, videotapes of family stories, music, or worship
3. *Taste*: favorite foods, fruits, hot foods, cold foods, thin foods, thick foods, guessing games using various tastes
4. *Smell*: spices; foods cooking, flowers, popcorn, cinnamon toast, evergreens, perfumes, cedar chips, ground coffee, peanut butter, lemon, bacon, tobacco, soaps, citrus fruits, after shave and other grooming supplies, baking bread, aromatherapy
5. *Touch*: massage; various temperatures; ice or snow; objects (e.g., pipe cleaners, feathers, pine cones, fur, other items from nature); lotions; various fabrics; "feely" bags filled with various items; empty cereal boxes; folding clothing, especially old baby clothes; sorting through costume jewelry; finding objects in sand or rice; worship-related symbols (e.g., a cross, rosary beads); shoestring activities

A "poke and see" activity often attracts the attention of a resident with minimal ability to respond. A zip-lock bag is filled with colored distilled water to which interesting items have been added, for example, shells. Position the bag's zipped opening in the bottom of a second bag of the same size and then zip up the second bag. The second bag acts as a safety bag in case the first bag with the water springs a leak. Leave enough space in the bag of water so the items can be moved around by poking them.

ACTIVITIES FOR BEHAVIORAL REFOCUSING AND EFFECTIVE INTERVENTION

Activities can enable the residents to respond with positive behaviors and are also effective and significant tools for reducing or eliminating negative or unwanted behaviors. A well-chosen activity can distract or refocus the resident from the unwanted behavior's antecedent and become a successful intervention.

> Samuel's anxiety always increased at shift-changing time. He saw the staff who had been with him during the day putting on their coats and preparing to leave. He felt afraid that he would be all alone. Where would he sleep tonight? The staff on the next shift did not seem as familiar and they

were too busy to pay any attention to him. A staffperson who sang with the residents in the activity room, away from the commotion around the nursing station, gave Samuel the comfort he needed to feel safe. The rest of the afternoon's activities were discussed so Sam realized that he would not be left alone because he was part of this group of residents. A possible catastrophic reaction was avoided.

The choice of activities can change residents' overall sense of well-being. Emotional feelings and responses, including physical manifestations of behaviors needing refocusing, can be positively affected by appropriate activities. Success requires an on-the-spot assessment of the resident and the situation (see Chapter 8).

ACTIVITIES FOR THERAPEUTICALLY REDUCING THE PREVALENCE, ONSET, OR INTENSITY OF AGGRESSIVE OR COMBATIVE BEHAVIORS

Aggressive and combative behaviors are reflected in the resident's physical response of striking out due to fear, anger, misinterpretations, or perceived challenges to personal survival. Violent residents are frightened residents. Activities can be used to help decrease residents' frustration and aggressive behaviors. These therapeutically selected activities allow for residents to use large muscle groups that imitate the physical movements often demonstrated during angry outbursts. The activity goal is to offer residents a positive outlet for their frustrations and anger rather than, for example, kicking or hitting another resident or staffperson.

    I. Physical activities: gross motor participation
      A. Aggression-reducing exercise program components
        1. Holding an exercise or fitness program three times a day: mid-morning, late afternoon, and after supper
        2. Using the same repetitive, structured format for each group of residents to lessen agitation caused by change while providing a sense of the familiar for facilitating success
        3. Having resident perform large muscle movements, especially those that are bilateral (both arms, for example, clasping an exercise weight, tube, or fabric strip) and that involve crossing his or her body's midline (e.g., clasping a beanbag with both hands going from the floor to the left of his or her body, across his or her body, and up to right side above his or her head, or pretending to be swinging a golf club)
        4. Having resident make fists and punch up, out, and down
        5. Incorporating counting with movements, encouraging voice loudness
        6. Encouraging the use of handheld objects for increased attention span and focus, for example:
          a. Plastic tubes used to hold golf clubs—cut or full length
          b. Colorful "fun noodles" tubes (usually used for children's play in water)

    c. Cardboard tubes from hangers with crepe paper streamers pushed in one end so there is visual and auditory stimulation while moving (e.g., a rodeo lariat, figure eights, snapping a whip, fly fishing, circles to the side)

    d. Therapy balls made from colored yarn pom-poms that can be held, tossed, kicked

    e. Scarves of various fabrics, sizes, colors

    f. Beanbags of various fabrics, sizes, colors

    g. Thera-Band or other stretchy cords

    h. Stretchy, one-size-fits-all gloves, splitting the pairs so each resident, for example, has one red glove and one blue glove so color cueing can encourage participation

    i. Lengths of fabrics, knotted together into a circle, with enough slack so residents can hold on to the fabrics and carry out the exercises together, obtaining the needed cueing from their neighbor's movement and mirroring each other

    j. Over-the-door pulleys with easy-to-grasp handles

  7. Building an indoor fitness trail with large motor activities or an outside fitness trail and activity area (see Appendix 7-2), or both

B. Throwing activities

  1. All sorts of balls (e.g., beach balls, therapy balls, foam products)

  2. Paper products (e.g., plates, airplanes)

  3. Soft plastic flying disks, beanbags, plastic horseshoes, ring toss

  4. Throwing objects into laundry baskets, for floor games, at clowns with holes for scoring, over nets, into basketball hoop

  5. Bowling

C. Hitting activities

  1. Using hands, plastic tubes for golf clubs, ping pong paddles or similar small paddles, feather dusters, large kitchen spatulas, plastic bats, plastic hammers

  2. Hitting objects, balls, or balloons that are soft enough so that they will not hurt if a resident is not able to protect himself or herself

  3. Using objects to hit and pop plastic bubbles in packing materials

  4. Using a plastic inflated figure with sand in the bottom that will right itself when hit (select a figure the resident knows, such as Mickey Mouse or a clown)

  5. Playing drums of all sizes, shapes—but under control unless activity is done one-to-one with a staffperson or a music therapist

  6. Hitting balloons or punching bag hanging from the ceiling

  7. Playing tetherball

  8. Playing a volleyball game with balloons

  9. Punching balls on an elastic band worn around the wrist

  10. Popping bubbles being made by a staffperson or another resident

  11. Playing table games that require hitting objects (e.g., using a miniature hockey stick to hit a puck)

D. Tearing and ripping activities

  1. Fabrics of all thickness and length, including old bed sheets

  2. Newspaper (to be later donated to local animal rescue shelters for bedding)

3. Used office paper for a ticker tape parade, confetti.
4. Pictures from magazines
5. Hook and loop fastener strips from each other (good auditory reinforcement)
6. Zipping and unzipping large, sturdy zippers (action is similar to tearing)
7. Tearing bread for stuffing or bird food, especially if the loaf has not been sliced and is stale
8. Tearing husk from corn, lettuce leaves from the head
E. Kicking activities
1. Beach balls, large foam balls, balloons, large beanbags
2. Count loudly when each resident kicks so residents awaiting their chance feel connected to the activity
3. Bubbles being made by a staffperson or another resident
4. Punch ball on a long elastic loop held in the hand or, if the resident is seated, loop the elastic over one ankle so the other foot can kick the ball
F. Foot stomping, dancing, and marching activities
1. Vary music, beat, tempo, and kind of dancing
2. Use dancing with partners as well as "chicken dance," country line dance, etc., that can be done by oneself or in a line holding onto the person in front of you
3. Marching (e.g., slow, fast, in place, high step)
G. Gross motor arm movement: parachute activities
1. Use a sheet or several sheets sewn together
2. Parachute: residents sit in a circle and hold onto the edges, raising and lowering the fabric
3. Place balls or balloons on the fabric to give additional eye stimulation and interest
4. Tie fabric pieces together, use like a parachute
H. Clapping activities
1. Vary intensity, body parts used, tempo, music augmentation, speed
2. Start simply and build up and then return to a quieter, simple pattern
I. Workout activities: Assess residents for use of an exercise bike, pulleys, weights, self-propelled treadmill, and so on (see Appendix 7-2)
J. Walking Club
1. Group residents by ability to walk and form a club that can have a name, roster, chart for distances walked, and club T-shirts.
2. Be creative and find places to walk such as a main hall, taking an elevator down to the basement level or up to another floor, walking that hallway, and then taking the elevator back to the original area
II. Verbal participation activities
A. Singing and yelling activities: Sing songs that call for yelling out, such as "Take Me Out to the Ball Game," "B-I-N-G-O"
B. Singing and clapping activities: For example, use sing-along tapes
C. Counting loudly activities
1. Try doing the multiplication tables, such as 3, 6, 9, 12, and so on.
2. Count in different languages

     3. Use clapping for setting the rhythm when counting, and words are more easily accessed for residents having verbalization limitations

III. Touch participation activities
  A. Massage
    1. Receiving or giving massage
    2. Assess residents for tactile defensiveness, perceived enjoyment or apprehension, location on the body to receive the massage, and any medical contraindications
  B. Rubbing activities
    1. Polishing large surfaces such as furniture
    2. Polishing items such as silverware, candlesticks, cars, shoes
    3. Using fabric squares or carpet pieces for low-functioning residents needing to release anxiety by rubbing
  C. Brushing activities
    1. Stuffed animals
    2. Real animals, especially large and patient dogs
    3. Tabletops, floors, sinks, fabrics, fur scraps, showers, tubs, etc.

IV. Normalization participation activities
  A. Household-type tasks: Dusting, washing and wringing out clothing and hanging it outside, sweeping, vacuuming, washing floors, cleaning large window surfaces, scrubbing shower stalls, sanding, husking corn, peeling vegetables, chopping vegetables and nuts, kneading bread dough, scrubbing pots
  B. Outside tasks
    1. Sweeping, raking, pushing a nonmotorized lawnmower
    2. Washing lawn furniture, cars, bikes
    3. Pulling weeds
    4. Digging gardens

ACTIVITIES FOR RESIDENTS WHO PACE AND WANDER

Residents who pace can have a determined self-perceived agenda. At times, the reason for the pacing can be identified by staff, at times not. Wandering appears to be more aimless, often an activity of exploration and discovery. When the pacing or wandering appears to be safe for the resident or others met along the traveling path, the resident can continue on his or her way. When more structure is needed, perhaps for assistance, promotion of safety, or if the pacing and wandering are upsetting for the resident or others, then the implementation of an activity can help calm or refocus the resident. Examples of activities for residents who pace and wander include

- Dancing
- Walking together with a staffperson to perform a task such as picking up laundry, delivering papers
- Walking as part of a walking club, set up for residents with similar walking styles, led by a staffperson daily
- Roaming rhythm band or choir

- Health club, exercise groups
- Normalization tasks such as raking, sweeping, mopping, carpet sweeping, vacuuming
- Holding familiar belongings while walking
- Pets to walk with or brush
- Quiet music or a busy box to encourage sitting down and relaxing
- Shoestring or wearable activities
- A plastic shopping cart to push along

ACTIVITIES FOR REFOCUSING "SEARCHING AND DISCOVERING"

Searching and discovering activities help to support the resident's need to rummage, pick up, and redistribute items found along the way. The challenge is when the bureau drawers, room, or activity area "stuff" that is being carried off does not belong to the resident. Therefore, having attractive and interesting objects that are safe and made easily available may help the resident to enjoy keeping busy without encountering negative feedback from others. Examples of activities for residents who enjoy searching and discovering include

- Having a never-ending supply of items to pick up and carry about
- Peg boards, racks, bureaus, closets, shelves, or counter space containing items the resident can carry off (e.g., cards, ties, scarves, yarn, baby dolls, stuffed animals, washcloths, artificial flowers, baskets)
- Busy box items for rummaging (e.g., small balls of yarn, artificial flowers, bows, little jewelry boxes, costume jewelry, pot holders, small stuffed animals, large seashells, egg beater, sponge)
- Rolling yarn, cooking, sorting activities, and tasks using hands
- A plastic shopping cart or laundry basket on a wheeled frame
- Supervised drawer or closet cleaning or having an area, such as a box or drawer, just for searching
- A cobbler-style apron with many additional pockets that can be filled with small items; a piece of bias tape sewed to each item and attached to the inside pocket helps to keep the items and apron together
- A purse, tote bag, or small suitcase filled with items safe for rummaging or "shopping"

ACTIVITIES FOR LONELINESS, SADNESS, AND DEPRESSION

Residents may experience withdrawal from the social setting when they are feeling sad, depressed, or lonely. Activities that can assist them to move from a quiet setting or mood to one of feeling nurtured, comfortable, and safe can help the resident to gain confidence in him- or herself. A gentle approach is needed, with a familiar and trusted caregiver, if possible. Examples of activities for residents experiencing loneliness, sadness, or depression include

- Listening to quiet music and then moving on, when appropriate, to music with a strong, uplifting beat

Alzheimer's Disease: Activity-Focused Care

- Singing familiar "oldies"
- Looking at pictures of happy children to foster memories
- Performing a simple task, such as folding a few washcloths; help residents if necessary and give praise or thanks
- Petting animals; if they are not available, use teddy bears
- Holding a baby doll or teddy bear
- Blowing bright pinwheels
- Eating and drinking familiar foods and beverages with pleasant odors such as raisin bread toast, gingerbread, coffee
- Having a manipulation board made of thick plywood, 18 in. × 24 in., with hardware firmly attached to help the "fix-it" man feel helpful; it may contain a faucet, door latch, door bolts, and so on
- Tea for two
- Normalization tasks
- Taking quiet walks with a trusted friend or staffperson
- Making phone calls to a family member or friend
- Hugs, massage, use of a rocking chair with a handmade afghan to wrap up in

HEALTH CARE PROVIDER AND STAFF ISSUES

Activities are everyone's job in a health care facility. Job descriptions can reflect the implementation of activity-focused care. Nursing assistants receiving specific activity training can use these skills during their daily caregiving as well as during quiet times in their schedule. An example would be after the supper hour in the evening before residents' bedtime. The activity department should be responsible for having the equipment and materials ready and easily available. It seems to work best if there is also a list of five or six activities that the nursing assistants can select from. This cross-training of the nursing aides will only be effective when there is total facility support for the program, especially from the nursing department. If activities are part of the job description, nursing department staffpersons should have their performance assessed in this area as part of their evaluation. In the late afternoons or early evening, if activity staff are not present, the nursing assistants can rotate 30- to 45-minute periods of activity duty as part of their regular caregiving assignment.

An activity therapist (see Appendix 9-8) should be present during resident care conferences. Using activity therapy report forms (see Appendixes 9-9 and 9-10), the activity therapist can clearly describe the selection, therapeutic benefits, and implementation of an activity for a resident. This will help family members and staff to understand the significant role of activities for residents with dementia.

Activity-specific policies and procedures supporting the overall goals of activities and their implementation may be required by surveyors. Examples are found in Appendixes 9-3 and 9-4.

Health care facilities are challenged to provide meaningful activities to all of their residents. This is a vast and complicated challenge. Alzheimer's disease and related dementias affect each resident differently. When these effects are combined with the resident's life story and remaining strengths, activities must become the focus for meaningful caregiving.

SUMMARY

The *American College Dictionary* (1953) defines "activity" as a "state of action; doing" or "a specific deed or action; sphere of action." Activity surrounds everyone 24 hours a day. Understanding and caring for persons with dementia require awareness and therapeutic response to "being" and "doing" activities. Residents are often more capable and able to participate in activities than caregivers think they are. Within a community of acceptance, residents are enabled to use activity as a bridge spanning from them to caregivers and back again. The activity, task, or action gives residents' lives integrity.

REFERENCE

American College Dictionary. New York: Harper & Brothers Publishers, 1953.

SUGGESTED READING

Alzheimer's Association. Activity Programming for Persons with Dementia: A Sourcebook. Chicago: Alzheimer's Association, 1995.

Bell V, Troxel D. The Best Friends Approach to Alzheimer's Care. Baltimore: Health Professions Press, 1997.

Bowlby C. Therapeutic Activities with Persons Disabled by Alzheimer's Disease and Related Disorders. Gaithersburg, MD: Aspen Press, 1993.

Chavin M. The Lost Chord: Reading the Person with Dementia Through the Power of Music. Mt. Airy, MD: ElderSong Publications, 1994.

Sheridan C. Failure-Free Activities for the Alzheimer's Disease Patient: A Guide for Caregivers. San Francisco: Cottage Books, 1992.

Zgola J. Doing Things: A Guide to Programming Activities for Persons with Alzheimer's Disease and Related Disorders. Baltimore: Johns Hopkins University Press, 1990.

A9-1
Activity Analysis Example: Using a Beach Ball

	Abilities and Benefits	Inabilities and Risks	Assistance
Cognitive-based responses	Increases mirroring ability	Cannot follow instructions	Break down task into steps
	Allows choice to participate in a pleasurable activity, to select the person to throw ball to	Agnosia: no response to name called, may try to eat the ball or squeeze the ball to pop it	Stand behind the person to receive the ball
	Stimulates ability to follow directions of one, two, and three steps, for example: 1. throw the ball 2. throw the ball to to John 3. bounce the ball then throw the ball in the basket	Increased environmental stimulation Cannot understand the activity	Review body parts to increase body image and motor planning (e.g., "hit the ball with your foot, your head") Bounce ball to rhythmic music Count ball bounces and tosses
	Increases spatial awareness		Vary complexity and number of steps to increase attention span and sequencing skills
	Allows resident to reminisce (e.g., kinds of ball games, professional teams)		
	Active participation increases reality versus delusion or hallucination		
	Stimulates conversation and verbalization		
	Increases counting and sequencing skills		

	Abilities and Benefits	Inabilities and Risks	Assistance
Physical-based responses	Increases eye-hand coordination (e.g., catching, batting, throwing)	Freezing (i.e., cannot release the ball)	Use hand over hand to assist participation
	Increases range of motion	Startled due to decreased vision or hearing, or both	Vary ball surface (e.g., rough, smooth, hard, soft)
	Increases strength and endurance through varied ball weight	Apraxia (i.e., decreased motor planning skills)	Vary weight and size of ball
	Increases healthy fatigue	May increase muscle or joint stiffness or post-activity soreness	Pass the ball around resident's body to increase trunk stability and balance
	Provides a positive outlet for physical restlessness, agitation		Bounce the ball so the sound alerts the resident
	Gross motor movement		Roll the ball when grasp response is limited
	Bilateral activity		
	Increased trunk stability		Throw the ball into a container to assess and reinforce spatial-perceptual confidence
	Eye-hand and eye-foot coordination		
	Increases sitting balance and movement away from resident's midline		Tap basket on the floor for visual or auditory clueing, or both
	Increases standing balance		Use a ball tee
	Stimulates intact senses		Use bumpers for keeping the ball within a given area (e.g., bowling)
	Decreases one-sided neglect		
	Increases kinesthetic awareness and rhythmic movement patterns		
	Increases response to touch through tactile stimulation		
	Increases laughter		
Psychosocial-based responses	Outlet for anxiousness, anger	Increased apprehension	Vary group size
	Shared activity, fun	Hoarding the ball, leading to cohort anger	Use ball for one-to-one interaction when needed
	Decreases apathy, depression		Set up teams, keep

Abilities and Benefits	Inabilities and Risks	Assistance
Team participation (e.g., feelings of belonging, bonding with others, making a contribution)	Difficulties waiting for a turn	score, have special shirts, hats, etc.
Meaningful activity (e.g., workout club)	May think activity is too childish, too much work, too frustrating	Adapt the game to ensure success
Helping (e.g., "Please carry this ball for me.")	Discouraged or embarrassed about doing the activity wrong or poorly	Cheer for all responses
Feeling of ownership		Provide opportunities for hard hitting or throwing ball that allows release of aggression, anxiousness
Increased cooperation skills		Consider making resident needing leadership recognition the team captain

A9-2
Reminiscing Kits

Kits of familiar items to see, touch, and smell are used by persons with dementia for reminiscing. Memories often are prompted by a specific item or a grouping of things used for a common purpose. Many of the kit's items can be donated, especially if the facility puts together a "wish list" for family members and volunteers. Making up the kits is a great way to involve everyone. Examples of kits follow.

Kitchen kit
  wire whip
  eggbeater
  egg timer
  spatula
  rubber scraper
  ladle
  sponge
  hot pad mitt
  pan scrubber
  vegetable brush
  bottle brush
  measuring spoons
  nesting plastic measuring cups
  rolling pin
  hand strainer
  tea strainer
  potato masher
  pastry brush

Toolbox kit
  level
  ratchet wrench
  monkey wrench
  pliers
  metal extension tape
  C clamp
  ruler
  wooden folding ruler
  square
  screwdriver
  paintbrush
  sandpaper
  toolbox

Sports box
  tennis ball
  baseball
  golf ball
  racketball ball
  tennis racket
  golf glove
  horse racing sheet
  ski goggles, gloves, hat
  horseshoe
  birdie
  binoculars
  croquet ball
  mallet
  small football
  helmet
  shoulder pads
  large sports bag

Sewing box kit
  buttons strung together
  darning egg
  large spools of thread
  tapes, lace rickrack
  tape measure
  real sewing box
  pin cushion

Jewelry box kit
  costume jewelry—pins, bracelets, large clip earrings, necklaces
  large and small jewelry boxes

Young girl kit
  empty perfume bottles
  large and small puffs
  ribbons
  large barrettes
  music box
  young girl purse
  change purse
  artificial flower corsage
  pretty handkerchiefs
  comb
  mirror
  sunglasses
  scarves
  doll
  opera glasses

Young man kit
  shoe buffer
  tie clip
  clip bow ties
  ties
  wallet
  empty after-shave bottle
  empty shaving cream can
  shaving brush
  handkerchiefs
  comb
  eyeglass frames
  watch
  belt
  keys and key ring
  sunglasses
  magnifying glass
  shoehorn

A9-3
Sample Policy and Procedures: What Is an Age-Appropriate Activity?

It is the policy of this facility

To define age appropriate activities as those activities in which residents with dementia *respond or interact* with purposefulness as related to their current level of function

To provide and facilitate activities for persons with dementia that do not infantilize or demean their self-image and quality of life

To provide and facilitate activities that relate to residents' former life roles and life stories

DISCUSSION

The interdisciplinary team, family members, and others involved with the resident should understand that the word "age" does not always refer to chronological age. Residents with dementia require activities that range from the most complex, such as making waffles, to the most simple sensory experience, for example, touching a soft plush stuffed animal. The chronological "age" assigned or "thought of" as being appropriate for a specific activity becomes an unimportant factor when the activity fulfills the objectives and criteria of a therapeutic activity:

The objectives of a therapeutic activity are to focus on the resident's abilities, not limitations; provide a purposeful use of time and a sense of belonging; enable an opportunity to support positive behaviors; offer a tool to reduce or eliminate negative or unwanted behaviors; and provide a vehicle for verbal and nonverbal communications.

The criteria for a successful activity include: modification, repetitiveness, multisensory cueing, safety, adaptability, dignity, cultural support, and fun.

Therefore, any age resident can find meaning and receive benefit from any activity that meets the objectives and criteria for a therapeutic activity.

PROCEDURES

1. Activities and materials used with residents will be assessed on an individual basis, in particular when determining and using activities, props, toys, and materials viewed as being for children.
2. Activities will be removed from childish boxes or containers and placed in baskets or appropriate holders that reduce the activity's toy-like appearance.
3. Activities should not stimulate regression caused by the resident's attempt to meet the expectation of the task or the person presenting the task.
4. An adult approach focused on the resident's dignity will be used when introducing and facilitating all activities, for example:
   "Please help me with . . ."
   "Please show me how to . . ."
   "Would you please make this for . . ."
5. If a resident responds to a specific activity that may be viewed as childish but is an important part of his or her therapeutic activity, the activity should be part of the resident's plan of care. For example:

   > Harry was a retired carpenter. He loved "fixing" all the furniture. Harry was content, happy, feeling actively and meaningfully involved when he used his toy plastic tool set, tool belt, and toolbox. He felt extremely helpful and important. The use of the plastic tools and kit were incorporated into Harry's care plan.

6. Optional procedure: An activity resource book can be developed with descriptions of activities and their therapeutic values.
7. Making the policy operational requires education. For example:
   staff training: all staff, management, housekeepers, etc.
   family training
   proactive interaction and demonstration for surveyors

A9-4

Sample Policy and Procedures: What Is a Life Work or Normalization Activity?

It is the policy of this facility to offer familiar life work activities to persons with dementia that provide a sense of meaning and purpose enabling active, voluntary participation. Examples include washing dishes, mopping, wiping tables and dishes, polishing silverware, cleaning windows, washing personal laundry, hanging up the wash, folding wash, folding baby clothes, folding fabrics, baking, "spring cleaning," sorting costume jewelry, raking, car washing, envelope stuffing, and polishing shoes.

DISCUSSION

Life work or normalization activities are the everyday "work" of life. They combine all the qualities of cognitive, physical, and psychosocial activities. The normalization activities can vary from the most simple to the complex (e.g., from stirring cookie dough to reorganizing a tool box). The selection of a life work activity or normalization task must meet the objectives and criteria for a therapeutic experience:

The objectives of a therapeutic activity are to focus on the resident's abilities, not limitations; provide a purposeful use of time and a sense of belonging; enable an opportunity to support positive behaviors; offer a tool to reduce or eliminate negative or unwanted behaviors; and provide a vehicle for verbal and nonverbal communications.

The criteria for a successful activity include: modification, repetitiveness, multisensory cueing, safety, adaptability, dignity, cultural support, and fun.

PROCEDURES

1. Life work activities should meet the following selection criteria:
   Occur within the context of work, self-care, play, or leisure, or a combination

   Individual specific: unique to each person; influenced by his or her life experiences

   Promote ability, pride, and dignity

   Can be adapted or modified to assure success

   Support positive behaviors and assist in refocusing negative or unwanted behaviors

   Are safe
2. Life work activities should reflect the resident's life story (see Chapter 3).
3. Participation is always voluntary.
4. Life work activities can become part of a resident's plan of care when appropriate.
5. Optional procedure: An activity resource book can be developed with descriptions of the activities and their therapeutic values.
6. Making the policy operational requires education. For example:
   staff training: all staff, management, housekeepers, etc.
   family training
   proactive interaction and demonstration for surveyors

A9-5
*Life Work Activity Examples**

**EACH ONE TEACH ONE: PRIDE IN ACTIVITIES
OF SHARING WISDOM AND SKILLS**

Purpose

To provide an opportunity of pride for a resident to successfully access lifelong knowledge that can be shared with others seeking to learn and enjoy his or her collective wisdom

Essentials

1. The resident's area of expertise is identified, taking the resident's cognitive, physical, and psychosocial abilities into consideration.
2. The resident is invited to share his or her skills and knowledge.
3. Staff or family support, or both, must ensure that the "teaching experience" is successful and offers the resident a positive experience of success and sense of accomplishment.
4. Staff are experienced in adapting, simplifying, and providing cueing and props for triggering memory, if needed, and are familiar with the resident's communication skills.
5. The subject or skill can vary and range from the tremendously simple to the complex. For example: "Please show me how to get the knot out of this sock," "Please teach me how to set the table, I always put the fork on the wrong side," "What kind of flower is this? Is it easy to grow? Does it need sun or shade?"
6. The "classroom" area and length of time for the class are carefully considered, again assuring the resident's positive experience.

---

*Life work activity examples are reprinted with permission from C Hellen. LifeWork Activities. In Alzheimer's Association (ed), Activity Programming for Persons with Dementia: A Sourcebook. Chicago: Alzheimer's Association, 1995. (This book can be obtained through Alzheimer's Association chapters.) Reprinted with permission from the National Alzheimer's Association.

7. The "students" are carefully chosen based on their sensitivity and understanding of persons with dementia and the topic or skill to be taught.

Process

1. Approaches with the resident could include
   "Please show me how to . . ."
   "Could you help me with . . ."
   "I need to learn about. . . . Can you teach me?"
2. Possible sources of "students":
   Staff, family and friends, other residents
   Clergy, scout groups working on badges
   School or day care children
3. Examples of subjects or skills for sharing:
   Piano or other musical instrument, singing favorite songs
   Ornithology, geography, travel, floral care and arrangements
   Reading poetry, simple handicraft, sport, cooking
4. Offering validation: "apple for the teacher" ideas
   Following the class or skill demonstration, ask if you are doing it right or repeat the information, asking if you have understood it correctly; have a "report card" for the teacher to fill out
   Compliment the teacher on his or her abilities and communicate the importance of the information to you
   Send a thank-you note or "Teacher of the Year" award

HANDS FOR OTHERS: PRIDE IN ACTIVITIES OF SERVICE

Purpose

To be a valued contributor, experiencing pride and feelings of accomplishment by actively participating in opportunities of meaningful service and "work" done for others

Essentials

1. Assess the resident's abilities and select an appropriate task.
2. Qualities of a service activity:
   Can support resident's strengths and positive responses
   Does not have a "due" time
   Can be broken down into simple steps
   Has meaning as a process or on completion, or both
   Can be started and stopped without compromising the outcome
   Can be adapted to individual, small-group, or large-group involvement

3. Match the resident to the task.
4. Assess outcome, and make necessary adjustments to ensure success.

Process

Adapt the following suggestions and create your own activities:

1. Service activities focused on cognitive abilities and skills:
   Select food coupons and cut out for staff to use
   Put together picture files for the activity department
   Create a scrapbook for the children's hospital
   Bake cookies for other residents
   Color pictures for kindergarten students
2. Service activities focused on physical abilities and skills:
   Tear paper for an animal kennel
   Walk trails in a nature center, picking up sticks and trash
   Plant and tend to flowers in a community area
   Dust and replace books in a library
   Shine silver, candlesticks, and so on.
   Unknot socks, twine, yarn
   Fold church bulletins or information for a mailing, stuff envelopes
3. Service activities focused on psychosocial abilities and skills:
   Set up a desk for resident greeter in a facility area
   Develop and implement a resident volunteer auxiliary, using name tags,
       pins reflecting hours served, recognition functions
   Plan and share a party for others

NEIGHBORLY CELEBRATIONS: PRIDE IN ACTIVITIES OF HOSPITALITY

Purpose

To facilitate the resident's pride and ongoing gift of offering hospitality enabled by socially focused activities

Essentials

1. Involve residents as much as possible in all aspects of the activity, using adaptations, simplifications, and identifying which parts are appropriately done by individuals independently, one-to-one, or in small or large groups.
2. Hospitality components:
   Planning and anticipation
   Sending invitations

Preparations (e.g., cleaning, decorating, food preparation, setting up party
   area)
Greeting guests
Event
Showing appreciation and closure
Cleaning up
"Thanks for coming" activities and reminiscing

Process

1. Ideas:
   Theme parties (e.g., seasons of the year, ethnic celebrations, senior prom,
      country fair, back to school, Special Olympics, hat day, clown day, hon-
      oring staff party, pajama party [it's fun])
   Family and intergenerational parties
   Teas (ask for donations and use real china and teapot)
   Holidays, holy days
   Seasonal celebrations (e.g., start of baseball season, Halloween, first day of
      spring, start of fall, snowman building party, longest day of the year, birth-
      days, anniversaries)
   "Let's go visit the shut-ins" (other facility residents)
   Traveling choir (e.g., sing to the bookkeeper, administrator)
2. Remember: keep it simple, short, and fun.

ORDINARY AND ORDERLY: PRIDE IN ACTIVITIES OF HOMEMAKING

Purpose

To be actively engaged in familiar, lifelong tasks central to everyday living that
facilitate memories to be revisited with pride

Essentials

1. Assess the selected activity for ability to modify and simplify, safety, and outcome, and match the activity to the resident's abilities, attention span, and
   interest.
2. Use familiar and repetitious activities that respond to the resident's long-term
   memory and past involvement.
3. Approach the activity by saying, for example, "This is really a mess, can you
   help me sort this silverware? I really need your help" or "I haven't had time to
   fold this laundry. Would you be willing to give me a hand?"

Process

1. Ideas:
   Folding wash, fabrics, baby clothes, ribbons, scarves, napkins, neckties
   Rolling underwear for placement in a drawer or footlocker-type tray
   Sweeping, dusting, washing, wiping, doing dishes, cooking
   Hanging up clothing, placing costume jewelry into sectioned boxes
   Matching socks, lids of various sizes for plastic containers
   Winding yarn
   Sanding wood
   Sorting very large nuts and bolts, silverware, cloth loops for pot holder crafts
      by color, tongue depressors from popsicle sticks, two or three sets of play-
      ing cards, pictures of various categories into sets (e.g., flowers, animals,
      cars)
2. Always thank the resident for helping, offering praise for the task done and
   validating his or her importance to you.

ON THE JOB: PRIDE IN ACTIVITIES OF LIFE'S WORK

Purpose

To build opportunities of pride reflecting the resident's participation and role in
life's work, formal and informal

Essentials

1. Identify resident's life family roles (e.g., sister, grandmother, uncle, aunt).
2. Identify resident's life work roles (e.g., boss, secretary, chemist, gardener,
   homemaker, cabdriver, military).
3. Choose elements of the role or work that favorably enable the resident's abilities and safety.
4. Simplify or adapt the activity to ensure success, using creativity and flexibility.
5. Assess before and after the "On the Job" activity, making necessary changes
   to the activity, approaches, timing, and so on.
6. Reflect on the activity with the resident, validating his or her former role and
   life work.

Process

1. Examples of activities and materials to enable pride in a job well done:
   Desk with files, drawers, office supplies
   Simple, safe machinery that can be taken apart and reassembled

Brochures to study, "place order" (e.g., car, home decorating, crafts, flowers, hardware)

Large, safe, and stackable items, often appealing to farmers and construction workers (e.g., plastic patio chairs, plastic cartons, rose cones)

Use videotapes of work (e.g., construction, fire engines)

Build busy boards of familiar hardware items that can be turned, unscrewed, etc.

Baseball cards for trading

Military insignia to sort and talk about

Use reminiscing boxes filled with work and hobby-related safe items (e.g., fishing, gardening, car care, house decorating, kitchen, sewing, travel, carpentry, farming, banking, bookkeeping)

Exercise equipment for a "workout club"

A9-6
Community Partnership Example Letter: Creating Meaningful Activity Opportunities for Nursing Home Residents

The following is an example of a letter that can be sent to community groups to foster support for nursing home residents' activities.

Dear Community Group,

Nursing homes are places to live; few residents are seriously ill. Research shows that close to 60% of all nursing home residents have dementia, mostly of the Alzheimer's type. These residents have limited memory, are often unable to wash, dress, or feed themselves, and can wander and be unsafe. However, residents with dementia maintain the same needs you and I have—to feel in control, to have a purposeful use of time, and to be loved and accepted.

The challenge, therefore, is to enable residents to be all that they can be within their ability level. They need to live in a community of acceptance that supports the contributions they are capable of and does not draw attention to their limitations.

Meaningful, purposeful activities provide the opportunities to involve the resident and bring the resident success. An activity should meet the following criteria:

• Meets the resident's needs: cognitive, physical, and psychosocial

- Focuses on the resident's ability
- Can be broken down into simple steps, modified, or adapted to ensure success
- Can be done independently, with assistance on a one-to-one basis, in a small group, or in a large group
- Is safe for the resident and for others

Residents with dementia are able to respond to activities that are familiar, simple, and repetitious. Activities based on past learning are seldom forgotten. Often, the most successful and accepted are "normalization" activities. These are task- or work-related activities that residents would be doing if they were living in their own homes. Folding wash, wiping tables, polishing shoes, sorting through the mail, or putting away silverware are examples. The residents want to "help."

Adapting activities and gathering materials for normalization activities requires time, patience, and love. Many of the projects are unavailable or too expensive to purchase. However, needed supplies, for example, neckties, socks, and pictures, are often easily donated.

Nursing homes need your support and help. Perhaps your church, synagogue, club, school, or civic group can make or gather the suggested items or equipment. In return, our Alzheimer's care center can offer you educational programs and volunteer opportunities. The ideas for meaningful activities are flexible and are opportunities for your creativity. They will present a challenge that will be received by the nursing home resident with great thankfulness.

MEANINGFUL ACTIVITIES FOR NURSING HOME RESIDENTS

Directions for activity project ideas to be made or put together from everyday items are listed below. Always keep safety in mind—some of the listed activities can only be used with supervision if the parts are too small.

1. Scrapbooks
   Scrapbooks are a great activity that can be enjoyed alone or with others, especially with a visitor or family member.
   Use a three-ring binder for the book.
   Cut up old or new file folders for pages.
   Select bright pictures that are easy to see.
   Be creative—use scripture verses, a map and travel picture, pictures of famous people, past and present, an old fashioned recipe, etc.
   Print a phrase under some of the pictures that would be descriptive or interesting to read; use a dark pen.
   Make a scrapbook based on a theme (e.g., winter, summer, school, travel).
2. Busy boxes
   Busy boxes are used by the resident to look at the items, hold them, sort them, etc. They help to distract the anxious resident and can also be used for low-functioning residents that cannot participate in more complex tasks.
   Use a sturdy shoe box or other box that will fit on a lap.

Put in items of interest: be sure they are safe, not small enough to be swallowed, and nontoxic.

Ideas for items: small balls of yarn, artificial flowers, bows, little jewelry boxes, costume jewelry, pot holder, small stuffed animal, large seashells, egg beater, sponge.

3. Reminiscing kits (see Appendix 9-2)

4. Poker chips

Covered poker chips are a great sorting task and can be used as a very simple activity, using just a few chips or a few patterns, or as a more complex activity.

Cover poker chips with contact paper; glue onto each chip to be sure it sticks.

Make 10–12 chips of each color or pattern.

5. Adapted bingo

Simplifying bingo by color and shape allows the resident to succeed.

Make bingo cards requiring four, six, or eight shapes.

Use 3×5 cards for each shape that will be selected.

Use a colored 3×5 card to "cover" the shape when residents have the one drawn.

Use poster board for the game board.

Plain colored contact paper is the best for the shapes because it does not fade as construction paper sometimes does.

6. Fabric boxes

Boxes containing pieces of fabric can be used for reminiscing or just sorting through, to be touched or stroked, and folded.

Use a lap-sized box.

Cut or tear various fabric pieces small enough to fit in the box and large enough to feel with both hands.

Use a variety of textures, colors, patterns, old and new fabrics (e.g., wool, burlap, drapery, old flannel shirt piece, lace).

7. Beanbags

Beanbags can be used for games, catching, and so forth.

Use strong fabrics, make bags large but able to be held comfortably in one hand.

Double sew all seams.

8. Matching and sorting colored file cards

This can be used as an "office work" activity.

Use file cards or colored paper in two or three different sizes.

Purchase a desk-type file box or similar realistic-type place that the cards can be sorted into.

9. Picture files—categories

Picture files can be used for reminiscing or sorting.

Purchase pocket file folders to hold pictures.

Label each folder (e.g., transportation, food, people, sports, kitchen).

Clip pictures from magazines, calendars, and so on.

10. Dominoes

Dominoes is a familiar game that can be simplified by the number of cards, players, and other modifications.

Make dominoes from file cards (e.g., a 4×6-in. card cut into thirds).

Mark each card to resemble a domino with a permanent marker, large dots.

11. Busy board with hardware

A busy board with hardware is a great activity for men.

Use a heavy piece of plywood 2 ft×3 ft.

Affix to the board safe hardware-type items that can be manipulated (e.g., door latches, door bolts, faucet).

All items must attach to the board in some way, even the parts, so they are not lost.

12. Flash cards

Flash cards can be used for word and math games.

Make cards of simple and complicated addition, division, multiplication, and subtraction problems.

Use 5×8 file cards and bold, black permanent pen.

13. Apron with many pockets

An apron with many pockets can be worn by the resident in a wheelchair.

Sew on bright pockets with safe items attached on a tape within each pocket that can be pulled out, looked at, and stuffed back in (e.g., yarn doll, artificial flower, pretty handkerchief).

14. Decorative pillows for beds with name tag sign

Residents with dementia have problems remembering which room is theirs; seeing their name outside the bedroom door often does not mean to them that the room is theirs.

A pretty, simple 14- to 16-in. pillow on the bed with their name on it might be the clueing they need to recognize their room.

Each pillow would have a felt name tag large enough so the first name could be written clearly with a permanent pen. This could snap or button into place so the name could be changed if needed.

15. Sorting activities

Sorting activities are perhaps some of the most meaningful activities because they are familiar.

If possible, the containers that the items are to be sorted into should be realistic, for example:

A laundry basket for socks; vary the sizes and colors

A simple box with rubber bands for playing cards

A kitchen plastic drawer bin for silverware

Bins for bolts

A box with a lid for buttons (small buttons can be sewn together with a strong thread or plastic fishing line, for safety)

A9-7
*Community Partnership and Collaborating Forces to Enhance Quality of Life: Much More Than Just Entertainment**

Although the thought of a resident chorus has often proved to be powerful and empowering, who would have thought that it could be so magical? Or, should it be asked, how could a performance group be so meaningful to persons with Alzheimer's disease?

Many have the misconception that persons with Alzheimer's disease are no longer able to participate in ongoing projects, such as a choral performance group. Some argue that residents with Alzheimer's-type dementia are unable to remember or retain what was rehearsed from week to week, let alone acknowledge that they are members of this special chorus.

In working within today's philosophy of activity-focused care, caregivers are reminded to focus on the strengths and abilities of their residents. Caregivers strive to find successful and meaningful outlets for each person on his or her own individual level, rather than emphasizing the negative or, worse yet, simply providing camp-like activities that hold little value or meaning.

It has been proved time and time again that music allows persons with Alzheimer's disease to participate successfully in the here and now. Music can be molded and designed to create an atmosphere free from failure, and music-based programming can heighten levels of both self-esteem and increased socialization. If music is truly one of the most effective interventions, why not form a performing

*With special thanks to Katherine J. Schellin, M.T.-B.C., and Sharyce Floss, A.D.C., assistant activity director of recreational therapy, The Wealshire, Lincolnshire, Illinois.

group of residents diagnosed with Alzheimer's-type dementia? If residents are treated as if they no longer have the ability to be included in a choir, they will in turn create their disability. If residents are encouraged to strive for achievement in such a group, they will display their own ability and accomplish their own success.

Performance groups, such as a resident chorus, can become a motivation to individuals with dementia. A performance group can assist residents in finding a life purpose. Residents can feel a sense of pride for belonging to an organization, reaping multiple benefits, including increased motivation, feelings of accomplishment and gratification, and a heightened sense of pride and belonging, all of which contribute to a sense of empowerment and self-respect.

In 1996, a choir called the Swingin' Singers was formed at The Wealshire in Lincolnshire, Illinois. This facility was one of the first of its kind offering a continuum of care for persons with dementia. Therefore, the choir was composed solely of persons with dementia at varying levels of abilities and inabilities. The goals of the choir were to create a truly meaningful, worthwhile group joining voices together in a chorus as one. Allowing for a successful, musical experience, increased socialization, increased self-esteem, and a heightened sense of self-respect and pride, the group began rehearsals and discussions of favorite musicals, including songs, styles, and artists.

Once the theme was arrived at, the magic began. First was a show on the history of Rodgers and Hammerstein musicals. Residents were asked to reflect on favorite shows and selections, memories were shared remembering attendance to those events, and historical data, collected by the music therapist, tied it all together. Residents read details from a script regarding the history of how shows, such as "Oklahoma" and "The Sound of Music," came to be. Two residents sang solos from "The King and I" and "Carousel." Staff created billboard signs to announce the different shows. Others danced to familiar melodies, such as "Give My Regards to Broadway," and together, with the residents, united as a team. It was a huge success.

Following this exciting debut, requests came from the administration for future performances. The Swingin' Singers performed for such events as the Fourth of July "Star Spangled Celebration" and the second anniversary party of The Wealshire. The success of these performances gave birth to the idea of an even bigger event: a collaboration of efforts between two different care facilities. Why not combine the talents of two separate facility choral groups to join as one? How inspiring and meaningful to join forces and increase opportunities for socialization, and what an incredible boost for residents' self-respect and self-esteem.

In this era of contractual creative arts therapists, the music therapist from The Wealshire, also contracting services to Gidwitz Place/Weinberg, a facility of The Council for Jewish Elderly, was able to begin rehearsals on an identical repertoire. Rehearsals began for an exhilarating show, a "Radio Days" musical extravaganza. Each rehearsal consisted of practicing a variety of old, familiar songs heard on the radio when radio was the number one form of entertainment. Rehearsals became part of the process. The emphasis was never on the techniques or actual performance of the task, but rather on the totality of the process being a fun, musically stimulating, and fulfilling experience.

After weeks of rehearsals, a script was added by staff members and residents to create an atmosphere of an old-time radio show. What began as an adventurous "experiment" became a top-notch musical extravaganza with all the trimmings. The two separate choirs rehearsed as one over a 2-month period and became adept with the nuances of each individual singing troop. Voila! Success and self-esteem, dedication to the "show must go on" philosophy, and magnificent pride in a job well done became the results of hard work from all concerned.

To underestimate any special population is counterproductive. The goals of all professionals should be to reach for the highest star and let naysayers wallow with less. Collaboration between different disciplines and separate facilities is not only realistic, but the way of the future. Combining a variety of talents and resources produces powerful outcomes that should be considered viable and valuable for true excellence in therapeutic programming of the future.

A9-8
*Activity Therapist Job Description Example**

Objectives:
Our objective is to remember at all times that each resident at The Wealshire is entitled to respect and the very best care available. By providing a stimulating, interesting, pertinent, and therapeutic activity agenda, we convey that respect. We make tangible the intangible concept of activity-based care.

Position Summary:
The activity therapist is an integral part of the team approach to resident care at The Wealshire, emphasizing quality programming and varied activity implementation under the guidance of the director of recreational therapy (DRT) or the assistant director of recreational therapy (ADRT).

Education and Experience:
Some college is preferred, as well as activity-related work experience.

Job Responsibilities:
The activity therapist has the following responsibilities:

- Daily implementation of activities at The Wealshire
- Individualization of activities to meet the specific needs of each resident
- Activity assessment and timely updates for the assigned residents
- Continued fine tuning of activities to optimize resident participation and enjoyment
- Obtaining knowledge about each resident from the resident, family members, other staff, observations, and records to assist in a comprehensive program plan
- Documentation of attendance and the use of such records to assess resident participation
- Sharing pertinent resident information with other staff members in an effort to enhance the team approach to care
- Brainstorming with other activity staff and the DRT/ADRT to constantly improve, facilitate, and invigorate activities at The Wealshire

---

*Courtesy of The Wealshire, Lincolnshire, Illinois.

- Assisting in scheduling new activities, special functions, holidays, etc., with the ADRT
- Instructing volunteers, new staff members, and any staff members as to the activity-based care concept and demonstrating specific techniques when appropriate
- Providing information to family members about resident progress in activities and soliciting advice when necessary to aid in resident participation
- Providing information to the DRT or the ADRT on the status of activities and their success or failure in an effort to provide excellence throughout the entire activity program
- Maintaining and organizing supplies and communicating supply needs to the DRT
- Assisting special-function staff and entertainers
- Escorting residents to the activity location or taking the activity to the resident
- Accompanying residents on special outings
- Representing the activity department during care plan conferences and therefore maintaining up-to-date information on each resident assigned to the activity staff member
- Attending inservices, seminars, and any learning opportunity requested by the DRT
- Providing the liaison necessary between all other staff and the DRT/ADRT with regard to residents' needs, desires, limitations, abilities, and individualization

A9-9
*Activity Therapy Care Conference Report Form**

Resident: _____ Date: _____

Staffperson: _____

Activity Component	Activity Example	Therapeutic Value	Implementation
Cognitive			
Physical			
Psychosocial			
Spiritual			
Music			
One-to-one			
Small groups			
Large groups			
Special programs			
Other			

*Courtesy of The Wealshire, Lincolnshire, Illinois.

A9-10
*Activity Therapy Care Conference Report Form Information: Therapeutic Value**

Listed are examples of activities and their possible therapeutic benefits.

Active games: Physical wellness, opportunity to increase body awareness, feeling of being in control, enjoyment in participation, possibility of being a team member and making a contribution

Beauty shop: Feeling validated, enjoyment of one-to-one attention, past life-role opportunity, opportunity to reminisce, pride, feeling attractive, opportunity to receive compliments from others

Bingo: Fun, remembered past activity of enjoyment, cognitive stimulation, opportunity to increase attention span, excitement connected with the possibility of winning, feeling equal to all the other participants (equal chance of winning), being part of a group of peers

Crafts and hobbies: Stimulus for creativity, sense of purpose and accomplishment, joy in the process and the completed project, validation, feeling needed, pride, display of past life talents

Cooking and baking: Sensory stimulation, cognitive challenges, joy in past life roles, sense of purpose and accomplishment, reminiscing, pride in the process and the finished product, opportunity to share with others and to reinforce hospitality abilities

Creative arts: Enjoyment, cognitive stimulation, creativity opportunity, pride in accomplishment, joy in participation, reminiscing, display of past life roles or talents

*Special thanks to Rachel Field, activity therapist, The Wealshire, Lincolnshire, Illinois.

Dance and movement: Physical wellness, increased body awareness, joy in active participation, feeling in control, ability to make choices, reminiscing, reminders of past life roles and experiences

Entertainment and special events: Reminiscing, delight in being entertained, cognitive stimulation, sensory stimulation, fun in participating in a special event, increased socialization, being part of a peer group sharing pleasure

Exercise and fitness: Physical wellness, increased body awareness, feeling in control, sense of accomplishment, awareness of positive outcomes, general well-being

Family or friend visit: Feeling special, validation, reminiscing, pride, feelings of belonging, joy in being accepted, opportunity to be a host or hostess, awareness of being a person of worth

Gardening: Sense of accomplishment, joy in nurturing, pride, purposefulness, reminiscing, connection with past life experiences, delight in seeing and enjoying the end product, opportunity to share with others the end product, pride in the process

Ice cream social: Area to exchange friendship and socialization, an activity of comfort, reminiscing opportunity, good arena for storytelling, opportunity to be a host or hostess by serving others, friendly place to entertain family and grandchildren

Intellectual and educational gatherings: Intellectual stimulation, being validated, reminiscing, opportunity to share ideas and hear other residents' opinions, feeling connected to the past

Intergenerational groups: Joy in being needed, accepted, being able to give and offer wisdom, being able to give and receive affection, pride and self-esteem remembered from past life's roles

Ladies' group: Reminiscing, pride, and self-esteem from past life roles and positions; delight in sharing stories and comparing experiences; feelings of being validated, safe arena to tell "ladies'" stories and experiences; pleasure in being a "member of the club"

Massage and relaxation: Relaxation and sense of well-being, reduction of stress, reduction of agitation, enjoyment in being touched, validation of self

Men's group: Reminiscing, pride from past accomplishments, esteem from past life roles and positions, safe arena to joke and tell "men's" stories and jokes, opportunity to discuss subjects of interest, such as sports and military experiences, feelings of being validated

Movie: Delight in being entertained, feeling part of a group and sense of belonging, challenged to think and follow the story line, sensory stimulus, encouraged attention span, relaxation

Music program: Reminiscing, provides enjoyment, sense of comfort and well-being, delight in the familiar, feelings of being connected with others, sensory stimulation

News and views: Intellectual stimulation, feeling "in the know," past normalization activity, participation in a past ritual (daily) type activity, opportunity to share opinions

Normalization activities: Sense of purpose, reminiscing, enjoyment of normalcy, joy from remembered past task, feeling of accomplishment and pride, sense of having worth

One-to-one: Feeling validated as a person of worth, intimacy of someone's undivided attention, arena to share feelings and thoughts, sense of companionship

Outdoor walking group: Sensory stimulation, opportunity to engage in physical well-being, feelings of freedom, reminiscing, joy in active participation, past lifestyle engagement

Percussion or drum circle: Opportunity to express emotions in an acceptable medium, feeling connected with the music, being part of a group, arena to express creativity

Pet care and therapy: Opportunity to nurture, arena to give and receive affection, sense of purpose, reminiscing, past normalization activity involvement, feelings of purpose, possibility of reducing stress and encouraging relaxation, feeling of being needed

Reading and writing: Intellectual stimulation, sense of accomplishment, joy from the remembered past, opportunity to reminisce, purposefulness, pride

Religious activities: Normality, togetherness and being part of a community, opportunity to remember past traditions and rituals, feelings of wellness and acceptance, feeling loved

Reminiscence: Opportunity to share stories and emotions, enjoyment in sharing about past life history and roles, feeling validated, pride in the past, pride in individuality, opportunity to receive support and caring over past life's difficulties

Resident volunteer: Feeling helpful, sense of pride and purpose, being needed, validated, joy in participating in past life roles or opportunities, feeling connected to a task of meaning

Self-initiated activity: Opportunity for self-motivation, sense of well-being, able to make choices, sense of being in control, accomplishment

Sensory stimulation: Opportunity to activate the senses, possibility of encouragement for basic responses, reminiscing, enjoyment of past life's experiences, validation, opportunity for one-to-one stimulation

Storytelling: Pride in being listened to, validation, reminiscing, enjoyment of past life experiences, feelings of creativity, accomplishment, delight in being the center of attention

Swingin' singers (performing group of residents): Pride, delight in being part of the group, sense of participation, excitement of performing for others, validation, opportunity for socialization and friendship, sense of community, overall well-being, accomplishment, delight in being the center of attention and having the ability to please others

Table games: Socialization, physical exercise, mental stimulation, joy in participation, reminiscing, delight in fun experiences from the past, fun of winning,
possibility of being a team player, excitement of competition

Tea and talk: Socialization, cognitive stimulation, opportunity to increase polite-
ness and listening skills, feeling part of a group, opportunity to share ideas, comfortable activity, joy from remembered past experiences

10

Expressions of Intimacy: Giving and Receiving Affection

Last night I heard an owl call my name
As a curtain of darkness descended from the sky
The gust of wind suddenly so still
Could it have been an owl who softly called Mil?

Perhaps it was my own beloved Joe
Remembering that I was his wife
Had his curtain of darkness lifted for a while
Did thinking of me bring back his wonderful smile?

Ah, Joe, what could God have had in mind
When you were robbed of all that once was you
Your intellect, your kindness and your giving
All the things that made our lives worth living

We can't give up but must go on instead
There is still so much that you, Joe, have to offer
With head held high you are a special man
I'll do my best to help you all I can

—Mildred Goodman Sampson,
Where Are You Joe? Losing a Love to Alzheimer's
(Self-published, 1997)

Mildred Sampson goes on to say in her writing, "Where Are You, Joe? Losing a Love to Alzheimer's," that "Intimacy is a private, highly personal feeling. Intimacy, at one time in our lives, was all consuming. Without explanation, each of us knew what the other was feeling; two souls with matching heartbeats."

The desire to be called by name and to receive smiles and kindness are all involved in the giving and receiving of affection. Mutual well-being is supported within the capacity of each person involved. Uniqueness is honored and vulnerability becomes a sacrament. Intimacy can have many definitions and expectations.

311

The intimacy between devoted spouses, supportive and loving adult children and their parent, friends reaching out to friends, as well as caring professionals for their residents, provides multiple meanings to the word "intimacy." The need to alter or vary the involved feelings and demonstrations of intimacy is challenged because the experience of dementia is a shared journey.

Intimacy is the sharing of one's deepest self with another, appreciating each others' uniqueness, vulnerability, gifts, and well-being.

Sexuality is the seeking of intimacy and connectedness, the desire for physical closeness and the uniting of attitudes, feelings, and behaviors. It includes sexual identity, the desire for closeness with others, and an inner closeness that calls forth one's personhood.

Expressions of intimacy and sexuality continue throughout one's life despite losses, illness, and life's circumstances, including the world around oneself and the world within. The giving and receiving of affection, starting with the mother and child relationship, evolves to include family, friends, peers, and lovers. In Mildred's beautiful tribute to Joe, she shares continued intimacy with him by being the "rememberer."

Always, there is heartfelt vulnerability, the possibility of loss, the chance of being misinterpreted. The basic calling to belong, to be desired, to share oneself with another is not diminished because of Alzheimer's disease. The boundaries of the need for intimacy may take on new shapes due to the cognitive losses, but deep within the expressions of intimacy, the desire to give and receive affection remains.

INCLUSIVENESS OF INTIMACY

We are all touched by and involved in the intimate aspects of day-to-day living. When a loved one is affected by Alzheimer's disease, undoubtedly the past definition of intimacy will be revised.

Married couples usually experience a change in their relationship as they journey together during the dementing illness of one of them. Roles change, blur, and at times become reversed. Losses are experienced and emotional responses can vary from love to anger. Often, there is little or no emotional or physical strength left after the basics of caregiving are attended to. Some couples weather the redefinition of their intimate relationship with limited stress. Others find the changes brought on by forgetfulness and self-centeredness experienced by the partner with dementia an overwhelming producer of loneliness (see Appendix 10-1).

As care moves to the nursing home, couples can experience continued challenges and changes to their previous marital relationship. The spouse with dementia may "find" a new intimate companion, perhaps due to a limited ability to remember his or her loved one (see Appendix 10-2). The sadness of visiting one's spouse can be escalated when he or she prefers the company of another resident and walks away. Difficult sexual behaviors may develop, causing the spouse and family possible embarrassment and concerns.

Other family members can have similar experiences. Adult children, grandchildren, and family friends can be devastated by the sexual or intimate acting out of their loved one. Fear of a possible requested discharge from the facility due to sexual behaviors concerns families.

Offering families a safe arena to talk about their loved one's expressions of intimacy can occur during the plan-of-care conferences. The implementation of expressions of intimacy guidelines (see Appendix 10-3) involve appropriate family members and the staff in decision making. The choices made by families can be discussed and a plan developed for their implementation whenever possible.

Family education provides opportunities for further insight and a forum for a realistic assessment of the situation and learning of appropriate interventions.

INTIMACY-RELATED RESPONSES: ENABLING STRENGTHS AND DIMINISHING CHALLENGES

Seeking intimacy is a basic human need. The giving and receiving of affection calls us forth to share in humanity. Dementia may alter the expressions of intimacy but the basic components of self-acceptance and desire to connect with others remains.

"Being intimate" with a person with dementia certainly does not mean jumping into bed together and having sex. Intimacy is in the mind of the beholder: the caregiver and the care receiver. The use of caring touch and nurturing is the cornerstone. Hugs; hand holding; rubbing of shoulders; applying lotion to arms, legs, and feet; gentle fingers smoothing the cheeks and forehead are all components of the intimacy of touch acceptance and belonging.

The essence of intimacy is also fostered in the realm of personal respect. Mutual tenderness, comfort, security, warmth, and communication are expressions of intimacy. Perhaps intimacy is found in allowing a thought to be expressed and completed without interruption or listening with full attention and facial support. Asking a question and waiting for the response brings forth the intimacy of valuing the resident's answer. Letting emotions be expressed and having feelings validated is the intimacy of having worth. The joy of the everyday found in meaningful activity, as well as shared memories, reduces loneliness and celebrates even the most simple connection between two persons. Intimate family moments and the communion of shared foods can often call forth the resident's abilities to enact a most basic essence of personhood, the intimacy of hospitality. Expressions of intimacy can facilitate and support a positive, affirming quality of life and joy in the sacredness of the everyday.

Residents with dementia can experience many benefits derived from the presence and awareness of intimacy in their lives: cognitive, physical, and emotional benefits (see Appendix 10-4). Examples of these types of benefits are as follows:

1. *Cognitive benefits*: A sense of well-being and normalcy, increased orientation to self, projected meaningfulness to life, encouragement of verbal and non-verbal responses, facilitation of social skills and stimulation of choices, enabling of reminiscing of enjoyed experiences and traditions from the past
2. *Physical benefits*: Outlet for caring touch to be given and received; promotion of sensory stimulation; positive energy outlet from being with another resident and walking, dancing; a link to reality
3. *Psychosocial and emotional benefits*: Increased confidence and self-esteem; feelings of being valued, pride experienced in being wanted or selected; having approval from others; feeling of being in control; sexually attractive, wanted and desired

As with all human experiences, expressions of intimacy can have a negative effect on the resident, leading to challenging responses. Examples are as follows:

1. *Cognitive challenges and risks*: Increased awareness of losses, decreased memory of appropriate social responses and boundaries that may add to overall confusion and disorientation, misunderstanding of the need for privacy for self and others, misunderstanding or misinterpretation of verbal or nonverbal responses from others may be perceived as an invasion of personal space
2. *Physical challenges and risks*: Inappropriate touching or physically invading the personal space of another resident, possible display of aggressive or combative behavior when frustrated or unable to display affection
3. *Psychosocial and emotional challenges or risks*: Feelings of inadequacy, increased stimulation of jealous responses, paranoia, depression, increased attempts to control others

USING AN INTIMACY PROFILE

Residents with dementia bring caregivers a past rich with experiences, strengths, and weaknesses. Information obtained before admission enables the staff to be prepared with an accountable plan of care. The plan will need constant revising, but the resident's past remains the same. The LifeStory Book (Chapter 3) can provide a wealth of information and acts as a rudder steering the way into the moving changes of dementia.

Asking family members for information about their loved one's giving and receiving of affection and expressions of intimacy reflects the understanding that sexuality is a continuing human expression and need. An intimacy profile (see Appendix 10-5) should be part of the pre-admission procedure when program or health care placement is being considered. Sensitivity should be used when talking with families about their loved one's sexuality and intimacy history. Obviously, asking them to tell you about their mother's sex life may be embarrassing and repugnant to the family. An intimacy profile can ease the process if caregivers are uncomfortable with discussing details.

> Ernie's penis was erect for 4 days. The staff did not know how to handle the situation and were refusing to go into his room to provide care. Very soon, Ernie's penis was the topic of conversation throughout the facility. It was decided to send Ernie to the community hospital's psychiatry unit. On arrival, a physician assessed the situation. Ernie had a penile implant that had become blocked. After treatment from a urologist, Ernie was returned to the facility. Ernie had not been able to tell the staff what was causing his erection. His niece had forgotten to report the implant during her uncle's admission. The admission procedure had not included any intimacy-related questions.

The profile will provide information on current responses to intimacy and behaviors as well as offer valuable data for reminiscing. If difficult behaviors have been experienced in the past, it is helpful to gain as much understanding and information about them to possibly avoid their continuance. For example:

> Millie slept in a double bed with her husband for 57 years. Since his death and the onset of Alzheimer's disease, Millie wanders at night in the nursing home and often climbs into bed with George. Having read Millie's intimacy profile, the staff realized, based on her years of marriage, that she was probably seeking a companion to share her bed. When a body pillow was placed in bed with Millie, she was content and appeared to feel that it was similar to the presence of a sleeping partner.

In a residential setting where the emphasis is on high-touch caring, the intimacy profile uses personal insights to call forth the resident's abilities and can also be a tool for refocusing challenging or difficult responses. The intimacy profile, when completed at the time of admission, becomes an integral instrument in the development of the resident's overall plan of quality care.

MASTURBATION: SELF-DIRECTED INTIMACY AND CAREGIVING INTERVENTIONS

"Solo sex" is another name for masturbation, fondling, rubbing, or stripping for self-exhibition. Personal values may lead some persons to unequivocally announce that any form of self-stimulation is wrong. Certainly, masturbation and its issues are subjects for discussion and educational consideration. The questions to ponder are what are the benefits to the resident involved in masturbation and what are the negative aspects. Perhaps the resident is bored and lonely and self-stimulation feels good. Masturbation may be a ploy to attract attention. Self-directed intimacy may be an activity of reminiscence bringing forth fond memories from the past.

Recommendations for responding to the masturbating resident are as follows:

1. Move the resident, without any shaming or teasing, from a public place to one of personal privacy so masturbation can continue if the resident chooses.
2. What is the rubbing "saying"? Check for a possible urinary tract infection, rash, clothing that is too tight, possible bladder prolapse, prostate problems, and discomfort due to position.
3. Check for safety from the use of objects, which may be used by women for masturbation (e.g., spoons or a call light).
4. Should ejaculation occur, use precautions for high-risk body fluids.
5. If masturbation continues for a considerable length of time or reoccurs every time the resident is not involved in activities of daily living, use a behavior observation form (see Appendix 8-2). Determine if there are antecedents, such as noise, specific other residents in the area, pre- or post-family visits, television show, and so forth, that might be triggering the continuous masturbation. Discuss the resident's medications with his or her physician. Develop a

plan of care as an appropriate response if self-directed intimacy is precipitating a medical problem (e.g., raw skin areas).

At times, the resident who is masturbating can respond to being distracted and will become involved in another activity. Suggestions for redirection are

1. Relocation to another place may be effective if an assessment of the current location where the masturbation is occurring has been made. For example, move resident from a noisy place to a quiet place.
2. Offer food, drink, or an interesting activity that calls for the resident's active participation.
3. Cover up the groin area to discourage touching—sort of "out of sight, out of mind." Examples:

   • Placing a lap board or a pillow over the resident's groin.
   • Using a plastic athletic cup supporter to "hide" the resident's scrotum and penis.
   • Attaching suspenders to slacks, skirt, or underwear to make it more difficult for the resident to strip off his or her clothing. This can be especially effective if suspenders are worn under the top layer of clothing but over underwear.
   • Filling a "fanny pack" with "yummies," interesting items to touch, hold, and fondle, such as cookies, in hopes that zipping the bag open and closed and removing the goodies may distract the resident from the genitals (place the bag over the groin area).

4. Residents may become distracted if they wear a bracelet of bells that sounds when the wrist is moved as the resident reaches for the genital area.
5. Select clothing that is difficult to take off. Do not put clothing on backwards that was not meant to be worn that way. A belt can be slid around to the back side of the resident rather than opening in the front. Overalls for either men or women can be effective.
6. Dress the resident in many layers, if he or she will not become overheated, to discourage stripping. For example, a slip over a T-shirt, a button-down-the-front blouse, a sleeveless sweater, and a sports jacket.
7. "Bridge" stripping activity by placing six to eight T-shirts on a doll or teddy bear and asking the resident to "strip" the doll or bear (see glossary at the end of this book).
8. If appropriate, consider X-rated movies or magazines as distractions.

OVERT OR HYPERSEXUALITY: ISSUES AND CAREGIVING INTERVENTIONS

Residents with dementia may exhibit intense interest in sexual activity, perhaps due to diminished ability to interpret their surroundings because of changes in their brain tissue, interpret the interest or actions of others, and appropriately comprehend their own emotional drives. The overly sexual interest may be targeted toward another resident, a family member, including spouse, other family members, or a staffperson. Difficulties arise when the persistent sexual behavior precipitates anger, disgust, confusion, or anxiety in others.

Possible causes or situations that trigger the resident to respond sexually include

- Medications that may increase the libido
- Fatigue, disruption of sleep patterns
- Need to go to the bathroom
- Loss of judgment, misinterpretation of people or the environment, or both
- Prostate problems
- Bladder or uterus prolapse
- Clothing that is uncomfortable, too tight, or wet
- Longing for touch, to have past memories fulfilled once again
- Past lifestyle responses

Examples of hypersexual responses are

- Grabbing, undressing self or another person, being naked in public places or exposing oneself inappropriately during daily caregiving
- Sexual gestures, masturbation, or remarks with sexual language content
- Insistent touching and fondling or forced bodily contact, including sexual activity
- Writing sexual words or drawing genitals on walls or in books
- Urinating or defecating in inappropriate places

> Agnes, age 73 years, would propel her wheelchair up to a man seated in the dining room awaiting his meal. She would reach over into his lap, unzip his pants, and fondle his genitals. At times, she attempted to perform oral sex. Distraction techniques were tried. For example, Agnes would be detained from entering the dining area until the food had arrived and the meal had started. She then shifted her sexual activity until after the meal was completed. Agnes would become angry and combative when she was pulled away from the man she had selected. The physician was notified and medications that were possibly increasing her libido were reduced. The staff began to involve Agnes in active exercise before meals so she was a bit tired and thirsty and therefore anxious for her own meal without stopping to be with a male resident. She also began to receive regular massage therapy that appeared to help satisfy her need to be touched.

Physicians contacted concerning situations of hypersexuality may try a course of medication to reduce anxiety or provide antilibidinal hormones.

Family support and education is usually necessary for dealing with hypersexuality issues. Family members can become fearful that their loved one will be asked to leave the caregiving setting. If hypersexuality occurs at home, family members should institute distraction techniques whenever possible. For example: John's wife of 54 years may need to say, "John, I know that you want to have sex with me this morning, but I am really hungry. Let's eat breakfast first." Perhaps, John will forget his sexual urges after a large breakfast and good walk. Alternatives to sexual intimacy, such as back rubs, dancing, and hugs, may help family members to cope.

Equally important, within a care setting, is staff education on handling the hypersexual resident, especially if the amorous attention is focused on them.

Caregiving suggestions include

I. Staff should establish a routine to use with a resident requesting sexual favors, touching, making sexual remarks, or using sexual gestures. Suggestions include the following:
A. Have a consistent approach for all staffpersons to use that includes the same words when addressing the resident.
B. If unacceptable behavior continues, use two staffpersons for the resident or use a caregiver of the other gender.
C. Plan ways to respond in emergency situations.
II. Be aware of verbal and nonverbal communications (e.g., how the caregiver uses his or her hands to touch, tone of voice, hand gestures, and eye contact).
III. Is the caregiver's clothing suggestive? Tight? Revealing? Appropriate for the position held as a hands-on caregiver?
IV. Help caregivers to monitor the use and position of their body during caregiving. For example:
A. Does the caregiver reach across the resident while assisting dressing, which causes her breast to be in easy reach?
B. When facing away from the resident to pick up an item, does the caregiver's "fanny" move into pinching or hitting range?

> Sally, the nursing assistant, reaches across Jim while he is stretched out in bed. She finishes pulling up his slacks and starts to zip them up and fasten the waist closure. Jim reaches out and squeezes Sally's breast. Sally responds by firmly telling Jim to stop touching her. By studying the antecedent to Jim's unwanted behavior, Sally realizes that she had inappropriately placed her breast within Jim's reach and that the touching of his slacks was being interpreted as a sexual advance. By repositioning herself more toward the bottom of the bed, she would have been out of his reach.

V. Make statements, not judgments, to the resident when his or her behavior is not acceptable. Scolding, arguing, teasing, or shaming are inappropriate responses that focus on the resident, not the behavior.
VI. When needed, define your role clearly (e.g., "Mr. Brown, I am your nursing assistant," "Mrs. O'Brien, touching me is not appropriate. Keep your hands to yourself, please," "Mr. Smith, stop, do not grab me").
VII. If possible, identify the antecedent or trigger that leads to inappropriate sexual behaviors. Consider
A. Time of the day or night
B. Activity (e.g., television, bathing before bedtime)

> Alex enjoyed more than 60 years of marriage with Esther. When she died, Alex entered a care center, and because of

Alzheimer's disease, he was placed in a special care unit. He was on the "P.M. bath schedule." During the bathing, he would reach out to stroke his caregiver's breast and tell her how he was looking forward to having intercourse with her. Having an evening shower before enjoying sex with his wife had always been Alex's pattern. Alex must have thought that since he always had the same caregiver, and always had his shower before going to bed, he therefore would like to have sex with this new person. Alex would become combative when his desires were not met. Changing his shower schedule to mornings helped to refocus this situation. Massage, men's activities, dressing Alex in clothing reminiscent of his former management position, and social parties helped to meet Alex's needs to give and receive affection and be proud of his maleness. This pride in his manliness was effective in reducing his need to "prove it."

    C. Environmental over- or understimulation
    D. Limited communication abilities: receptive and expressive
    E. Gender or cultural issues
    F. Inability to "read" the resident's nonverbal cues (e.g., limited facial expressions due to the Parkinson's-like symptom of facial masking or from medications)
    G. Agnosia (i.e., inability to integrate or the misinterpretation of information received through the senses)
VIII. Bathing hints for reducing sexual acting out:
    A. Bathe the resident with loose-fitting clothing on or wrap the resident in a large beach towel to allow the caregiver to keep the resident covered while bathing by reaching down from the top and up from the bottom.
    B. The caregiver places his or her hand over the resident's hand, and then by hooking the thumb to hold onto the resident's hand, guides the resident's hand when doing the genital area so the contact is between the resident's hand and his or her own body.
    C. Have safe objects for the resident to hold during bathing so he or she is less likely to grab the caregiver (e.g., a washcloth, empty plastic shampoo bottle, sponge).
  IX. Night wandering and looking for someone to crawl into bed with may be just a need for comfort, warmth, and the fulfillment of past memories of years of a shared bed with a loved one. If this activity becomes a problem, a body pillow placed in the bed at night may help to decrease the urge to seek companionship.
   X. Think ahead. For example:

Tony is verbally abusive and could be combative. MaryKay has recently started to make friends with Tony and they enjoy eating meals together. The staff observed that when MaryKay is with Tony, his behavior is more gentle. The activity department started to seat Tony and MaryKay together for programs because for the first time, Tony was not disruptive and appeared to be enjoying the activity. In between activities, the staff would encourage Tony and MaryKay to sit together. In other words, MaryKay had the ability to calm Tony down and reduce his difficult behaviors. Why, then, would the staff be shocked or surprised when they found Tony in MaryKay's bed? The staff had not really thought through the ramifications of their own needs to have Tony be an easier resident for caregiving.

In reality, hypersexuality occurring in residents with dementia is not very common. Because many caregivers are uncomfortable talking about or responding to expressions of intimacy, it is assumed that the resident is acting out or oversexed. Human nature may label the resident who is sexually acting out but is liked as "cute." However, the same behavior demonstrated by a disliked resident wins that person the label of "dirty old man." Behaviors are most often the resident's method of communication. This includes sexually related behaviors. Answering the question, "What is the behavior saying?" can help to identify the resident's need. For example, vulgar swearing could be a call for "help" that the resident is not feeling well. At other times, the expression of intimacy may be an attention-getting activity. A resident who is identified as having sexually inappropriate behaviors requires caregivers to use problem analysis skills in selecting interventions that enable the resident to maintain dignity. Another question to ask is, "Whose problem is it?" The intimacy-related behavior may be a problem to the family member or caregiver, but not to the resident. It is hoped that all involved can embrace intimacy and its many expressions as a natural part of life, even when, and especially when, one has dementia.

GUIDELINES FOR INTIMACY EXPRESSIONS IN CARE FACILITIES

Harry and Jane are in bed together, naked.

Jack takes Deborah into his room and urges her to perform oral sex.

Charles keeps touching Annette's breast, and she is angry.

What are appropriate actions? What's right? What's wrong? The highly charged subject of intimacy elicits feelings from all involved persons reflecting their culture, their gender, and their world view. Respect, dignity, well-being, and well thought out responses become the key components for guiding care.

The Omnibus Budget Reconciliation Act of 1987 created a patients' bill of rights stating that the resident has the right to "associate and communicate privately with persons of his or her choice, including other patients." If the resident is not cognitively challenged, the bill of rights is to be respected and implemented.

What about the resident with dementia? The situation immediately becomes more complex. Does this resident understand the complexities of the expressions of intimacy, with its positive merits or negative aspects? Lichtenberg and Strzepek (1990) described three conditions of informed consent for assessment of institutionalized dementia patients' competencies to participate in intimate relations.

These are: (1) voluntary participation, (2) mental competence, and (3) awareness of risks and benefits. The questions to ask are whether the resident can avoid exploitation and whether the expression is an authentic choice. In other words, can the resident say "No" when he or she wants to?

Other considerations for assessing the resident's decision-making capacity concerning the intimate involvement may look at

- How are intimate situations experienced, received, and remembered?
- Are intimate situations related to personal values and past life experiences?
- Can alternatives be accessed? On a consistent basis? With consistent outcomes?

It is not the role of the nursing home to block residents' efforts to be involved in meaningful relationships. However, realistic thought must go into assessing situations of intimacy. Awareness of family members' responses, especially when they hold the durable power of attorney for health care, are equally important. For example, Bertha, arriving to spend time with her husband, might be totally incensed to see him walking down the hall holding hands with Josephine. The question becomes, when does the nursing home respond to intimate relations? At the "hand holding" period, or when two residents are in bed together? Because there is no way of knowing the tolerance level for each family member, it is suggested that staff of the nursing home respond following a 48-hour period of intimate behavior between two residents, including evidence that the two residents have been seeking each other out for companionship.

The implementation of expressions of intimacy guidelines (see Appendix 10-3) starts with two major emphases. First, the residents involved are distracted from each other if possible while contact is made with the family member holding durable power of attorney or the family member that is the resident's legal representative. The facts are described to the family, withholding the name of the other resident involved in the expression of intimacy. Families are told that their wishes for responding to the situation will be considered, their loved one will be monitored, and they are invited to attend a plan-of-care meeting for further planning. Second, documentation occurs during this period by recording exactly what was seen to have been the intimate situation. This begins the initial course of action to be documented on each resident's plan of care and requires a multidisciplinary response involving all staff on all shifts that have contact with the residents. The residents' attending physicians are also notified, reporting the occurrence as a "change of condition." All contacts with the physician and family members are documented.

Residents' intimacy profiles are consulted and expanded if more information is needed. For example, information on past experiences of intimacy, possible relationship to the time of day or night, possible use of or responses to sexual gestures or language, and identification of possible behavioral triggers are explored. The residents are assessed as to their abilities to meet the criteria for informed consent.

The plan of action may lead to involvement of the facility's ethics committee. It is suggested that the state ombudsman working with the care center also be called in, informed, and asked to participate in the care conferences or the ethics committee meeting. The ombudsman helps to monitor the upholding of resident rights.

The addressing of intimacy issues must also consider the following elements:

1. *Other residents*: For example, Jim and Jane kiss and fondle each other during mealtimes. Henry and Susan also share the table and find this behavior unac-

ceptable, they have stopped eating well, and are asking for the staff to do something about Jim and Jane.

2. *Other family members*: For example, Henry's daughter is also uncomfortable about the hugging, petting, and stages of undress that Jim and Jane are exhibiting in the activity area. She complains to the staff.

3. *Staff*: Uncomfortable with addressing older residents about their behavior and embarrassed by the sexual content, the staff would rather ignore what Jim and Jane are doing. The staff feel angry and, at times, disgusted, but they do not know what to do. Additionally, some of the staff think Jim and Jane's behavior is okay, others do not.

Because there are so many components involved in care issues involved with expressions of intimacy, it becomes difficult to have any sort of blanket policy and procedure. Each situation requires individualized attention. The guidelines in Appendix 10-3 at least offer a system to put into action. The guidelines provide a menu of considerations to be examined and therefore help to address the uniqueness of each situation. A policy and procedure may not offer the same kind of flexibility. It becomes obvious that personal values, feelings, and beliefs surround all outcomes. The bottom line calls on all involved to reflect on the giving and receiving of dignity for all involved: residents, family, and staff.

HEALTH CARE PROVIDER AND STAFF ISSUES

Expressions of intimacy occurring within a health care setting produce a plethora of complex dilemmas. These dilemmas can include the involved residents, involved family members, other residents, other family members, staff, and regulatory and other licensing bodies.

David and Margaret spend much of the day snuggling, kissing, and petting. However, they are not discerning as to the location of their lovemaking. The dilemma of this situation is

1. David, a widower, is a gentleman and becomes deeply hurt if his "manners" are attacked. His family does not mind that Dad has found a special friend.

2. Margaret, a widow, has an underlying psychiatric delusional problem that leads her to become instantly angry. Her family acknowledges the situation but wants the door to be open whenever she is with David.

3. When Margaret explodes in anger, it is aimed at David, who cannot understand what he "did" to set it off, especially since Margaret's ability to express herself is limited. David displays evidence of feeling very hurt during these times. He also is angry when he wants the door shut when Margaret is in his room. He responds to staff by saying, "I'm 78 years old and no kid is going to tell me what I can do and what I can't do." At times of Margaret's tirades, David is overwhelmed. David has begun to appear more confused.

4. Other residents in the area are angry at the couple, feel that their behavior is "disgusting," and want them moved away. In fact, some residents will not share a table at mealtime because of the heavy petting.

5. Family members voiced their concern about the situation to administration.

The staff followed the expressions of intimacy guidelines (see Appendix 10-3) by contacting each family and also the residents' physicians. It was difficult to name which part of the dilemma concerned the staff the most. They were embarrassed over the couple's behavior but at times when Margaret was with David she was easier to handle. On the other hand, the staff disliked what Margaret's temper was doing to David, who had always been very calm and gentle. The staff were also aware of other residents' discomfort when the sexual scene was intense, as well as their own embarrassment.

The outcome of the situation required every staffperson's cooperation. It was decided that each time David and Margaret were petting or kissing, they would be approached by a staffperson who would say, "David and Margaret, that behavior is not appropriate in this public place. I want you to get up and leave this area, now." Some staff had difficulty approaching the couple and their discomfort was recognized. Therefore, if they were the ones to see the couple being inappropriate, they could go immediately to ask another staffperson to make the statement. In time, the couple began to curb their amorous public displays, and the other residents relaxed, as did the staff. Issues, therefore, involved not just David and Margaret, but the other residents, family members, and the staff as well. Each sexual dilemma requires a team approach that recognizes the sensitivity of the situation.

Issues also affecting the health care provider are

- Possibility of family-enacted legal action
- Residents being moved from the facility
- Marketing (i.e., effect on inquiry tours)
- Staff quitting because of personal responses to the residents' intimate behaviors toward each other or to them

Another set of issues arises when the health care facility is caring for spouses with dementia (see Chapter 2). The guidelines for expressions of intimacy, as well as individual resident's rights, require staff, along with the couple's family members, to look at the sexual issues if it appears that one spouse is overwhelming or being forceful with the other.

Spouses that are separated, with one living in the community, are permitted to have sexual experiences, in private. When the spouse living in the care facility has a roommate, the challenge to assure privacy takes clever thinking on the part of the staff and monitoring of the area. Problems occur if the staff observe or hear actions that lead them to think that the visiting spouse is taking advantage of the spouse living in the facility. The care center is responsible for the resident and must assure that his or her rights are being safeguarded. Again, this is an opportunity to call in professionals, involve the ombudsman representative, and bring together the ethics committee. There are no easy answers, but together the team and responsible family members can work out a plan of care. The ultimate challenge is when the abusing spouse holds the legal papers of support for his or her spouse and wants to continue the conjugal visits.

The emotionally charged subject of intimacy is too often ignored, perhaps due to thinking that "it will go away." Feelings about the subject range from "it's a natural part of life" to "not here, not while I'm around." Concerns may range from the husband who fears that his wife might be raped because she cannot defend herself to the staffperson also concerned about personal safety while bathing a strong, sexually acting out male resident to the dismayed embarrassment of a granddaughter being asked for sexual favors by her grandpa.

Health care centers that offer opportunities to discuss these concerns and feelings, as well as other issues related to sexuality and intimacy, provide an extremely important service to families and staffpersons. Informed speakers, videotapes, and educational games can provide not only the needed information but also allow opportunities for attendees' feelings and concerns to be expressed.

SUMMARY

Residents and their family members can encounter complex issues surrounding intimacy and sexuality throughout the course of dementia. It is hoped that all involved will find a comfortable way to address these issues with understanding and sensitivity.

The experience of providing health care for residents with dementia must acknowledge that sexuality and intimacy issues are occurring and be willing to step up to the issues involving residents and their intimate giving and receiving of affection. Understanding the "measuring" of what is a consenting adult with dementia will be an ongoing subject to be studied and discussed. The use of guidelines as shown in Appendix 10-3 can provide a method for processing concerns.

The topic of sexuality and intimacy for persons with dementia will continue to be sensitive, ethical concerns will continue to be a dilemma, and personal feelings will continue to color outcomes. As a basic human need, intimacy will continue to be an integral part of who we are: man, woman, young, old, well, ill, with or without Alzheimer's disease.

REFERENCE

Lichtenberg PA, Strzepek DM. Assessment of institutionalized dementia patients' competencies to participate in intimate relationships. Gerontologist 1990;30:117–120.

SUGGESTED READING

A Thousand Tomorrows: Sexuality, Intimacy and Alzheimer's Disease [videotape]. Chicago: Terra Nova Films, 1995.

Ballard EL, Poer CM. Sexuality and the Alzheimer's Patient. Durham, NC: Joseph and Kathleen Bryan Alzheimer's Disease Research Center, Duke University Medical Center, 1993.

Cooper AJ. Medroxyprogesterone acetate (MPA) treatment of sexually acting out men suffering from dementia. J Clin Psychiatry 1987;48:368–370.

Hellen CR. Intimacy: nursing home resident issues and staff training. Am J Alzheimer's Dis 1995;10:12–17.

Kuhn DR. The changing face of sexual intimacy in Alzheimer's disease. Am J Alzheimer's Care Res 1994;9:7–14.

Kyomen HH, Nobel KW, Wei JY. The use of estrogen to decrease aggressive physical behavior in elderly men with dementia. J Am Geriatr Soc 1991;39:1110–1112.

Philo S, Richie MF, Kaas MJ. Inappropriate sexual behavior. J Gerontol Nurs 1996;22:17–22.

A10-1
*The Changing Face of Intimacy**

When a married person develops Alzheimer's disease or a similar dementia, the couple faces enormous challenges. Nearly every aspect of the relationship is tested by the diminished abilities of the impaired partner and the healthy spouse's increased caregiving responsibilities. The expression of intimacy, particularly sexuality, is one of the main aspects of marriage that the disease often changes.

Although a number of chronic diseases, and the medications to treat them, have been identified as causes of sexual dysfunction, little is known about the impact of Alzheimer's disease on sexuality. This topic has received scant attention in the professional literature.

Data from a few studies of people with Alzheimer's disease indicate that sexual dysfunction may be commonplace. For example, a 1991 study of 30 couples in which one partner had Alzheimer's disease reported only 27% were still sexually active compared to 82% of an elderly control group. A 1990 study of 55 men with Alzheimer's disease who had an average age of 70 years reported 53% were impotent; this percentage is considerably higher than expected for this age group.

And in a 1989 study, 22 of 26 wives of men with Alzheimer's disease reported that the disease had affected their sexual relations with their spouses. In this study, eight men with Alzheimer's had little or no interest in sex and four became more interested in sex. Ten of the wives lost interest even though their husbands continued to want sex. The reasons for the loss of sexual functioning are not yet fully understood, but a number of factors are involved.

For the impaired person, structural changes in the brain and nervous system may account for sexual dysfunction. Also, coping with the disease-related changes in memory, thought, and behavior are stressful for the person with Alzheimer's. Psychological reactions, such as depression and anxiety, are fairly common, too, and are known to contribute to sexual dysfunction in the general population as well.

The healthy spouse's desire for sex may be affected by the personality changes in the impaired partner: forgetfulness, repetitious questions, short attention span, and annoying behaviors. For instance, a person with Alzheimer's disease may forget how to make love or may immediately forget when it is over. Consequently, the healthy spouse may feel rejected or angry.

---

*Reprinted with permission from D Kuhn. The changing face of intimacy. Rush Alzheimer's Disease Center News, 1993;winter:1.

Or a healthy spouse may fear "taking advantage" of a willing partner with Alzheimer's disease and feel ambivalent about engaging in sex.

The ongoing emotional and physical demands of caring for a demented partner are also likely to inhibit sexual desire. As a result, mutually satisfying sexual activity may decrease as a priority in the relationship or may no longer be possible to achieve as a couple.

Occasionally, people with Alzheimer's disease are overly interested in sex. This hypersexuality may include aimless masturbation and frequent attempts to seduce others. Such behaviors are symptoms of the disease and are likely related to brain damage, rather than maliciousness. Furthermore, such behaviors may signal the need for attention, reassurance, and closeness instead of the need for sexual gratification. Touching, hugging, and other forms of affection my help meet this end.

Because sex is a private matter, there is usually a reluctance to discuss it with others. However, it may be helpful to seek the advice of a professional. One's doctor should always be notified for possible medical intervention in cases of persistent sexual aggressiveness. The healthy spouse, in particular, may need accurate information, support, and counseling to cope with changes in the sexual aspect of marriage.

Of course, sexuality is only one expression of the gift of love. Even if sex in a relationship is lost due to Alzheimer's disease, other expressions of love and affection may continue to thrive. Respect, care, companionship, and intimacy may take on new and deeper meaning. A special grace marks those who have learned to live with the disease and continue to find meaning in their marriage.

The heartbreak of Alzheimer's disease may be offset by the fulfillment often experienced in keeping the commitment to love "for better or worse, in sickness and in health."

A10-2
The Joy of Life: Compassionate Relationships*

Do you remember your senior prom? The thrill of being "chosen," the delight of feeling special, the sharing of laughter and fun? Winnie and Mo, King and Queen of The Wealshire's Senior Prom, reigned with a regal countenance of happiness and well-being.

Caring for persons with dementia focuses on connecting with their well-being, offering respect and promoting remaining abilities. Interwoven within a supportive environment is the joy of friendships and relationships. The intimacy of giving and receiving affection becomes a basic care component.

Should we be surprised when two residents, such as Winnie and Mo, "find" each other and share a special relationship? The answer must be "no" if indeed caregivers strive to create a loving and safe place for residents with dementia to live. The beauty of compassionate connectedness with one another affirms oneself as a person of worth, one who is valued. Persons with dementia do not lose their abilities to seek nurturing opportunities, for fulfillment of their own self-esteem and needs, as well as the bliss of giving affection to others.

There must be no room allowed for responses from others of teasing or shaming. Certainly, there are concerns experienced by families and care center staff about resident relationships and special friendships. Are the residents involved widowed or do they have spouses? Is the expression of intimacy a shared joy or not appreciated by one of them? Does the relationship allow for enhanced individuality or does domination or control become an issue? Do we discourage friendships because of the possibility of changes due to the progression of Alzheimer's in the future and possible hurt feelings? Are the resident rights mandated by federal regulations being supported? What is the response from the residents' families? Other residents? And what is the response from staff?

It is hoped that family and staff can communicate with each other with understanding and respect for the inherent joys surrounding delicate situations of shared affection. Being in touch with one's own thoughts and values concerning relationships regarding intimacy and older persons with dementia is imperative. What happens and how do families and staff respond if the intimacy of affection moves to sexual intimacy?

---

*Reprinted with permission from CR Hellen. The joy of life: compassionate relationships. Rush Alzheimer's Disease Center News, 1996;spring:4.

Can our personal bias, cultural mores, and perceived expectations of "appropriate behaviors" be reframed to reflect the residents' happiness? In the midst of so many difficult and delicate questions, let us focus on what persons with dementia, such as Winnie and Mo, are offering to teach us. They display for us the joy of a caring touch and gentle words. The meaning of being present to one another is shown by listening with acceptance to shared thoughts, enjoyment of the moment with laughter, the mutual tenderness of held hands and loving eye contact. But most of all they gift us by demonstrating life's essential joy of being a valued partner in a compassionate relationship.

A10-3

Expressions of Intimacy Guidelines for Persons with Dementia Residing in Care Facilities

I. Issues of intimacy will be addressed during the admission assessment process
   A. Families will be encouraged to create a LifeStory Book (see Chapter 3)
   B. An intimacy profile (see Appendix 10-5) will be completed, with data to include:
      1. Resident's current awareness and intimate activity
      2. Past expressions of intimacy, including touch, sexual activity, hugs, sleeping arrangements, sexual preference, any reasons to suspect abuse, current memories of intimacy (positive and negative)
II. Responding to self-expressed or self-directed intimacy
   A. Respect of the resident's dignity and privacy issues will be supported by the staff
   B. Issues of physical well-being and appropriate distractions or interventions, or both, will be assessed and used
III. Responding to issues of intimacy between a resident with dementia and a cognitively alert resident
   A. Resident rights will be used when responding to the cognitively alert resident
   B. Intimacy guidelines will be used for the resident with dementia
   C. Family members of each resident will be informed and invited to attend a plan of care for their loved one that will address the intimacy expression
   D. Staff will respond appropriately to the abilities and needs of each resident while maintaining the resident's self-esteem and personhood
IV. Considerations for responding to intimacy between residents with dementia
   A. Activate considerations following a 48-hour period when two residents have been together or sought each other out and have been touching, holding, or stroking each other

B. Distract residents from each other, if possible, during information gathering and reporting period
   1. Monitor the residents and their whereabouts during this period
   2. If possible, without upsetting the residents, find meaningful activities they could individually participate in
C. Document observations only
   1. Check with all staff, use a behavior observation form if necessary (see Appendix 8-2)
   2. Develop initial course of action for each resident's care plan
   3. Inform all staff, all shifts involved with the residents
D. Inform responsible family member
   1. Describe facts, withhold other resident's name
   2. Ask how family member wishes to have the intimacy expression handled or monitored
   3. Invite family member to attend a care conference and set the date
   4. Document the outcome of the conversation with the family of each resident
E. Inform attending physicians of affected residents
   1. Report as "a change of condition," because of the noted change in the resident's behavior
   2. Ask for input, review medications for the possibility that they are increasing the resident's libido
   3. Document conversation with each resident's physician
F. Expand the residents' intimacy profiles
   1. Gather more in-depth information than provided in admission information from the families of the residents
   2. Include information such as past and present sexual gestures, language and behavioral triggers
   3. Invite staff to add their observations, if appropriate
G. Assess residents' awareness of sexual expression and conditions of informed consent. Use Lichtenberg and Strzepek's (1990) three conditions for informed consent:
   1. First informed consent: voluntary participation, not physical or psychological coercion, is action an authentic choice?
   2. Second informed consent: mental competence of decision
   3. Third informed consent: awareness of risks and benefits, who is initiating, whom is involved, what needs, wants, or outcome does the resident express, can the resident avoid the sexual advances of the other resident?

   In other words, can the resident say "No" if he or she wanted or needed to?
H. Further plan of action
   1. Hold a team meeting or plan-of-care conference that includes all disciplines
   2. Assess resident rights, competency issues, and family issues
   3. Institute a behavior profile (see Appendix 8-1), behavior observation form (see Appendix 8-2), behavior analysis form (see Appendix 8-3), and sensory profile (see Appendix 5-2)
   4. Involve the physician when appropriate
   5. Check medications for possibilities of increasing the libido

6. Incorporate family suggestions whenever possible
7. Involve facility's ombudsman to assure that resident rights are being upheld
8. Address unresolved issues to facility's ethics committee
9. Put plan of care into effect
10. Provide inservices for staff about the plan's approaches and interventions and their participation
11. Require a consistent staff approach
12. Monitor the involved residents

I. Provide family information and support
    1. Respond to the families' needs for education, understanding, support
    2. Address issues such as visiting, appropriate resident interaction, behavioral refocusing

J. Require staff to receive sensitivity training about expressions of intimacy, residents with dementia, ways to offer support to their families and personal issues
    1. Use videotapes, games, and discussions to enable staff to express their personal issues and responses about the residents they work with and their expressions of intimacy to each other or to the staffperson
    2. Offer special caregiving interventions
    3. Problem solve regarding specific residents and concerns and acceptable approaches and refocusing techniques

REFERENCE

Lichtenberg PA, Strzepek DM. Assessment of institutionalized dementia patients' competencies to participate in intimate relationships. Gerontologist 1990;30:117–120.

A10-4
Expressions of Intimacy: Analysis

	Abilities and Benefits	Inabilities and Risks	Assistance
Cognitive-based responses	Provides sense of well-being, normalcy, ego strength, nurturing; increases orientation to self; projects meaningfulness to life, encouraging the thoughts required to "give" to someone rather than self-centeredness; encourages verbal and non-verbal responses; facilitates social skills; stimulates choices; facilitates reminiscing of enjoyed experiences and traditions; method to attract attention	Makes resident aware of losses, past significant others, situations; decreased understanding of total environment and persons, socially acceptable boundaries and etiquette; decreased memory for appropriate responses; adds to confusion, disorientation, not knowing where resident is; misunderstanding or lack of recognition of others and their significance; not able to use sound judgment or understand consequences, or both; decreased understanding of need for privacy for self or others, or both; perceived invasion of personal space; misunderstanding or misinterpretation of verbal and nonverbal responses from others; cannot use verbal wishes or concerns;	Assess what the intimate behavior is "telling" you; focus on strengths, abilities; give verbal reassurance that you care and will be there to give support; use communication skills to increase understanding; use a consistent routine to give assurance and facilitate response; encourage acceptable expressions; promote meaningful activities and a purposeful use of time; allow choices to encourage sense of being in control; use activities that encourage friendships, reminiscing of life stories, shared favorite poetry; encourage former life "roles"; spend quality time with resident when he or she is the absolute focus of your attention; use resident's past experience

	Abilities and Benefits	Inabilities and Risks	Assistance
		inability to interpret body "messages," use of verbal obscenities	of expressions of intimacy as a guide for appropriate current caregiving; understand appropriate use of endearing terms for each specific resident, including family nicknames or meaningful words, especially if English is not being spoken; use a consistent approach for inappropriate expressions of intimacy, do not scold or belittle; use distraction or redirection techniques when necessary (e.g., offer food, sit with resident, ask resident to help you with a task); use a strong but not chastising voice; use cueing and task breakdown techniques for orientation
Physical-based responses	Resident can demonstrate caring by touch, word, action; is an energy outlet (e.g., walking together, dancing); is a method to decrease stress; response to affirming touch; use of touch as link to reality; promotes sensory stimulation; outlet for expressing sensory needs or desires	Displays of aggressive or combative behaviors; touching or invading physical space of another resident, or both; inability to integrate responses to touch, body part movement in a meaningful way; decreased sense of body image, possibly leading to abrupt, inappropriate, or unsafe situations; use of physical obscenities; misinterpretation of environmental overstimulation	Validate self and achieve maximum attractiveness through clothing and grooming; use clothing that is difficult to take off if inappropriate strippingtakes place; show physical affection (e.g., hugs, back rubs, lotion rubs, shake hands in warm greeting each time you pass by if tolerated); use caring touch when communicating, speak at the resident's eye level; use activities that stimulate friend ships by active games,

	Abilities and Benefits	Inabilities and Risks	Assistance
			holding hands in a circle game, passing objects one to another; try to pinpoint the antecedents of desired physical expressions; provide a safe environment; use more than one staffperson when appropriate; assess resident's care needs in terms of caregiver's gender; allow privacy when appropriate; facilitate privacy with a spouse when appropriate; assess physical health for problems and needs; assess for sensory deficits, especially hearing and vision
Psychosocial-based responses	Increases confidence, sense of comfort and familiarity, feeling useful; increases self-esteem; enables recognition, approval from others, sense of dignity, feelings of being valued; builds pride, feelings of being sexually attractive, wanted, desired, being part of a supportive peer community; able to "receive" from others, feeling of being in control, ownership; is a vehicle to act out expressions of fear or boredom	Feeling of inadequacy, frustration of not knowing what is expected of him or her; increased stimulation of jealous responses, not wanting to share companion with others; paranoia, increased attempts to control others; facilitates depression, misinterpretation of emotional stimulation	Address resident rights through intimacy guidelines; use consistent, familiar trained staff; be knowledgeable in the meaning of intimacy expression in relationship to the resident's gender, cultural, and ethnic background; protect dignity (e.g., privacy for masturbation); reassurance of self-worth, give respect, build trust, emotional closeness; use praise and verbalize acceptance, give compliments; do not argue or confront; provide companionship; use activities that stimulate friendship and

Abilities and Benefits	Inabilities and Risks	Assistance
		increase socialization (e.g., parties, sharing, holding hands for circle games); offer family support in understanding the resident's expressions of intimacy; assist in discussing realistic expressions

Alzheimer's Disease: Activity-Focused Care

A10-5
Intimacy Profile

Name: _____ Date of birth: _____

Married: _____ Number of years: _____

Widowed: _____ Number of years: _____

Sexual preference: Male: _____ Female: _____

1. Describe expressions or demonstrations of intimacy within the last 6 months and with whom. Concerns? Problems? Specific sexual behaviors?

   _____

   _____

2. Any reason to suspect occurrences of sexual abuse? Describe. _____

   _____

3. Any reason to suspect a sexually transmitted disease? Describe. _____

   _____

4. Describe intimacy history
   A. Demonstrations of affection given and received (include use of touch, hugs, ways of showing affection verbally and nonverbally, demonstration of inappropriate touching, displaying personal body areas): _____

      _____

   B. Marriage relationship and history (include details such as strengths, joys, difficulties, and sadness related to being married, what kind of bed they had, how affection was demonstrated, possible triggers leading to appropriate or inappropriate sexual responses, or both, describe each marriage if more than one occurred): _____

      _____

   C. Being single: demonstrations of intimacy. Describe. (Include details of strengths, joys, difficulties, and sadness.) _____

      _____

   D. Being divorced: demonstrations of intimacy. Describe. (Include details of strengths, joys, difficulties, and sadness.) _____

      _____

Name and relationship to the resident: _____

_____

Date: _____

11

Spirituality: Compassionate Connectedness and Well-being

Personal faith journeys enhance spirituality in later years. Sometimes, the words "spirituality" and "religion" are used interchangeably, but they take on a meaning of their own for persons with dementia. Spirituality is the essence of all that we are "within," our inner light, the hope, strength, and search for meaning that radiates from our holy and divine-centered self. Dementia can never diminish this very personal divine light as it connects us with ourselves and one another. Religion is the upholding or demonstration of spirituality in a more open or public way, experiencing beliefs, rituals, teachings, community, and a shared essence of divinity. The practices and rituals offered by a personal or organized religion can extend an opportunity to persons with dementia that calls them forth to be connected with their familiar and remembered faith journey. A person's well-being finds spirituality and religion united in the affirmation of life, providing an intimacy of the divine within and integrated throughout everyday moments, revealing that all of life is sacred.

APPRAISING SPIRITUAL WELL-BEING AND NEEDS

Residents with Alzheimer's disease continue to respond to their faith and inner needs through long-remembered rituals that connect them with the present. There is a centering, a simplicity that enables a sense of wholeness and being in control. Joy-filled memories can be sacraments. Reaching out to residents invites caregivers to identify their personal source of divine strength. The door to connecting opens when caregivers can surround each person with love by honoring and fulfilling their spiritual needs, including

- To have self-worth and personal faith journey upheld
- To experience the sacredness of daily life's offering of dignity, meaning, and purpose
- To sense the presence of the divine, within ones capability to understand, as honored

- To be tenderly held in loving arms that enable loss and trying circumstances to be transcended
- To be surrounded with the glories of love, thanksgiving, and forgiveness
- To be called into community, with a divinity and with one another

Considerations to be included in appraising a person with dementia's spiritual well-being and needs can be formalized in an assessment tool (see Appendix 11-1). This assessment tool can be adapted to include relevant items related to specific religions, clergy involvement, pastoral care programs, care settings, and activity support.

THE CLERGY, CARING CONGREGATION, AND CONFUSED WORSHIPPER*

> "Help me, help me," Joseph calls out during worship. A still-ness hangs in the air while the congregation listens and watches what will happen next. The pastor responds, "Bless you, Joseph, we all can help each other." The worshippers set-tle back in their seats, lifting up Joseph and his family in their prayers and surrounding them with love and understanding.

Helping clergy, worshippers, and members of a faith community and the person with dementia to come together upholding one another's search and implementa-tion of spiritual wholeness can be a challenge. The "Joseph's" of our lives have much to teach us. They help us to learn how to talk without using words, how to be open to the giving and receiving of love, how to trust a person's goodness, and how to see beyond all that is viable into a world of feelings. "Joseph" introduces us to our child within by welcoming us into his simple activities. We learn about the immense pain of separation from self, but he also shows us an indefatigable strength to persevere. We are challenged to be loving even when we are unrecog-nized or pushed away. We are called to be creative and respectful of human dig-nity. "Joseph" offers us communion with ourselves, our community, and our divine center.

CLERGY SUPPORT FOR PERSONS WITH DEMENTIA AND THEIR FAMILIES*

Clergy are in a unique position to offer support and assistance. They also can model acceptance and build the bridge enabling their worship community to continue their outreach of care. However, it is often taken for granted that clergy and caring persons know how to interact and give ministry to all persons in all situations.

---

*Adapted from C Hellen. The "C" connection: the confused worshiper with dementia, the clergy and the caring congregation. Aging and Spirituality. American Society on Aging Newsletter of the Forum on Religion, Spirituality and Aging. 1994;VI:1, 4, 8.

Alzheimer's Disease: Activity-Focused Care

This is an unfair assumption because lack of knowledge or experience can lead to discomfort, embarrassment, or misunderstandings. Persons ministering to residents are called to become comfortable with silence and simplicity and to re-evaluate their personal definitions of dignity, trust, worth, health, and aging.

The clergy can help in the following ways:

1. Clergy may be the first to recognize the problem of dementia, especially when there is denial in the family. They are in the position to encourage a valid diagnostic workup. Clergy may be called on to alert out-of-town family members or those not in close contact with their family member.

2. Clergy may be the first people willing to talk honestly about the memory loss problems with "Joseph," offering support and facilitating planning for the future. This can include the various needed legal decisions such as the living will, power of attorney, and life support wishes.

3. Clergy can model a sense of comfort and acceptance during the worship service if a behavior is not appropriate. For example, if "Joseph" gets up and wanders back and forth in the aisle, the pastor might reach out his hand and invite "Joseph" to stand or sit by him. At other times, it may be best to just ignore "Joseph" if he is not disruptive. Certainly, there are many factors to take into consideration: the familiarity of the congregation with the person with dementia, the structure and ritual of the service, the consideration of the concerns and needs of the worshipping congregation, and the abilities of "Joseph" to be redirected.

4. Clergy can encourage normalization for "Joseph," such as continued participation in the choir, congregational committees, social events, and outreach ministries.

5. Clergy can implement the invitations to the Alzheimer's Association or other knowledgeable speakers for helping the congregation to understand the changes they are seeing taking place in "Joseph." Information and understanding of the disease are needed as he becomes more forgetful and confused rather than having him become the object of ridicule and rumors because of behavior changes. Clergy can offer their facility as a place for support groups.

THE CONGREGATION'S SHARED COMMUNION OF LOVE AND SUPPORT*

The worshipping community can extend supportive caring to persons with dementia and their families by breaking through their often felt sense of helplessness created from not knowing what to do. This often leads the families of persons with dementia to experience isolation when their loved one has Alzheimer's disease.

---

*Adapted from C Hellen. The "C" connection: the confused worshiper with dementia, the clergy and the caring congregation. Aging and Spirituality. American Society on Aging Newsletter of the Forum on Religion, Spirituality and Aging. 1994;VI:1, 4, 8.

Members of the congregation can help in the following ways:

1. Members can use simple sentences when talking with "Joseph" that can help to reinforce his self-esteem by "telling" him how glad they are to see him. Sometimes, reaching out a hand and using a gentle touch while saying, "You are safe here with me; I will worship with you this morning," is helpful. Kind words and a caring smile can help to reduce "Joseph's" ever present fear of ineptitude.

2. A familiar friend can be ready to lead "Joseph" from the service and involve him in a meaningful activity, if needed. This can focus on a former role such as sorting envelopes in the office, checking out the building's maintenance needs, moving books in the library, helping with child care or classes, or attending to tasks in the kitchen. The important point is to simplify the activity into easy steps and always promote the person's abilities. It may be that just walking around could be helpful, or finding a quiet place for a cup of coffee.

3. Members can assure safety. The congregation can monitor the environment for potentially hazardous items (e.g., cleaning supplies and tools), make sure that stairways are well lit and with full handrails, and use a non-skid strip and a bright color to contrast the lip of each stair. Spatial-perceptual difficulty can be experienced by persons with dementia, precipitating falls both up and down stairs. Have signage for way-finding; the confused person can become lost within the building. Use a picture of a toilet as well as the word "toilet" or "bathroom" on the washroom doors. Just having the words "men's" or "women's" may not be meaningful when "Joseph" is looking for the toilet.

4. Members can develop a plan for assisting "Joseph" if he is living alone. Family members living away may not be aware of his increasing forgetfulness and inability to care for himself. Inappropriate hygiene and clothing selection plus a significant weight loss or gain can signal the need for help. If the person is totally alone, key persons in the congregation can contact care providers for assistance. Many congregations have a parish nurse or other ways to implement care management. Provide a Safe Return bracelet from the Alzheimer's Association (1-800-272-3900). At times, "Joseph" may become lost going to or from worship. He may lose the ability to understand time and venture off to services at times when no one is present in the building.

5. The congregation can write up a list of volunteers ready to help the family caregiver. This could include assistance with transportation, meals, and errands, and providing respite in the home so the caregiver can attend services alone or have a needed break. When the time comes that the family can no longer bring their loved one to the formal worship services, enlist volunteers to bring the service to them.

6. Members can be ready to continue caring support if "Joseph" goes to a care facility. He and his family still need the love of the spiritual community. Bring brief worship services to him (e.g., use familiar Bible stories, prayers, and hymns). Friends from the congregation become to "Joseph" a window to the spiritual world within and offer a safe bridge of compassionate connectedness to others.

THE CONFUSED WORSHIPPER*

Residents with dementia often can sense the peace of the worshipping community. Usually congregations find that the behavior of a person with dementia is almost always appropriate during services.

The confused worshipper can be assisted and supported in the following ways:

1. Have "Joseph" enter worship after the music begins or just before the service starts. This allows for the needed cueing and supportive environmental factors to promote familiar comfort. Select a seat on the aisle that allows for an easy retreat from the service or use a certain familiar seat that "Joseph" has always used in the past.
2. Have significant items of worship available to be held in his hands. "Joseph" can become focused and have his attention span extended when holding safe objects such as a prayer book, rosary, hymn book, church bulletin, or Bible.
3. Snacks, such as cookies and cut up fruit, can be brought to the service by the caregiver or friends to be used for refocusing "Joseph" if signs of apprehension or agitation are noticed. Having a "busy box" of small balls of yarn to be wound, paper clips to be untangled, or a simple scrapbook of religious cards, sayings, and scripture verses available, if needed, can also help to reduce anxiety.
4. Encourage the use of name tags. Persons with dementia can read late into the disease process, although they may not always understand. If members of the congregation wear name tags with large, bold printing, knowing someone's name may become a lifeline to the forgetful person.

CREATIVE MINISTRY: UNITING AN ALZHEIMER'S CARE CENTER AND A LOCAL CONGREGATION

Defining the Need

Residents residing in retirement homes, assisted living, and long-term care centers often rely on local congregations for their pastoral care needs. Some homes are fortunate to have their own pastoral care support. As clergy and interested laity reach out to their nearby facilities, there are opportunities to bring the two groups together in a meaningful and mutual exchange.

Alzheimer's care programs greatly appreciate assistance in meeting the spiritual needs of their residents. Involvement might include adapted worship, scripture study, special event celebrations, music, and companionship.

Local congregations also have needs. Experienced care center staff can offer the local congregation and its members information about caring for persons with

---

*Adapted from C Hellen. The "C" connection: the confused worshiper with dementia, the clergy and the caring congregation. Aging and Spirituality. American Society on Aging Newsletter of the Forum on Religion, Spirituality and Aging. 1994;VI:1, 4, 8.

dementia, including practical hands-on ideas and appropriate activities. Training can also provide assistance on how to visit residents, communicate, and create meaningful worship. The ability of clergy to know how to call on persons with dementia and to worship with them is often taken for granted by a care center, when in reality, clergy often appreciate all the help and training they can get.

Putting the Ministry Into Action

Staff can identify the faith traditions of their residents and approach a local congregation to request a shared ministry. Sometimes, there are several residents from an area church or synagogue so there is already an interest in learning and sharing with each other. Another suggestion is for the care center to host a "clergy breakfast" for local congregations and give a presentation on the spiritual needs of persons with dementia and how a compassionate connection would be of benefit.

The local congregation might create a task force to assess interest and to identify persons willing to be involved. This task force would then meet with care center staff and develop a calendar of shared events.

Opportunities for sharing ministry include the following:

I. Scheduled opportunities for the care center staff to come to the congregation to share dementia care information. Sharing information would also include setting up a caregiver resource phone number and a staffperson for members of the congregation to contact when they need advice on diagnostic centers, daily care issues, and support groups.

II. The care center can put together a descriptive "wish list" for the congregation to respond to. This could include worship and friendly visitor needs. Especially valuable is a listing of specific activity items that would appeal to various ages and interests within the congregation and could be specifically made for the center. Examples are (see Appendix 9-5 for descriptions of how to make the following items):

A. Scrapbooks with bright pictures and phrases for reading
B. Busy boxes of safe, interesting stuff to touch and hold
C. Reminiscing boxes based on themes
D. Adapted bingo (e.g., using colors, shapes)
E. Boxes of fabric of varying textures, colors
F. Beanbags for tossing games
G. Picture files by categories for reminiscing
H. Busy board with familiar hardware
I. Decorative pillows for bedrooms
J. Aprons with many pockets with taped-on safe items
K. Large flash cards with letters or math problems
L. A wooden tie rack and ties
M. Boxes of gathered supplies for sorting
N. Place mats and tray favors
O. Seasonal decorations made by children
   1. Cards and notes
   2. Birdhouses and feeders

III. Opportunities can be planned and scheduled for clergy or various laity groups, or both, to come to the care center for shared activities and worship. Staff would help with the planning and implementation of these programs, which could be open for various groups within the congregation, including opportunities for all ages to participate.

The possibilities for shared ministry are endless. Perhaps in time residents will be invited to join the congregation's worship and celebrations. It is important to have various opportunities for the congregation that include projects that can be done within the congregation without having to visit the care center or have contact with the residents as well as hands-on, active participation with each other. This allows everyone's comfort level to be respected.

CREATING A PRAISE, THANKSGIVING, AND WORSHIP CENTER*

A praise, thanksgiving, and worship center within the health care facility can provide a spiritual and interactive place of holiness, welcoming the residents to touch, listen, see, smell, and taste the essence of their remembered experiences of worship.

If possible, select an area where the center can be permanently set up so residents know where to find it. Ideas could include a quiet corner, a card table set up at certain times, a wall display using shelves or a pegged rack to hang items on, or perhaps a resident's room when appropriate. Other variations might be objects placed in a labeled drawer or in an attractive box able to fit on a lap or lap table. Awareness of the safety needs of residents must be considered as the worship center elements are selected.

Using a religious, spiritual, and sacred center assessment (see Appendix 11-1), focus on each resident's abilities and needs in relationship to participation with the center. This would include suggestions for time of day, length of time, one-to-one versus small group interaction, and any adaptation needed to ensure a positive experience. Care should be taken to assess for possible negative responses and inappropriateness of the center as an activity. Identify the resident's goals or outcome measures, or both, that you hope to enable by using the center.

Gather objects for residents' interaction. Suggestions include

- Prayer books, Bibles, Bible story books, pictures
- Scripture written out on large cards with large print or scripture cards
- Sacred symbols, icons, rosary, battery-powered candle
- Prayer vestments, stoles, kepa, tallis
- Dreydel, miniature menorah, mezuzah
- Kiddush book or cup, matzo cover
- Hymn or sacred books of music

---

*Reprinted with permission from C Hellen. Activities of Compassionate Connectedness and Well-being. In Alzheimer's Association (ed), Activity Programming for Persons with Dementia: A Sourcebook. Chicago: Alzheimer's Association, 1995. Reprinted with permission from the National Alzheimer's Association.

- Tapes of sacred music, prayers, readings that can be played on a cassette player or individual player with earphones
- Meditation aids (e.g., pictures of a sunset, sunrise, babies, flowers, large shells)
- Foods of the holidays and holy days (e.g., matzo, gefilte fish)
- Items exuding aromas of the holidays and holy days

Observe residents' responses and make necessary adjustments to the center, which could include needed assistance, facilitation, or termination of the activity. The center can be an interactive activity with others or an opportunity for the resident to experience the sacred alone, both of which can enable the center's mission of supportive spirituality and personal well-being.

ACTIVITY-FOCUSED ADAPTED WORSHIP SERVICE GUIDELINES

Creative approaches to worship focus on old learning and familiar experiences. Storytelling is an effective method to unlock memories of past rituals and celebrations. Simplifying ceremonies or sermons and leading the resident to follow or participate spiritually require step-by-step methods of involvement.

Rituals, long remembered by persons with dementia, play a role of facilitating connection of the sacred self to the caring community. Prayer can become ritual-like when, for example, prayer before meals and prayer at the end of the day mark the passage of time. At times, new rituals are appropriate. Examples would be a service of welcome when coming to a care facility or a ritual of blessing for one's room, its contents, and roommate. Rituals from the past often become a magic web to gather in feelings, memories, and a sense of being surrounded and enveloped in the loving arms of love, acceptance, and safeness.

The worship experience becomes an arena for the expression of feelings and emotions. Few other opportunities encourage or allow for these silent or verbal displays of sadness, grief, or loss, as well as joy and contentment. Understanding methods of facilitating appropriate communications and acceptance of a diminished attention span challenge the worship leader. Promoting positive behaviors and adaptive procedures to reduce or decrease inappropriate responses takes worship into the sphere of meaningful activity.

The following are guidelines for activity-focused adapted worship:

I. Prepare yourself
  A. Be ready to express love and caring, respect, and dignity for all
  B. Be ready to receive the love and presence of the residents: presence is their offering of their soul
II. Simplify
  A. Focus on one thought, theme, or topic you hope to share
  B. Use props such as pictures, items, poems, short readings
  C. Use familiar prayers, music, hymns, readings
III. Worship table or altar and setting
  A. Use visual and sensory props and symbols of faith, flowers, candles, etc., to help focus residents on the worship experience
  B. Select the worship space carefully so you can reach out and touch those present during the service (e.g., have rows of residents on each side of the

room but facing toward the center so they can see each other and the person conducting the service can walk up and down a space left in the center of the room)

    C. Wear symbols of the faith, if appropriate

IV. Service format

    A. Have music playing in the background as residents arrive

    B. Start with a familiar gathering prayer, and use the same one for each service

    C. Celebrate the day God has given, the day is where the resident lives, the day is a sacred place

    D. Celebrate the assembled residents

    E. Ask residents to share the past week's joys and sorrows

    F. Ask residents if they have a concern or need that can be lifted up by the group in prayer, bring concerns into an understandable context, connecting all of life with the ordinary and its sacredness

    G. Sing the first verse of a hymn, consider using the same one for each service, have the words printed in large print

    H. Read scripture from a familiar source, such as the King James version of the Bible

    I. Provide a meditation or homily (5–10 minutes) using a storytelling mode that calls forth the worshippers to feel connected and involved by including opportunities for sharing, the passing of items to be touched or held

    J. Allow time for silence

    K. Theologizing and the use of abstract or complicated thoughts are too complex to invite the worshipper's attention or focus

    L. Nonverbal communications are often the understood essence of the worship experience

    M. Use a prayer of celebration that brings together the main thoughts of the meditation and makes them a personal blessing for all present

    N. Sing again, the first verse of a hymn, again considering using the same one each week

    O. Have a closing prayer of peace and encouragement, one of going forth as a beloved person of great worth

    P. Touch or shake hands with all residents, calling each one by name and giving each a personal blessing as you thank them for their presence

ACTIVITY-FOCUSED WORSHIP EXAMPLE: HOLY HANDS*

This service activity is to create a tactile and visible symbol for connecting a resident's love and work for others by reflecting on the past and validating the present. The prayers, for example, can reflect Bible readings from Psalms that call out for God's care and other scripture that talks about being held by God or being held in His hands.

---

*Adapted with permission from C Hellen. Activities of Compassionate Connectedness and Well-being. In Alzheimer's Association (ed), Activity Programming for Persons with Dementia: A Sourcebook. Chicago: Alzheimer's Association, 1995. Reprinted with permission from the National Alzheimer's Association.

Move among the residents and reach out to hold their hands and talk with each resident about their hands, feeling their strength, and acknowledging the shape, lines, and skin texture as you enable the reflection of the past and present use of their hands. This requires you to know each resident's life story so you can assist his or her memory of past tasks and accomplishments (see Chapter 3).

Hands cut from construction paper can be used to symbolize the resident's hands. Each hand can have a hole punched in it with yarn attached so it can be worn around the neck, or the hands can become part of a wall collage. Decide with the resident the words and information that could be written on the hands (e.g., "These hands baked hundreds of pies for church suppers"; "These hands have held seven children, 21 grandchildren, and 16 great-grandchildren"; or "These hands built small engines and helped to run the factory"). Help the resident to decide the placement of the finished activity (e.g., to be hung in a private or public place or to be a gift for the family).

Another possibility is to create a handprint using finger paints or tempera and good quality paper. The hand is placed lightly into the paint and then positioned onto the paper, pressing down firmly and then lifted up directly, not rolled out of position. A soft clay or dough made out of flour, salt, and water can also be used (mix 4 cups flour and 1 cup salt, adding enough water to form a firm ball that can be rolled or patted out to receive the handprint). If clay is used, the hand is pressed down firmly and far enough into the dough to make a clear outline when lifted out. Attach a wire loop to the back side of the clay carefully and allow plaque to harden.

During the worship service or activity, take the opportunity to reminisce with the resident about his or her hands as a symbol of personal well-being and connectedness with others.

ACTIVITY-FOCUSED WORSHIP EXAMPLE: TO BE CALLED BY NAME*

This service activity is to provide the delight, honor, and deep-felt feeling of being called by name and included in a caring community. For example, use scripture readings reflecting on being called or named by God. Ask residents to share their name with the gathered. Take time to talk about how they received their name, whether they liked the name throughout the years or would have preferred another name. Offer words of praise and thanksgiving for each resident and his or her name by reflecting on the resident's individual gifts and strengths.

Validating and reverencing residents' worth by calling them by name can be done in several ways. A name tag can be made and placed on the resident. If the worship area permits, the resident can make his or her own tag, decorating it with stickers or drawings or leaving it plain. Residents with dementia can often read for a long time. Name tags become a source for increasing communications, by helping residents address activity companions, tablemates, roommates, strolling friends, and others by name. Names can be placed in a soft plastic convention badge. When not being worn, the name badges can reside on a "family tree" banner made of felt for all to see and admire.

---

*Adapted with permission from C Hellen. Activities of Compassionate Connectedness and Well-being. In Alzheimer's Association (ed), Activity Programming for Persons with Dementia: A Sourcebook. Chicago: Alzheimer's Association, 1995. Reprinted with permission from the National Alzheimer's Association.

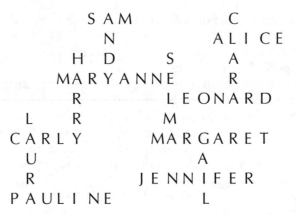

```
        S A M              C
        N              A L I C E
      H D    S          A
    M A R Y A N N E      R
        R        L E O N A R D
      L     R        M
    C A R L Y        M A R G A R E T
      U              A
      R              J E N N I F E R
    P A U L I NE          L
```

Figure 11-1
Example of a "name scrabble."

Another way to honor residents' names is to create a "name scrabble." File cards that have been cut into squares (e.g., 3 in.×3 in.) can be used. Each letter or the resident's name is written with a bold, dark marker on a square. The cards can be all one color, or a variety of colored file cards can be used, but use only one color per name. Select a large wall or bulletin board area for applying the squares using double-sided tape. Start with longest name and build out from this name, connecting all residents' names. The response to seeing all the names being connected will often be, "See, we are a family" (Figure 11-1).

SERVICE OF REMEMBRANCE: CELEBRATING OUR FRIEND*

This service activity is to provide a gathering for friends to celebrate a deceased resident's life, thereby offering a ritual of connectedness and closure while reinforcing the living residents' awareness that they too will be lifted up in celebration and remembered when they die.

The celebration can be facilitated by a caring person or persons. Examples of facilitators include pastor, nursing assistant, activity therapist, housekeeper, and administrator.

Plan to involve the resident's family and invite them help design and participate in the service whenever possible. Select an appropriate place for the celebration. This could include holding the service in the chapel area, a dining-activity room, or perhaps it could be a service for the former roommate and therefore the bedroom might be appropriate.

The timing of the celebration as soon as possible following the resident's death helps the other residents remember their friend. Be flexible on length of time (15

---

*Adapted with permission from C Hellen. Activities of Compassionate Connectedness and Well-being. In Alzheimer's Association (ed), Activity Programming for Persons with Dementia: A Sourcebook. Chicago: Alzheimer's Association, 1995. Reprinted with permission from the National Alzheimer's Association.

minutes suggested) and select the best time when residents and staff are the most available and able to respond to the celebration's caring connection of remembrance. Select residents you think would want to attend; roommates and mealtime tablemates are especially appropriate.

Create a worship center or altar by using props such as pictures of the resident, his or her life story book, flowers, battery-powered candles, favorite music and hymns, and, when appropriate, the symbols of faith. A program, for example, entitled "Celebrating [resident's name] Program," with a brief life story can be put together. This can include pictures of the shared life at the facility, words and music that will be said and sung during the service, and, if possible, a photocopied picture of the resident being celebrated.

Open with a favorite and familiar song that helps residents feel comfortable and a part of the gathered caring community. Introduce yourself and say a few words about the resident's life being celebrated. The celebration's design is to be based on recognizing the best possible program that supports the abilities of the attending residents and therefore should be open and flexible so they can choose to participate. Invite residents, family, and others to share personal memories. Many times, staff wish to say a few words. Remember that this is a celebration and familiar songs can be included, such as "Let Me Call You Sweetheart," or, "The More We Get Together," or readings from love sonnets or poetry can be used along with the more traditional aspects of worship. Suggestions include familiar readings, songs and hymns, and using symbols reflecting the deceased resident that offer visual cueing of appreciation for a life lived, personal value and strengths (e.g., a flower for beauty, a book for wisdom, a basket of cookies symbolizing the gift of a smile and hospitality shown for others [cookies can be shared at the close of the celebration], and a candle for the inner light of love for family and caring for others).

The closing of the service of remembrance can include singing, perhaps by holding hands with each other, and a blessing for the departed friend as well as one for the worshippers.

HEALTH CARE PROVIDER AND STAFF ISSUES

Health care providers can reach out to their residents and offer spiritual support, but it must be done in a sensitive way. Each resident has his or her own personal spiritual life history. Dementia may or may not affect residents' current-day response to religious services of any kind. Care should be taken that residents are never brought to a service or religious meeting if they do not wish to attend or, perhaps, if their family does not wish them to attend. The resident's rights must be protected.

Having religious opportunities within a care center is important. Examples are Friday services, mass, Christian services, Bible or religious studies, prayer groups, and hymn sings. The activity could be posted and, as residents enter, they could be reminded what the nature of the spiritual activity is going to be, then invited to stay if they wish. The bottom line is that the facility and the staff should be sensitive to residents' individual differences and wishes.

Providing a spiritual service that does include the word "God" may provide for the needs of many of the residents. These can include references to many different religions. The music can be a combination from religious writings as well as secular. For example, "My Country 'Tis of Thee," or, "I'm Forever Blowing Bubbles," can be "just as spiritual" when sung with feeling as a traditional hymn when the singing is enjoyed by residents with dementia. These services are often conducted by an interested staffperson or family member.

The health care provider does need to monitor the religious services offered by staff, family members, or volunteers. The concern centers on the possibility that persons with strong religious points of view may become zealous about their faith, possibly leading to evangelizing the residents. Services should be pleasant, not insistent.

Health care providers can open their doors to the clergy and the laity of the resident's former congregation. Clergy and laity should be encouraged to come and continue their connection with the resident. Providers can also host clergy training, perhaps by having a breakfast followed by information on dementia and suggestions for the clergy ministering to persons with dementia.

Pastoral care staff are not available in many health care facilities. Staff often enjoy being involved in the spiritual activities within a care center. Offering the residents spiritual activity can take a variety of formats. Staff may want to be part of the service, do the scripture reading, sing, or lead the service itself. Staff may also want to be involved with a memorial service when a loved resident has died. Other ideas are evening vespers, prayer groups, prayer circles, blessings before meals, and prayer before or just on going to bed.

Some care centers set up Bible studies or prayer groups for the staff. Scheduling may be a challenge and it is up to the center as to the times, as well as whether the activity is during work hours.

Health care providers, sensitive to the spiritual needs and uniqueness of their residents as well as their families, and the staff that care so deeply about them both, can be appreciated and respected. Compassionate connectedness unites us all.

SUMMARY

Caregivers ministering to residents are called to become comfortable with simplicity and shared silence and to re-evaluate their personal definitions of dignity, trust, worth, health, and aging. The routines of caregiving can take a ritual form that becomes intertwined with ministry between the caregiver and the resident. The poignant giving and taking and the offering of unconditional love and trust can become a grounding for redefining faith and inner values. The touch of hands, the rituals of bathing and dressing, the sharing of food, and the ability to see the divine within each other become a shared sacrament. Understanding, knowledge of the cognitive, physical, psychosocial, and spiritual aspects of dementia, and a deep love for what Quakers describe as "that of God within everyone" empowers shared experiences of well-being and spirituality.

Spirituality, therefore, can be a centering focus and a source of comfort for the person with dementia and his or her loved ones. Compassionate connectedness comes from one's positive sense of self, meaningful interaction with activity and others throughout the day, opportunities to reach out and do for others, and being surrounded by the warmth of a caring community of friends. "Being with" enables the spiritual self to enter into the sacredness of each day, and worship takes on new meanings and becomes an inner light for the yearning self, an activity of grace and acceptance.

SUGGESTED READING

Alzheimer's Association. Activity Programming for Persons with Dementia: A Sourcebook. Chicago: Alzheimer's Association, 1995.

Fischer K. Winter Grace: Spirituality for the Later Years. New York: Paulist Press, 1985.

Hellen C. The "C" connection: the confused worshiper with dementia, the clergy and the caring congregation. Aging and Spirituality. American Society on Aging Newsletter of the Forum on Religion, Spirituality and Aging 1994;VI(1):1, 4, 8.

Hopkins E, Woods Z, Kelley R, et al. Working with Groups on Spiritual Themes. Duluth, MN: Whole Person Associates, 1995.

Moore T. Care of the Soul: A Guide for Cultivating Depth and Sacredness in Everyday Life. New York: HarperCollins, 1992.

Murphey C. Day to Day: Spiritual Help When Someone You Love Has Alzheimer's. Philadelphia: The Westminster Press, 1988.

Richards M. Meeting the spiritual needs of the cognitively impaired. Generations 1990;4:63–64.

A11-1

Religious, Spiritual, and Sacred Center Assessment of Compassionate Connectedness

---

Resident: _____ Date: _____

1. Faith History
   A. Religious denomination choice and connection (past and present): _____

   B. Former worship community (name, address, pastor): _____ _____

   C. Level of involvement (services attended, committees, positions held, likes or dislikes, including scriptures, sacred music, sacraments, etc.): _____ _____

   D. Past sources of spiritual strength other than in formal religious settings. Describe. _____ _____

2. Current Faith Awareness and Spiritual Support
   A. Personal connection and perception of a higher power. Describe.___ _____

   B. Remembrance of past faith and worship experiences: _____ _____

   C. Current awareness and responses to worship, religious activity: ___ _____

   D. Present sources of strength, hope, and connectedness: _____ _____

E. Responses to and choices of spiritual activities: _____

Clergy visits. Describe likes and dislikes. _____

Religious services. Describe kind, place, number of participants, inactive or active involvement (e.g., choir, readings). _____

Sacraments. Describe responses, likes and dislikes of familiar and unfamiliar. _____

Rituals and symbols of faith. Describe likes and dislikes. _____

Scripture readings, discussions. Describe likes and dislikes. _____

Prayer opportunities (one to one, small group, large group): _____

Creative arts opportunities (literature, poetry, art, dance, drama, writing, nature, crafts): _____

Sacred music. Describe type, where, when, how. _____

Religious or spiritual videotapes. Describe likes and dislikes. _____

Service projects and activities for others. Describe. _____

Signature and position: _____

12

Terminal Care: Final Storm Weathered

A CHERISHED SENTINEL

Frequently death strikes swiftly
severing the thin line between
now and then, like a conifer
snapped by raging wind.

Quietly grief heals the sudden
pain, and love restores the
broken landscape. The living
accommodate, and move on.

Occasionally death strikes slowly.
Beginning at the top, it creeps
down life's tree until only a snag
remains, rooted, but bereft of green.

Then grief can't heal until the
loved ones let the snag become a
cherished sentinel, marking
memorable days and storms weathered.

—Arthur O. Roberts,
The Evangelical Friend, 1990;23:17

It is difficult to define the "terminal stage" of Alzheimer's disease; perhaps it is the time of the "cherished sentinel." The presentation of symptoms attributable to the dementia can be variable. Little is known about when, why, and how specific functional abilities are lost during the progression of dementia-related illnesses. It is as though the brain can no longer tell the body how it is supposed to respond.

Cohen et al. (1984) described the sixth and final psychological stage of dementia as being "separation from self":

At this point, individuals are capable of reacting to certain things that happen in their environment, but do not have the ability to be active in their environment. The family accepts the patient as greatly changed and a "different person." The major needs of the patient are to be comfortable and secure. During this period patients seem almost part of another world, unable to communicate or to act, yet they may still remain important persons in the emotional lives of their families.

Some residents become ill with symptoms leading to pneumonia or other systemic problems for 2–3 weeks before death. Others may remain in a nonresponsive state for months. Certainly, medical professionals have experienced surmising that a resident with dementia would expire within a few days, for example, due to refusing food for an extended period, only to find the resident starting to eat again, often with gusto. Family members often face an emotional roller coaster and a prolonged anticipatory grief experience.

It is equally difficult to describe the myriad of decisions facing families, physicians, and nursing home staff during the final period of caregiving. There are numerous legal issues affecting both family members and professional caregivers. Ethical considerations and legislative laws are changing, making the issues complex and, at times, confusing.

The intention of this chapter is not to attempt discussion of complicated legal or ethical questions. However, the issues involved in terminal care include decisions concerning the offering or withholding of the following active medical interventions:

- Resuscitation: Cardiopulmonary resuscitation? Respirator? Do not resuscitate?
- Aggressive workup for medical or emotional problems
- Transfer to acute care setting or hospital
- Treating acute, life-threatening problems
- Use of blood products
- Use of intravenous procedures
- Use of medications
- Tube feedings: food, hydration
- Gastrostomy feeding
- Forced feeding with syringes
- Fever and pain management

FAMILY GRIEF: SADNESS WITHOUT END

Comforting family members journeying with the resident through the final days requires health care professionals and caring staff. The family is now faced with the reality of death. They have been experiencing "anticipatory grief," perhaps for years. Often, grieving over the cognitive losses of their loved one has colored their days ever since the diagnosis of Alzheimer's was made.

Grief has many faces and is displayed in a variety of ways. Feelings are expressed or kept within the privacy of the heart. Families come to the terminal care period

Alzheimer's Disease: Activity-Focused Care

of their loved one with many emotions. Past experiences of dealing with loss now affect the current situation. It is hoped that the family will welcome and accept the offered help and support from the many persons who care, both during the experience of the resident's dying and after the death (see Chapter 13).

PAIN: RECOGNIZING AND RESPONDING TO THE MESSAGE

How should caregivers interpret the resident's moaning, crying, or restlessness? What is the message behind these symbols for words? Is the message pain? Pain is usually due to sources other than dementia. Experienced nurses and caregivers, who know the resident, can often pick up on the small changes that appear to be a response to pain. In Alzheimer's disease, the ability to communicate with words is often lost in the terminal care period and the use of nonverbal language cues are relied on. All demonstrations of pain should be explored for possible causes.

"Messages" of pain may include

- Negative sounds or noise that has a coloring of anger, hurt, or pain, often expressed faster than normal vocalizations
- Facial responses such as frowning or grimacing, sad expressions or looks of worry, hurt, wrinkled brow, mouth turned down, sadness, tears, crying
- Increased restlessness and thrashing while seated or in bed, fidgeting, squirming
- Rubbing or pulling at a body part as though the resident wishes he or she could pull it off and throw it away
- Overall worsening of behavior
- Body positioning with increased rigidity and extension, knees pulled up
- Hands clasped or in fists

"Messages" that all is well and pain may not be present include

- Contented sounds or vocalizations with a lyrical sound
- Facial responses of relaxed mouth, eyes open and tracking movement or sound, smooth brow, unclenched jaw
- Sitting or lying with body parts relaxed or with minimal movement, normal muscle tone
- General peaceful look and response to persons and the environment

Residents with dementia may not be able to interpret pain and therefore they do not demonstrate its presence. For example, a rib fracture might completely consume a resident who is able to comprehend the pain and can show its existence with vocalizations, body movement, or facial responses. A rib fracture occurring in another resident might go totally unnoticed when the resident is unable to "play out" its existence because of cognitive changes. It is hoped that this resident has nursing staff trained in picking up the most subtle clue and responding appropriately.

Pain may or may not be a significant factor during the terminal care period for persons with dementia. Medical supervision and caring response can help residents that do experience discomfort. Hospice care is dedicated to helping the resident to be free from pain and therefore is often selected by families concerned for their loved one's comfort.

HOSPICE: FINAL DAYS WITH A CARING TEAM

Hospice is a palliative treatment available when the disease itself is beyond cure and the resident is recognized by the attending physician as having 6 months or less to live. Although this is a difficult determination to make, physicians are able to most often be correct. The physician will certify that the resident is terminally ill.

Hospice care focuses on the care and management of the resident's comfort and pain level. The American Hospice Foundation, based in Washington, D.C., states in its brochure *Alzheimer's Disease and Hospice*:

> Hospice is a philosophy of care that treats people, not diseases, and neither hastens nor prolongs dying. Hospice affirms life and regards death as life's final task. Hospice professionals can develop a plan of care to meet the specific needs of persons with Alzheimer's disease. While the patient benefits from the best in medical care, both the patient and family are offered psychological, social and spiritual support.

Hospice benefits, usually covered under Medicare, can be used in the resident's home or can follow the resident into a care facility and continue services. Residents living in a care facility can also use hospice. Most hospice services involve a multidisciplinary team. When service is provided in a nursing home, the home's staff also interact with this team. Included on the team are nurses, nursing assistants, physicians, social workers, pastoral care services, bereavement counselor, and volunteers. Additional team members could include nutritionists, physical and occupational therapists, and other therapists as needed.

The decision to use hospice services rests on the family. Social services, working closely with families, are usually the one to inform family members about hospice services. It appears that some families are less likely to use services when they are content with the care being provided to their loved one by a nursing home. The hospice team and the facility's team must work together and support each other if the program is to be viable and successful. Conflict is not appropriate during this sensitive time of caregiving to the resident and to family members.

TERMINAL CARE CONSIDERATIONS

Caring for residents during the late stage of dementia requires flexibility and a focus on the resident's responses. The daily schedule changes to include more attention to medical and nursing-related caregiving. Mealtimes and promotion of adequate nutrition and hydration often become the central activity of the day. Social activities require more one-to-one attention for the resident to be able to interact. Naps are common, often while seated as well as in bed. The overall milieu of the environment is subdued, if possible—one of peace.

Even with the difficulties surrounding the definition and magnitude of terminal care interventions, valuable information is available to enable residents, families, and staff to respond and cope to the best of their abilities. Research and experience are widening the range of intervention options. Active dialogues, depending on personal ethics, will continue to challenge the balancing of life-sustaining actions with personal directives.

All aspects of care are reflected in the end stage of Alzheimer's disease. These include

- Medical needs and responses to impending death
- Psychosocial issues
- Communication
- Activities of daily care
- Eating and nutrition
- Mobility
- Behaviors
- Activities
- Spiritual support
- Death

The resident's experience of the ending of life, the family's responses and needs, and the effects of staff's caregiving enter a shared place that calls forth life's sacredness. Certainly, the resident, family, and staffpersons are affected deeply, as each in his or her own way struggles for inner peace, dignity, and the upholding of quality-of-life convictions.

MEDICAL ISSUES AND IMPENDING DEATH

Goals for medical management of the resident with terminal dementia needs vary. The challenges of end-stage care require family members and caregivers to recognize that the resident will not improve. The resident's comfort is supported by relieving pain and other distressing symptoms.

Resident's Experience

- The terminal care period may last a few days or more than a year.
- The resident is totally dependent on others for care but may respond to hand-over-hand care.
- The resident is unable to self-direct or initiate responses.
- The resident may experience inability to respond to any or all of the following: touch, sound, visual field, taste, odors.
- The resident has severe memory loss and inability to comprehend.
- The resident has decreased abilities or total inability to control body movement or functions.
- The resident has an increased possibility of skin ulcerations and skin tears.
- The resident has an increased risk for pneumonia and depressed immune system.
- The resident has increased oral secretions that cannot be coughed up and may require suctioning, or dry mouth due to mouth breathing or medications, or both.
- The resident may experience weight loss, even when intake is normal.
- The resident may experience hyperorality, in which nonedibles and most items placed in the resident's hand go directly into his or her mouth.
- The resident has an ongoing risk for dehydration.
- Caregiving can be difficult due to a primitive response that causes the resident's arms and legs to resist passive movement (called *paratonia* or *gegenhalten response*).
- The resident may experience sudden jerking, irregular muscle responses (myoclonus).
- Due to resident's restlessness in bed, railings may need to be padded.
- Caregivers may need to consider using a temperature-controlled water mattress or an alternating pressure mattress for supporting the resident's skin integrity.

- The resident's arms and legs may become cool to the touch.
- The resident's breathing may become shallow with periods, up to 30 seconds, of no breathing.
- There may be increased sleeping off and on during the day, and the resident may be difficult to arouse.
- The resident is aware of self only, and has decreased orientation to others and ability to recognize family.
- The resident may continue to be mobile but often is in a wheelchair or is bedridden.
- Death may be precipitated by a systemic illness, broken hip, etc.
- The resident may not show response to others but will usually show response to unmet needs such as hunger, pain, or unsafe environment.
- The resident may be moved from an intermediate care unit to an intensive nursing and skilled care area.
- The resident may be moved from a special care unit if unable to meet specific program criteria.
- The resident's response to care often is determined by the staff's expectations and philosophy. For example:
    Encouraging the resident to be present in the social environment
    Having a dedicated determination to keep the resident alive rather than offering palliative, noninterventional medical care

Family's Responses and Needs

See Chapter 13, Family and the Dying Resident.

- The family may move the person with Alzheimer's disease to a nursing home for increased medical care.
- This is a time for making decisions and advanced directives, if not already made (e.g., do not resuscitate, palliative care, medical intervention, symptom control, comfort support, hospitalization, nutrition and tubes).
- This is a time for revisiting decisions already made. These can be influenced by medical professionals recommending extensive medical interventions, and often result in the family feeling guilty if "everything" is not done for the resident.
- The family may consider hospice care options.
- The family should talk with the resident's physician about what to expect and how problems will be handled during the course of terminal care and decline.
- The family may elect to prearrange funeral plans.
- The family may consider a decision to authorize a brain autopsy.

Staff's Caregiving

- The staff should have social services available to provide information and support to the family.
- The staff should be offered support and information about the stages of grief (of the resident, his or her family members, and their own personal grief as caring staffpersons) before and after death.

Alzheimer's Disease: Activity-Focused Care

- Regulatory and legal policies and procedures should be in place for terminal medical care and support.
- Staff should deliver care, drawing on extensive staff training and experience.
- Consistent staffpersons familiar with the resident should be used.
- If requested, there should be a working arrangement with a hospice.
- Pastoral staff should be used to support resident, family, and staff.
- The facility should have a close, working arrangement with a hospital that is familiar with and understanding of Alzheimer's disease care (see Appendixes 12-1 and 12-2).

PSYCHOSOCIAL ISSUES: EMOTIONAL SUPPORT AND PRESERVATION OF PERSONHOOD

Compassionate touch and caring offers the resident emotional support and respect. Being present with the resident and comfortable with the shared silence can enable family and staff to journey together through the final days.

Resident's Experience

- The resident may appear depressed or emotionally unresponsive.
- The resident continues to need touch, acceptance, love, and safety and security.
- The resident exhibits decreased socialization or interest in others.
- The resident usually has limited tolerance for groups.
- The resident becomes annoyed by too much noise or activity by others.
- The resident may be unable to track visually, acknowledge others, recognize others.
- The resident may be withdrawn, "in his or her own world."
- The resident is unable to make choices between more than two objects.

Family's Responses and Needs

- The family experiences increased sadness and disappointment due to not being recognized or acknowledged during caregiving, visiting, or when bringing gifts.
- The family may need to redefine personal goals for visiting and may need to be encouraged to visit with "props" such as food or a flower to hold. They should continue to touch the resident to show caring and to offer him or her a sense of worth and value.
- Residents receiving love and attention from family members will usually also receive more attention from staff.
- The family member should develop an ability to become comfortable with "silence" with the resident who cannot talk to or with the family member.
- The family may experience or feel that the loved one is a different person (e.g., "This is not my mother, so I'm going to call her by her first name.").
- Family members should set aside time to take care of themselves.
- The family may benefit from professional emotional support.

Staff's Caregiving

- The staff should convey emotional and supportive responsiveness to the resident and family.
- The staff should continue to include the resident in social situations and activities, if tolerated.
- The staff should continue to dress and groom the resident appropriately.
- The staff should spend one-to-one time with the resident, using sensory input such as lotion, perfume, touch, massage, and hugs.
- The staff should continue talking with residents as though they understood every word (e.g., thanking them for being cooperative, thanking them for drinking their juice, and giving them step-by-step descriptions of caregiving procedures).

COMMUNICATION: "TALKING TOUCH"

Communications continue through the terminal-care period. Words, music, touch, humming, holding the resident, and rocking all become an open door for connecting with the resident in a meaningful, often adaptive and wordless language of love and support.

Resident's Experience

See Appendix 4-2.

- The resident will experience the "words" that compassionate touch conveys.
- The resident can communicate consent to caregivers in subtle ways.
- The resident may communicate through "geriatric rap" (i.e., ongoing verbalization that makes sense if you listen carefully, as the immediate surroundings and happenings might be related in a songlike way, although sometimes the sung words are reflections from the past).
- The resident may have incoherent verbalizations or word perseverations, such as, "help me, help me, help me," or, "here, here, here, here."
- The resident is usually nonverbal except for occasional words or limited phrases.
- Even if caregivers are unable to judge what the resident understands, residents still should continue to receive respect and adult, not childlike, conversation from others.
- The resident may try to speak, often in a foreign language if English was not his or her primary language.
- The resident may demonstrate facial grimaces or hand or arm gestures.
- The resident is often able to share feelings and awareness through nonverbal means and body language.

Family's Responses and Needs

- The family should continue talking with the resident, not asking questions but relating familiar family stories or describing present events, reading favorite poetry, scriptures.

Alzheimer's Disease: Activity-Focused Care

- The family should touch and use nonverbal communications. They should face the resident at eye level and try to attract his or her attention before speaking.
- Family members should continue to identify themselves at the start of the visit and occasionally during the time together (e.g., "Mother, I am Susan, your daughter.").

Staff's Caregiving

- The staff should realize that touch "talks" and use the opportunity to exhibit caring and love to the resident through touch, but they should also use care when contact is made with sensitive skin.
- Staff will be able to "hear" the resident's response to rough or insensitive care.
- Staff should have a speech therapist available for assessments, if appropriate.
- The staff should talk during contact with the resident, describing the caregiving process or other subjects the resident might find interesting, even though the resident does not acknowledge the conversation.
- The staff should sing around the resident, especially old familiar songs.
- The staff should be aware of personal body language and how it has positive or negative effects on the resident.
- The staff should continue giving smiles and hugs throughout the illness, even if the resident is bedfast.
- The staff should use knowledge from extensive training to observe the resident for subtle changes. They should watch facial expression as a communication predictor of the resident's current health and needs.
- The staff should provide a model for families on how to "visit" with the resident, even if meaningful conversation cannot take place.

ACTIVITIES OF DAILY CARE: ENABLING DIGNITY

Activities of daily care are the most personal opportunities for the supportive communication of love and respect for the resident. During the days of terminal care, residents can intuitively know they are safe and accepted when activities of daily living are offered with gentleness. See Chapter 5.

Resident's Experience

- The resident is dependent on others but may respond to hand-over-hand caregiving.
- The resident may have contractures or rigidity, or both, making activities of daily living care uncomfortable or painful.
- The resident may exhibit involuntary resistance and tensing in the arms and legs as a response to passive movement by the caregiver during bathing, dressing, and overall caregiving.
- The resident often responds favorably to a tub bath for relaxing, soaking, and bathing.
- The resident may refuse oral care, only allowing swabs or a washcloth to wipe teeth.

- The resident becomes totally incontinent of bowel and bladder with susceptibility to constipation, bowel impaction, and urinary tract infections.
- The resident may develop skin integrity problems that often lead to reddening
and skin breakdown. Skin may tear easily when touched. The resident may
quickly develop severe decubitus that responds poorly to treatment.

Family's Responses and Needs

- The family should provide larger, soft clothing with a loose elastic waist.
- The family should select cotton fabrics to decrease odor retention.
- The family should supply clothing or underwear that opens down the back, but
not with uncovered zippers or raised buttons.
- The family should provide undershirts instead of bras.
- The family should have available kneesocks, sweaters, and other warm cloth-
ing, as the resident may feel cold.
- The family should bring in loose-fitting socks to prevent ankle or foot swelling.
- If comfortable and wanting to participate in activities of daily living care, the
family should be encouraged to ask staff how and when to be involved.

Staff's Caregiving

- The staff should have knowledge and expertise in safe transfer maneuvers and
skills for positioning residents.
- The staff should continue to dress and groom the resident attractively, even when
he or she is in bed, with clean hair, shaved face, and makeup neatly applied.
- The staff should focus on keeping the resident clean and dry, observe for skin-
care needs, and report any reddened pressure areas.
- The staff should have an occupational therapist available to adapt clothing, and
to address eating and dressing modifications, if appropriate.

NUTRITION AND EATING: DEMONSTRATION OF CARING

Eating and mealtimes are always opportunities to offer the resident experiencing
late-stage dementia compassion and respect. Special health needs often require specific dietary interventions. All changes usually have a serious impact on the resident's abilities to eat and drink safely and effectively, thereby affecting his or her
well-being. See Chapter 6.

Resident's Experience

- The resident has decreased desire to eat and drink; therefore, mealtimes require
a caring and compassionate approach and patience.
- Eating becomes the daily focus; mealtimes may take up to 2 hours each.
- The resident should have food and drink continuously offered, even when he
or she refuses to eat.
- The resident usually loses weight, despite eating sufficient calories.

- The resident needs close monitoring of feeding due to increased risk of choking.
- The resident may need the consistency of food changed because of increased chewing and swallowing dysfunction.
- The resident may or may not be able to swallow.
- The resident may refuse totally to eat for a period and then start again for no apparent reason.
- The resident may clamp mouth shut and refuse any food or drink.
- The resident may need feeding through a syringe or tube feeding, if appropriate to his or her plan of care.

Family's Responses and Needs

- The family should understand that the refusal to eat often is due to the dementing illness, and should be prepared to participate in the decision to implement or withhold feeding through tubes.
- The family should determine whether it helps or not to be present at mealtime.
- The family should become knowledgeable about the resident's eating problems and the seesaw response of eating and not eating.
- The family should bring in a favorite food that is not generally available to the resident, especially an ethnic or holiday specialty.

Staff's Caregiving

- The staff should have knowledge and expertise in feeding residents with end-stage dementia.
- The staff should evaluate for all factors affecting eating (e.g., medicines, limited taste responses, obstructions, throat ulcers, or conscious effort on the resident's part).
- The staff should exhibit willingness to be patient and realize that mealtime takes an extended period.
- Staff should offer smaller meals, more often.
- The staff should have knowledge of the Heimlich maneuver in case the resident chokes.
- Staff should offer cold food, such as ice cream, in between spoonfuls of other food to encourage eating and swallowing.
- Pureed food that can be placed in a high-protein shake may be given when the resident refuses to let a spoon be placed into his or her mouth.
- The staff should have a speech therapist available for swallowing assessment.
- The staff should have a dietitian available to assess the resident's food consistency and suggest ways to promote increased calorie intake.

MOBILITY: ASSISTED AND PASSIVE MOVEMENT

Promoting safe mobility and range of motion helps residents with terminal care needs to move whenever and however possible. Careful attention is required for the resident incapable of self-movement skills. The family and staff unite to support movement and proper body positioning as a necessary component for the resident's overall well-being. See Chapter 7.

Resident's Experience

- Contrary to former thought, if ambulating is promoted, the resident may remain mobile in the terminal stage until up to a week or two before death or the onset of an illness precipitating death.
- If the resident is mobile, he or she may experience perceptual dysfunction such as walking into door frames or tripping over furniture legs or objects that stick out.
- The resident has increasing susceptibility to falls, decreased trunk flexibility, problems getting in and out of chairs, and poor balance; he or she needs encouragement to continue being mobile for as long as possible.
- If chairbound, the resident often will slouch or slide down out of the chair, lean to one side, or bend forward from the waist.
- When immobile, the resident may need total assistance for transfers and repositioning every 2 hours, or more often if needed. The resident may do better in a recliner-type chair or with a tray table on a wheelchair so the arms can help support the trunk.
- The resident has an increased tendency for contractures, especially in the shoulders, elbows, hands, hips, and knees.
- If inactive for several days, the resident often is not able to resume mobility.
- Terminal care residents are rarely able to recover mobility after breaking a hip.

Family's Responses and Needs

- The family can encourage the resident's mobility and range of motion by promoting exercise with activities such as a balloon toss or another game.
- The family can learn how to facilitate passive range of motion or assisted range of motion.
- The family may need to express concerns and participate in the plan of care because of the resident's failing ambulation and increased risk of falling.
- The family can give their opinion concerning the use of restraints as a safeguard intervention.
- The family can use lotion and massage fingers, hands, arms, and legs.

Staff's Caregiving

- The staff should have physical and occupational therapists available to assess mobility needs and to promote restorative services when appropriate.
- The staff should have an understanding and knowledge of the implementation of restraint-free positioning devices or methods to safeguard the resident and maintain the best possible positioning, such as wedge pillows to prevent sliding from a chair.
- The staff should be able to use restraints correctly if prescribed by the physician (e.g., use a geriatric chair for a constantly pacing resident in need of a therapeutic rest period).
- The staff should use range-of-motion techniques at least once a day.
- The staff should position the resident to reduce contractures.
- The staff should move the resident out of bed daily unless medically contraindicated.

- The staff should consider the positive, negative, or annoying aspects of splinting or adapted devices before using.
- The staff should use a variety of seating possibilities each day. For example, start the resident out in a wheelchair, transfer him or her to a regular chair at mealtime, and then to a recliner after meals.

BEHAVIOR: CHALLENGING DEMONSTRATIONS

The resident's behavior during late-stage care may include demonstrations of his or her need to touch, grab, and make noises. Behaviors often provide the resident with an opportunity to exhibit inner thoughts and needs. Safety and reassurance become the focus of behavioral refocusing interventions. See Chapter 8.

Resident's Experience

- The resident experiences behavioral responses affected by mood instability.
- The resident may hit, bite, scratch, or grab and hold on tightly to persons, doorways, or things.
- The resident has an increased tendency to grab at any stimulus and not understand how to let go.
- The resident may moan, shout, or swear.
- The resident may be in constant movement (e.g., wiping or moving his or her hands on tables or clothing; swaying side to side; tapping the table or lap; chewing fingers, clothing, or nothing; grimacing; or moving feet or legs).
- The resident may masturbate or play with genitals, strip off clothing.
- The resident may put everything in his or her mouth.

Family's Responses and Needs

- Family members need understanding, support, and acceptance when their loved one is calling or acting out. They should realize that this is often part of the progressive dementia.
- Family members need reassurance that their loved one will continue to receive good care even when his or her behaviors make caregiving difficult.

Staff's Caregiving

- The staff can model for the family ways of interacting with the resident even though difficult behaviors are being exhibited.
- The staff should incorporate the knowledge and experience needed to understand behaviors and appropriate interventions.
- The staff should show patience even for repetitive calling out or noises, and understand distraction techniques and the use of repetitious tasks, such as folding washcloths, to reduce undesired behaviors.
- Safety should be provided for the resident, other residents, families, and staff.

ACTIVITIES: HONORING SIMPLICITY

Creating and promoting safe, simple activities offers residents a means to focus, be engaged, and feel connected to the moment. Activities that can be enjoyed through the senses and the implementation of familiar normalization tasks can enable the resident to feel accepted and nurtured. See Chapter 9, Shoestring and Wearable Activities for Resident with Short Attention Spans and Sensory Stimulation and Activities for Late-Stage Dementia Care sections.

Resident's Experience

- The resident may continue to experience activities passively despite a limited demonstration of alertness.
- The resident may need hand-over-hand guidance for exercising and large-motor responses to activities.
- The resident will respond to music with a strong beat such as marches or "Sing Along with Mitch."
- The resident will hold objects tightly and often will not give them back.
- The resident has fleeting attention span, if any.
- The resident can be nonresponsive to all sensory stimulation.
- The resident may fade in and out of activity participation, taking little naps throughout the day.

Family's Responses and Needs

- The family should be encouraged to accompany the resident to church services and musical programs when visiting.
- The family can bring a friend when coming to visit or invite a more talkative resident to join the visit.
- The family can bring bright, cheery decorations for the bedroom for sensory stimulation.
- The family can supply and play cassettes of favorite music, hymns, or songs.
- The family may put together a family album to show when talking about the past, even if resident does not "see" the pictures or respond (see Chapter 3).
- The family may bring a pet to be patted, touched, and enjoyed by the resident.

Staff's Caregiving

- The staff should bring resident to activities, if tolerated, and do not leave him or her alone in the bedroom unless he or she needs "quiet time."
- The staff should carefully swing resident's arms to music, use hand-over-hand exercising, and offer one-to-one activities.
- The staff should introduce soft objects to hold, such as a teddy bear or, if accepted and appropriate, a baby doll.
- The staff should play music on a tape player or radio; try a headset.
- The staff should be aware of the music's mood and its effect on the resident.
- The staff should use brightly colored objects, such as balloons, to attract attention.

Alzheimer's Disease: Activity-Focused Care

- The staff should touch and hug the resident, and stroke his or her face and hair.
- The staff should continue to groom the resident.
- The staff should have recreational, music, or occupational therapists, or all, available to promote sensory stimulation and other therapeutic activities.

SPIRITUAL SUPPORT: COMPASSIONATE CONNECTEDNESS

Upholding the resident's spirituality throughout the final days helps surround the resident with compassionate caring. The resident, family, and staff may often seek spiritual support as a way to say final good-byes. See Chapter 11.

Resident's Experience

- The resident often continues to respond to familiar religious music, prayers, rituals, and symbols.
- The resident may continue to find comfort in worship services.
- The resident may be able to say parts of familiar prayers or chants.

Family's Responses and Needs

- The family often needs, benefits, and appreciates support from clergy.
- The family often finds pleasure in taking their loved one with them to religious services.
- Clergy may be helpful with end-of-life decision making.

Staff's Caregiving

- The staff appreciate clergy coming to spend time with the resident and the family.
- The staff often like to be included in bedside prayers.
- The staff may benefit personally from supportive pastoral care.

DEATH: CREATION OF A "CHERISHED SENTINEL"

Death may strike slowly or quickly, but it always brings, as stated in Arthur O. Robert's poem, *A Cherished Sentinal*, tales of memorable days and storms weathered. Family members and staff gather to share the grief.

Resident's Experience

- Immediate cause of death is often from pneumonia, dehydration, infection, or malnutrition.
- The resident often needs medical support, such as oxygen for comfort, just before death.
- After being in a comatose-type state, the resident often dies of pneumonia or systemic infections.

Family's Responses and Needs

- A family whose members live far from the dying resident may want to select a hospice that has an end-of-life sitter and vigil service so the resident is not alone.
- Family members are often "surprised" by their loved one's death, and say that they did not expect it. Usually, they need support, hugs, and understanding. Each family member experiences death differently, depending on many factors (e.g., past coping with death or difficult situations, past relationship with the resident, relationships within the family).
- If comfortable, family members may want to be available to grieving staffpersons who want to talk about the resident and may want to cry with the family.
- Family members may need to have understanding for staffpersons who are uncomfortable being with them when their loved one has died.
- The family may want to decide if they want contributions made to, for example, the Alzheimer's Association or the facility.

Staff's Caregiving

- Pastoral care services should be available for the resident, family, and staff.
- If possible, staff should be sure that the family knows when death is exceedingly imminent.
- The resident's mouth and lips should be kept moist; a room humidifier should be used.
- The staff should plan with the family, before the death, how they want to be called (e.g., Do they wish to be called just before death so they can come to the bedside? Are calls in the middle of the night all right?).
- The staff should allow the family to stay with the resident during the final days or hours, respecting their need for privacy and providing needed meals, use of the phone, and other basic facilities. If at all possible, a roommate should be moved to another room during the last few days or hours.
- The staff should use great care and sensitivity when phoning family members who were not present when the death occurred.
- The staff should be available to be with the family, if requested.
- The staff may need support and understanding as they grieve for the loss of the resident and "loss" of the family with whom they will no longer be involved.
- Staff should be allowed time for good-byes.
- The staff should allow the family to stay with the resident for as long as they wish after the resident's death.
- If an autopsy has been planned, staff should have the details worked out so that it can take place as soon as possible.
- The staff should help the family in gathering the resident's possessions or pack them for the family, if requested.
- A memorial service should be held for the other residents and staff, if appropriate. The family members should be invited to participate or attend if they would like to be present (see Chapter 11, Service of Remembrance: Celebrating Our Friend).
- Social services should be available for bereavement support for the family and staff.

AUTOPSY: THE OPPORTUNITY OF GIFTING OTHERS

The decision to have an autopsy is often made long before the time of the resident's death. At times, the decision is made by the resident during the early years of Alzheimer's disease and should be in writing. A durable power of attorney for health care or the resident's guardian can also make this decision. All paperwork must be completed before death occurs to ensure proper handling.

At present, an autopsy of brain tissues is the most accurate way to diagnose the type of dementia affecting the resident. Other reasons for an autopsy include assisting with research and to have accurate health records for the family for future reference.

Alzheimer's Association chapters can provide families and facilities with concise, helpful information about the autopsy procedure, how the tissue can be used, and what possible outcome to expect, including an accurate diagnosis.

Families who had intentions of following through with an autopsy sometimes change their minds, even when all the paperwork before death is in place. This is certainly the family's perogative and their wishes must be supported.

HEALTH CARE PROVIDER AND STAFF ISSUES

Has the staff shared in creating the late-stage care mission and objectives? Staff grieve, often deeply, for their residents and the families. The expectations of the family members should be clearly defined so staff can provide the end-of-life wishes. At times, the choices made by family members are extremely difficult for the staff to personally understand or respect. The family is ultimately the decision maker. Staff should have a willingness to accept diverse family behaviors and reactions during end-stage care and the resident's death. Staff may benefit from social services support, especially when their personal or cultural belief system conflicts with family directives. Usually, staff dislike "giving up" on a dying resident.

Just before the resident's death, staff who have a special caring relationship with the dying resident should be asked if they wish to be contacted if they are not on duty. If possible, allow staffpersons to sit with the dying resident to provide presence and comfort. Staff may also desire to have time to sit with the family members during this time.

At the time of death, gather staff to say good-bye, perhaps with prayer or holding hands in silence. If possible, offer staff time to be with the resident alone if they choose. Also, ask staffpersons if they choose to prepare the body or not, respecting their decisions. Enable staff to attend the resident's wake or funeral, if they choose.

Health care provider issues center on end-of-life decisions and the provider's response in honoring them. If a facility has specific issues related to the dying resident, they should be made very clear to family members at the time of admission. The family, experiencing the imminent death of their loved one, will feel anguish, frustration, and anger if there are any "surprises" from the provider around the preferred care offered.

Providing hospice care within the health care setting is becoming a viable choice for family members. Several hospice providers should be available so the family can make an informed decision. Another option is for the development of a terminal care or hospice special care unit within a facility. Teamwork and staff training, with tremendous support and nurturing from pastoral care and social services, are the key components for success.

If the family has decided that they wish to have an autopsy, this information should be on the resident's chart along with precise procedures to follow in contacting the designated hospital system providing the pathologist. Family members will be extremely disappointed and angered if the autopsy process is not facilitated in a timely manner. Be prepared that family members might change their minds just before or after the death and cancel plans for an autopsy.

A resident's death affects everyone within a health care facility. At times, mourning is "doubled" because the resident's family has been part of the facility's "family" and they, too, will be missed.

SUMMARY

Caring for the person needing terminal Alzheimer's care calls forth the caregiver's strength to have courage and, most important, to have presence. Presence reflects one's inner self . When the resident is dying, the simplicity of one's inner self that reflects a caring peace offered to the resident is the greatest gift.

The community of residents, family, friends, and staffpersons is touched and often diminished when a "Cherished Sentinel" passes from their circle.

REFERENCE

Cohen D, Kennedy G, Eisdorfer C. Phases of change in the patient with Alzheimer's dementia: a conceptual dimension for defining health care management. J Am Geriatr Soc 1984;32:11–15.

SUGGESTED READING

Brechling B, Kuhn D. A specialized hospice for dementia patients and their families. Am J Hospice Care 1989;4:27–30.

Groher ME. Dysphagia Diagnosis and Management (3rd ed). Boston: Butterworth–Heinemann, 1997.

Kitwood T, Bredin K. Towards a theory of dementia care: personhood and well-being. Aging Soc 1992;269–287.

Kovach CR (ed). Late-Stage Dementia Care: A Basic Guide. Washington, DC: Taylor and Francis, 1996.

Kovach CR, Wilson SA, Noonan PE. Effects of hospice interventions on behaviors, discomfort, and physical complications of end-stage dementia. J Alzheimer's Care Rel Dis Res 1996;11:7–15.

Mace NL. Dementia Care Units in Nursing Home. In DH Coons (ed), Specialized Dementia Care Units. Baltimore: Johns Hopkins University Press, 1991;55–82.

Volicer L, Hurley AC, Lathi DC, Kowall NW. Measurement of severity in advanced Alzheimer's disease. J Gerontol 1994;49:M223–M226.

Volicer L, Rheaume Y, Brown J, et al. Hospice approach to the treatment of patients with advanced dementia of the Alzheimer type. JAMA 1986;256:2210–2213.

A12-1
Alzheimer's Patient Hospital Transfer Information

Name: _____ Transfer date: _____

From: _____ Phone number: _____

Prefers to be called: _____

Right-handed: ____ Left-handed: ____

Awareness and orientation (attention span, task simplification): _____
_____

Communication, approaches, language: _____
_____

Physical movement or mobility: _____
_____

Eating (needs and behaviors): _____
_____

Bowel and bladder (needs and behaviors): _____
_____

Dressing, hygiene (approaches and assistance): _____
_____

Psychosocial support: _____
_____

Behaviors (responses and assistance): _____
_____

Safety concerns: _____
_____

Activity support: _____
_____

For more information, phone: _____

Name and position: _____

Time and date: _____

A12-2
Alzheimer's Patient Hospital Transfer Information Explanation and Worksheet

The purposes of the patient transfer form include the following:

- Use as a quick follow-up report to the hospital after nursing home discharge; all information on a one-page fax to be added to the patient's chart or posted at the bedside
- Augment the standard nursing home transfer form
- Inform hospital staff of specific caregiving and support information as it relates to patients with dementia
- A useful tool to "speak for" the resident—who usually is not able to speak for himself or herself
- Promote the continuation of caring, supportive approaches and care interventions by the nursing home before discharge
- Provide a resource person for the hospital to contact

AWARENESS AND ORIENTATION

- Ability to know where resident is, why
- Ability to respond to needs (e.g., use of the call light)
- Specific methods of using clueing verbally, nonverbally, and visually to increase understanding
- Use of reality orientation versus therapeutic fibs

COMMUNICATION, APPROACHES, LANGUAGE

- Verbal skills and inabilities
- Need to simplify words and sentences and to give one-step directions

- Use of yes or no questions or choosing between two items
- Use of touch—expected responses
- Nonverbal abilities
- Ability to understand staff's nonverbal intervention
- Include the communication assessment profile for residents with late-stage dementia, if appropriate (see Appendix 4-2)

PHYSICAL MOVEMENT AND MOBILITY

- Walking or gait patterns, dysfunctions
- Ability to sit down and stand up from chairs
- Body awareness
- Wheelchair mobility
- Ability to reposition body or move by command, problems
- Upper extremity and lower extremity abilities and inabilities
- Range-of-motion needs and suggestions

EATING: NEEDS AND BEHAVIORS

- Food consistency requirements
- Usual behaviors, approaches
- Ways to simplify food, utensil, and tray presentation
- Length of time to eat
- Specific help needed
- Safety—choking
- Food likes and dislikes
- Food adaptation suggestions

BOWEL AND BLADDER: NEEDS AND BEHAVIORS

- Ability to follow directions, kinds of assistance needed
- Routine (e.g., timing, habits, nighttime needs)
- Key words (especially if English is not primary language)
- Inappropriate toileting behaviors
- Type of incontinence product used, if appropriate

DRESSING AND HYGIENE: APPROACHES AND ASSISTANCE

- Need of assistance, task simplification
- Useful clueing methods
- Bathing preferences
- Oral care approaches
- Assistance needed to dress, groom appropriately

PSYCHOSOCIAL SUPPORT

- Usual responses to others, including race and gender biases
- Use of talking or singing, or both, during caregiving as a distraction technique
- Other distraction technique suggestions
- Validation support suggestions
- General mood information
- Ways to support self-image, give comfort
- Religious affiliation suggestions

BEHAVIORS: RESPONSES AND ASSISTANCE

- Specific behaviors (i.e., triggers, antecedents, interventions)
- Timing of behaviors to be refocused
- Distraction technique suggestions
- Anticipated responses

SAFETY CONCERNS

- Mobility and positioning challenges
- Eating unsafe items
- Spatial-perceptual dysfunctions
- Use of restraints
- Issues of safety with staff, other patients
- Elopement issues

ACTIVITY SUPPORT

- Simple tasks to give sense of well-being, purposeful use of time, meaningfulness
- Activity support in response to positive or negative behaviors, or both, such as activities to reduce or refocus combativeness and yelling and pacing

13

Family Caregivers: Needs, Partnership, and Support

The family's journey through the decline of their loved one's cognitive and physical abilities is often a long and involved struggle. Emotions, responses, hopes, joys, and sadness become like a roller coaster ride for all persons involved with the resident with dementia. The ambiguity of good moments or days in contrast with difficult periods becomes a challenge. Even the times of being or not being recognized by the resident wrench the hearts of caregivers because they never know what response will be forthcoming. The resident often looks well physically, which causes outsiders to question the caregiver's talk about incompetence or medical system failures.

Family members often experience isolation from friends, frustration, anger, exhaustion, and loss of patience. They strive to understand what is happening to their loved one, and they struggle together against the progressive dementia.

Family members may experience difficulty accepting the diagnosis of Alzheimer's disease or related disorders. They maintain an inner hope that the resident does not have dementia as physicians cannot be absolutely positive until the brain tissue is studied. Families may sometimes look for signs that the resident is getting better or hope that a cure will be found in time.

During the resident's middle to late stages of dementia, the family usually does their best to give care and cope with their own grief. They are forced into problem solving from the simplest dressing task to complex issues such as toileting, safety, and mobility. New roles and approaches need to be learned. Men may have to learn how to prepare meals and do tasks their wives at one time handled independently. Women may need to learn about family finances or, in some situations, learn how to drive. Caregivers are put into the position of making decisions regarding appropriate care, and often place themselves at risk emotionally and physically.

Families often choose to continue caregiving in their home. They have strong emotional ties and beliefs that strengthen their inner satisfaction of being able to provide hands-on care. Adequate support by family members and friends enable them to succeed. Caregiving is demanding and hard work. Caregivers need positive attitudes, confidence in themselves, and the insight to realize that caring for themselves is imperative (see Appendix 13-1). They may turn to respite help or other professional services in the home, especially at night so they can sleep.

Other families choose not to continue as caregivers or because of various circumstances find themselves considering alternatives.

GRIEF AND LOSS

Residents with dementia are continuing the journey of Alzheimer's along a path that travels through change and diminishing abilities. Family members also travel along this sometimes sad journey. Grief can be an appropriate emotional response to the experience of loss. It is unique to the person experiencing it. Anticipatory grief can occur before the death of the loved one with dementia. It is often called "preparatory grief" but it is just as real and poignant as the grief after the death of a loved one.

Symptoms of grieving for a family member with Alzheimer's disease affect one's physical, emotional, and spiritual well-being. Greater difficulties are experienced when the family has dysfunctional relationships among its members. Histories of abuse or excessive anger, unrealistic expectations about the resident's abilities or inabilities, limited support from within or outside the family, and the refusal to seek medical or care assistance compound the emotional complexities experienced by the family members. Typical experiences of loss, grief, and change for the family members may include

1. *Changes in the family member's relationship with the resident*: personality changes; difficulties with communication and understanding each other; role reversals and changes in previous relationship; need to take on decision making; weathering of the resident's behavioral challenges and emotional changes; and possible embarrassment or need to make excuses for the resident

2. *Changes in the family member's previously held dreams of the future with the resident*: experiencing changes in the person the resident used to be; challenges to rebuild the plans of today as well as for the future; changes in financial support for the future; disappointment of putting aside personal plans to be able to tend to the present situation of caregiving for a loved one with a progressive brain disease; grieving lost opportunities to share family joys

3. *Changes in the family member's daily life living*: days lived that focus around the resident and caregiving; becoming isolated from friends and social support; possibility of becoming overinvolved in resident care; feelings of limited time for personal interests; role ambiguity

4. *Changes in the family member's personal well-being*: possibility of depression; risks of overwhelming fatigue; feelings of being overwhelmed or alone on the journey of dementia caregiving; manifestation of physical health problems; need to be listened to and validation of his or her personal caregiving story; need to have options that offer a safe arena to process feelings, grief, and needs

MAKING NURSING HOME PLACEMENT DECISIONS

Certainly, the words "nursing home" have been lurking in the back of caregivers' minds since they first suspected their loved one's deteriorating mental abilities. Again, the roller coaster of emotions takes place as attempts are made to weigh the myriad of factors involved in long-term care placement. Many times the decision-making process is lonely, and the caregiver feels overwhelmed by the burden of responsibility. Sometimes promises made, such as, "I will never put you in a nursing home," haunt the family as they attempt to handle perhaps this most difficult crisis of caregiving. Not being able to follow through on this promise increases the caregiver's anxiety and sense of guilt (see Appendix 13-2).

When the decision to place a resident is being considered by a family that is a merged family of adult children due to a second or third marriage the issues become more complex. If at all possible, the goal is to achieve a consensus from all the family members. When this united support for placement is not possible, however, the individual family members sometimes appear to struggle during and after the placement. These family members often prove to be demanding and unrealistic in their relationship with a care center and its staff.

Suggestions to Ease Nursing Home Placement

Open communication with all members of the family is helpful before, during, and after placement in a nursing home. Social service staff may need to suggest individual or family therapy if appropriate. Staff benefit from training in sensitivity about family losses and grieving and how to offer support.

Social service agencies, departments on aging, hospitals, libraries, and senior citizen centers are a few of the professional resources available to help with the decision-making process. The Alzheimer's Association takes an active role in supporting caregivers with information and accounts of personal experience.

Decision-Making Factors

Resident

1. Ability to participate, enjoy, and benefit from the Alzheimer's program.
2. Incontinence, immobility, combativeness, hazardous behaviors, overall safety being compromised by diminishing awareness and poor judgment, and day-night reversal of sleeping patterns are the most common problems leading to the decision to place the resident in long-term care.
3. Poor hygiene that might lead to serious medical problems.
4. Weight loss, poor nutrition.
5. Noncompliance with medical needs (e.g., an insulin injection or cooperation with eating a diabetic diet).
6. Decreased skills and difficulties in caring for one's self or being uncooperative with caregiver.
7. Combativeness, physically or verbally abusive.
8. Lack of caregiving support, perhaps due to dysfunctional family relationships or being apart geographically.

Caregiver

1. Compromised physical wellness: decreased strength, health problems, exhaustion
2. Emotional stress, anxiety, depression, or fear
3. Concern over one's own quality of life and meaningful activities
4. Positive or negative past experiences of coping with illness
5. Willingness to seek help
6. Cultural norms affecting caregiving
7. Lifestyle incompatible with being involved with caring for an ill or needy family member

Support from Family and Friends

1. Family relationships, sibling support or rivalries, family history
2. Cultural background influences on caregiving, past models of handling stressful chronic illnesses, coping with losses, resolving grief
3. Geographic, financial factors

Financial Considerations

1. Complex because of a variety of issues: personal income, long-term care insurance, state laws and reimbursement, a nursing home's specific admission requirements, and other factors.
2. Decisions can be influenced by consideration of money spent for in-home assistance or day care and how much money is left for later entry into the nursing home of choice; this is often a delicate balance.

Continuum of Services Available

1. Options and care alternatives can vary greatly depending on location: could include respite care at home or in a facility; day care, sheltered care, or early-stage care within a facility; small group home; foster care; or bed-and-board home.
2. Time to become acquainted with options and assess their appropriateness should be taken, if possible, before a crisis that might require immediate decision making.
3. Many books, pamphlets, and the Alzheimer's Association may give assistance.

NURSING HOME'S RESPONSE: BUILDING THE BRIDGE

Nursing homes with a commitment to caring for persons with dementia can become a resource and support for families facing placement decisions. Family caregivers often ask, "When will I know it's the right time? When my loved one no longer knows who I am?" These often repeated questions can be the start of a close relationship between nursing home professionals and the family. The emphasis on support before resident admission will benefit all of those persons involved in the process.

Honest Description of Services

Staff in the nursing home must be honest about the care their program can offer as well as what they cannot provide. For example, some families may jump to the conclusion that since the Alzheimer's program is so excellent, their loved one will receive almost one-to-one care for activities of daily living and other activities. Being realistic should begin at the start of the relationship between the family and the nursing home. Unrealistic expectations become painful for both the family and the caregiver and open the door to distrust and disappointment.

Preadmission Support Factors

1. Recognizing caregivers' need for support and their grief over the loss of their loved one's cognitive and communication abilities as the dementia progresses. Being able to offer support for all of the family members, especially if some are from out of town.

2. Helping caregivers by encouraging them to take care of themselves physically and emotionally. Suggesting professional counseling, if appropriate.

3. Understanding the stress of selecting a nursing home as the family seeks to find the "best"—one that truly understands dementia care.

4. Willingness to be a resource and answer questions or solve a crisis via the telephone or in person while "waiting until it's the right time" for placement.

5. Inviting caregivers to attend educational or support group functions at the nursing home.

6. If possible, visiting the incoming resident for a home evaluation. This assessment becomes an opportunity to validate the caregivers and learn the approaches and techniques they have used with their loved one. Families generally have given excellent care to the resident and a health care professional's confirmation that they have done a wonderful job is tremendously important. The preadmission assessment decreases admission stress not only for the family but for the nursing home staff as well (see Appendix 13-3).

> Frances had been a successful artist and her apartment was filled with her paintings. During the home visit, the director of Alzheimer's care from the nursing home was able to compliment Frances on her great talent and ask her daughter about caregiving procedures. After this visit, the daughter videotaped her mother in the apartment while she commented about each picture. It was only as the daughter watched the video that she realized the depth of her

mother's impairments, physically and cognitively. The daughter discovered that each question she had asked Mom she had answered herself because her mother was not able to find the words or showed an inability to understand and follow the conversation. The daughter gave the facility the tape just before admission day. The staff who viewed this film appreciated its valuable information about Frances, including her history, word-finding and communication dysfunctions, socialization skills, and motor problems. Staffpersons expressed concern for the daughter who needed support because she probably was not fully aware of her mother's limitations.

7. Being available for a preadmission assessment to help caregivers decide about the timing of the placement.

8. Completing required documents, including designation of a durable power of attorney. One person should be named as the "responsible party."

9. Alerting the family to the possibilities that their loved one might appear to "improve" with placement in the care center. At times, the improvement is actual. Organized and nutritious meals, social events encouraging engagement, and meaningful activities may bring out the resident's abilities previously not used. Staff working 8-hour shifts have more energy and often more ability to engage the resident and enable overall well-being.

ADMISSION DAY: SUGGESTIONS ON GETTING THE RESIDENT TO THE HOME

"Do we tell Dad what is going to happen before the admission? When? How often? Not at all?" These are all good questions. The answers vary depending on "Dad" and family relationships, awareness and remembering ability, current ability to cope with change, and the distance to the facility. Rarely, in actuality never, should a resident think he or she is "going for a ride" and then get "dropped off" at the care center. Admission day is usually challenging enough without having the new resident totally outraged with the family as well as the care center's staff.

Families often ask, "How will I ever get Dad into the facility on admission day?" Staff at the care center should sit down with the family and plan a strategy. Looking first at the incoming resident's life story may offer suggestions. Examples might be telling Dad that he is wanted to be a volunteer in his specialty area and that his assistance is really needed or that he has the opportunity, by living in this specific community, to attend a club focusing on his past line of work or leisure interest. Issuing membership cards to the care center's exclusive club may be helpful. If the incoming resident has a positive experience with physicians, the explanation for admission might be along the lines of the doctor wanting to run some tests or asking for admission because of the need to monitor a specific situation. If nothing is working, it might be helpful to "blame the doctor." For example, "Dad, the doctor has called and he is requiring that you check into his facility so he can keep an eye on your health."

Alzheimer's Disease: Activity-Focused Care

When the resident is flying from a distant location to an airport near the care center, the preadmission plans will include suggestions for the family members involved with the resident and the flight.

Guidelines for travel by plane include the following:

1. Plan the flight to reflect the resident's best time of day. This is usually in the morning.
2. Carefully plan with the airline the following requests:

   Reserve a seating area for two, the resident by the window, toward the front of the plane, so he or she is not so overwhelmed by all the people on the flight.

   Arrange for curbside meeting with a wheelchair even if the resident is able to walk. Usually, long distances need to be traveled in the airport. The chair will also help to keep track of the resident. Tell the resident that he or she has just qualified for this special service or just won a contest from the airline and this is the reward.

   If the resident can walk onto the plane, have the resident be seated when the plane is full and about ready to leave. Waiting within the terminal may be helpful because the resident can be wheeled around or walked about during the waiting period rather than being placed into a seat on the plane and not able to move. Certainly, the flight itself will challenge the resident's ability to sit in one place.

   Arrange to have the flight attendants know about the resident's needs. Having suggestions written down to give to the attendants is helpful. Include favorite beverages and snack suggestions, as well as the appropriate name to use to address the resident.

   Prearrange with the attendants that the resident can use the first class toilet rather than walking all the way to the rear of the airplane.

   On landing, plan for immediate dismissal from the plane. Again, have a wheelchair waiting for the resident's use, if appropriate.
3. Suggestions for the caregiver:

   Do not plan a flight time that will cause the resident to rush.

   Help the resident to dress in comfortable clothing that is easy to remove for toileting needs.

   Rest well before the day of the flight, if possible. Being stressed will only complicate the situation and the resident will probably have increased negative responses to the flight.

   Be sure that the resident has a Safe Return bracelet on or some sort of identification in his or her pocket in case the caregiver and the resident become separated.

   Be prepared! Carry on an all-purpose bag of goodies. Include changes of clothing, snacks, magazines, something to read of interest to the resident, a simple project to involve the resident such as junk jewelry to sort, cards to look at, playing cards, crayons and a picture to add color to for a favorite grandchild, a small photo album, a cassette player with favorite music and earphones.

   Seek help from the resident's physician. If appropriate, the doctor can suggest medication that can reduce anxiety before, during, or after the flight. Be practical and use it if difficulties are anticipated.

ADMISSION DAY: FAMILY MOURNING

Caregivers have described the actual day of admission as the "worst day of my life," or later said, "Admission day was more difficult for me than my loved one's funeral." Often, loneliness and emptiness fill the caregiver's heart before the admission. The caregivers are sometimes sadly surprised that these feelings may become more intense during placement of their loved one.

> Tom's suitcase for the nursing home had been packed carefully by his wife, Joan. The staffperson and Joan placed the clothing in the bedroom closet. Tom was wearing a new sweatshirt with the name of the university from which he had graduated many years ago. He watched as his Boy Scout Merit Badge sash with his Eagle award was unpacked lovingly by his wife. Even though she was exhausted, Joan was overcome with sadness at having to place her husband in the nursing home. She wanted so much for the staff to realize the wonderful person her husband had been. She later was able to talk about her grief and the effects of the actual day of placement.

Admission day may be experienced as an end that is really not an end. A nursing home can plan ways to reduce admission day stress, including the following:

1. The day before admission, have any necessary paperwork signed and invite the family to bring in personal items to decorate the resident's room and bed, and hang up and put away his or her clothing.
2. Remind families to mark the resident's clothing with his or her name before admission.
3. Encourage admissions to take place mid-morning when residents usually are at their best and lunchtime makes a natural break for the family to leave.
4. If possible, limit or do not permit admissions on weekends because "regular" staff often are not present.
5. Check the resident's room just before the actual arrival to be sure that it is clean and ready, with no surprises.
6. Offer a symbolic ritual of admission to the resident and the family (e.g., a blessing of the room or presentation of a gift or flower to have in the new room).
7. Suggest that the caregiver bring a family member or a friend at the time of admission, but not more than a total of three persons.
8. Encourage the family to have a pleasant event planned for admission day such as going out for lunch after placement or dinner that evening.
9. Help the family determine when their first visit should be and how to phone to inquire about their loved one, including whom to ask for.
10. Remind the family that relocation is stressful, not just for the resident, but also for them. The "First Month Syndrome" might happen: resident unrest, anger, blaming, or overall increase in confusion. An adjustment period is normal for the resident as well as for the family.

Alzheimer's Disease: Activity-Focused Care

If the family or caregiver chooses to move the resident to another facility, they often experience the stress and grief of admission all over again. Stress is increased, for example, if the resident is on the waiting list for the nursing home that the family "really wants." While the resident has been at the first home the family members have "built up" their expectations about the second placement, and these expectations often lead to disappointment. Residents sometimes can appear to lose their abilities after a move, perhaps due to the changes in staffpersons and the unfamiliar environment.

CAREGIVING PARTNERSHIP: STAFF AND FAMILY

Inviting the caregiver and family members into a partnership with the nursing home staff continues the bridge between caring for their loved one at home and having permission to continue caregiving in the facility. The decision to form a partnership should be supported by administration first, then staff for it to be successful and meaningful, facilitating cooperation and interdependence. Families are sometimes suspicious and disappointed with nursing home care and the staff, thinking that they certainly cannot provide appropriate care because they do not know how to do it the way their loved one would understand. It is also very difficult for the caregiver to realize that the one-to-one attention he or she was able to provide is not available. A staffperson may have 6–12 residents to care for.

Uniting staff and families in partnership is a challenge and an opportunity for both. Each needs reassurance and a caring touch, for they are only human. Families may experience feelings of guilt and that they are abandoning their loved one. Staff may think that the family is unrealistic and demanding. At times, sharing the caregiving is not well defined and leads to control issues. Families can be unsure of their role as continuing caregivers, not knowing where to find answers to their many questions. Not knowing what to expect further complicates the relationship. Residents with caring family members who visit often receive the most staff attention. Perhaps this is because the family is modeling that their loved one is special.

Families should feel that the staff accept them no matter how their loved one responds to nursing home care.

> Margaret dreaded visiting her mother because she was combative and usually was yelling or crying. Her mother's actions embarrassed Margaret, and she was afraid that the staff would think that she was an awful person because her mother was so difficult. It hurt deeply that the staff did not ever know her "real" mother. It took time for Margaret to accept the staff's assurances that they loved her mother even though she was a challenge and that they were interested in supporting and caring for her also.

Staff sometimes can be puzzled by a family member's response to his or her loved one.

Louis was deeply frustrated because of his wife's illness. He could be heard yelling at her during visits. When the staff started to hear occasional sounds of skin being slapped, they had to intervene and limit Louis' visits with his wife to public areas rather than alone in her bedroom. The staff told Louis of this directive in a direct, nonjudgmental way and helped him to realize their responsibility for his wife's care and health.

Staff and family should have honest communication.

The staff could not understand why Jennifer rarely came in to visit her father. He seemed like a nice man, charming and fun to be with. When she did come, the staff delighted in sharing with Jennifer that they thought he was a wonderful, cooperative man. They said how much they enjoyed having him on the unit and how lucky Jennifer was to have such a fine father. Jennifer appeared angry and hurt by their remarks, which confused the staff and made them all the more protective and caring toward her father. In time, Jennifer was able to share that her dad had not always been charming; in fact, he had been abusive to her and her mother. This honest communication allowed the staff to understand the relationship and provide more support to Jennifer. They became more aware that their remarks to Jennifer about her dad's friendly ways needed to be decreased. The staff continue to demonstrate their acceptance of Jennifer's father for the person he is now.

A care center staff that has stretched the truth or misrepresented the type of care or programs being offered in the home will have difficult family-facility relationships. Families will forever comment, with strong feelings, "You promised. . . ." Realistic facility tours and information provided for families inquiring or placing a loved one must reflect the actual abilities of a health care provider.

If small children are part of the family experiencing the nursing home admission of a loved one, the children's feelings also should be considered. Perhaps the new resident is a cherished grandmother who has been part of the child's immediate family, maybe the loving person who tucked the child into bed each night. The family should be open and honest with the child about the grandmother's forgetfulness, the disease, and the need for long-term care. Letting the child ask questions is important. Answers lovingly shared can help to ease the child's sense of loss. Checking with the local chapter of the Alzheimer's Association might find that there is a support group specifically for young children. Another information source is fiction that demonstrates the loved one's changing care and needs from a child's perspective (see Suggested Reading). Names of appropriate books are also available from the Alzheimer's Association or the local library. Children should hear that they are still much loved by the resident. Helping the child to have an activity-focused visit at the home is meaningful because the child can bring papers from school and various projects to share. Involving the child during visits at the home can be a joy-filled experience. Examples would be exercising together, sharing treats and snacks, participating in sing-alongs, and taking walks together. Usually, children are quite sensitive and creative in sharing their world with a loved one with dementia.

NEW FAMILY ORIENTATION PROGRAM

Offering family members an orientation program during their loved one's first month at the nursing home can help to ease the transition they are experiencing. Goals include helping the family to gain knowledge about dementia and its effects on their loved one, to become familiar with the facility's mission and program objectives, to gain a realistic expectation of how the program works, and to gain information about key staff and what they do and how the family can address their concerns and questions.

The new family orientation should be held monthly, usually in the early evening, for 2½ hours. If attendance is a problem, the evening session can be rotated with an orientation held on a weekend afternoon every other month.

The program for the orientation can vary if the families present have some specific questions. The main focus is to increase families' adjustment to the facility and to extend the invitation for partnership. It appears that families, having participated in an orientation program and received this special attention, including "how the facility works," may have fewer adjustment problems and fit more easily into the program with their loved one.

DEVELOPING A FAMILY MENTOR PROGRAM

Some families have great difficulty adjusting to having their loved one in a nursing home and may experience anxiety, especially during the transition period of usually 2–6 months. On the other hand, there are families who have successfully made the transition and think that they are truly partners in caregiving with the staff. Asking these families to be a mentor for a new family allows them to share their personal expertise and wealth of experience. They can offer positive suggestions as well as being able to understand the difficulties the new families are having. Mentor families will be able to feel that they are making a significant contribution as they reach out to nurture those less able to cope.

Families receiving the mentor assistance appreciate hearing from their peers rather than receiving information only from staff. They often receive practical information, hints, and suggestions that the staff are not even aware of that can help them adjust to the transition.

Staff can help to identify family members willing to act as mentors and assist in matching them with new families. A team of a family member and staffperson can work together to facilitate the mentor program. After the family member and the mentor are introduced, they take over from there and arrange the time and number of meetings. This program might not appeal to all family members but having it available is important. Very often more can be accomplished with a mentoring program than having the family only rely on the staff for interventions, knowledge, creative care ideas, and overall nursing home adjustment.

PARTNERSHIP IN ACTION: FAMILY COUNCIL

A family council is not created by a health care provider; its origin and development come from the family members themselves. Care partnership is no easy task. Willingness to communicate must be a basic commitment for both the administration and a family council. Support from the provider is needed for the council to be a viable organization able to reflect its mission statement and carry out its purposes. The following example is from The Wealshire (a dementia-specific facility in Lincolnshire, IL) Family Council's Mission Statement and Purpose*:

> *Mission Statement of The Wealshire Family Council*
>
> To join in partnership with The Wealshire to insure that our family members are treated with the care, dignity, love and respect they deserve.
>
> *Purpose of The Wealshire Family Council*
>
> To serve as resident advocates.
>
> To promote better communication between the families and The Wealshire staff and management.
>
> To provide family support, education and resources.
>
> To create a forum to consolidate ideas in order to establish and direct achievable goals.
>
> To provide volunteer support when appropriate.

Examples of family council meetings and activities include the following:

1. Each department's director can be invited to attend a meeting. This get-to-know-you session is helpful to all, if both family members and staffpersons are willing to listen and care about the meeting's outcome. Each director can share about the program or care area he or she is responsible for, what has been going on, and plans for the future. Family members can offer suggestions, ask questions, voice complaints, and, it is hoped, see themselves as a helpful part of the solution.

2. An annual meeting with administration and directors to discuss philosophy of care, plans, and goals for the year becomes a source of shared information for the families, enabling them to feel connected to the facility as valued team members.

3. Monthly meetings can be held at different times and days, including an occasional weekend morning or afternoon. The agendas are well advertised and all family members are invited to attend. Some meetings are for families only and others have invited speakers, usually staff (e.g., activity therapists and their program, including how family members can assist with outings and special events; behavior refocusing and how the restraint reduction program relates to

---

*With permission from The Wealshire Family Council, Lincolnshire, Illinois.

Alzheimer's Disease: Activity-Focused Care

dementia care; how the nursing assistants and the family members can work together better).

4. Special meetings can be called with family council permission. For example, a researcher who wants to inform family members about his or her study and needs to ask for assistance.

5. All new family members can be invited to join the council and offered a council guide with the dates and times of all meetings as well as the names, addresses, and phone numbers of council members and officers.

6. An employee holiday fund can be established and facilitated. Donations are solicited by and made through the family council. Working with administration, the council develops the guidelines for distributing the money (e.g., gifts to all employees working at the facility since a certain date). The council handles the distribution of the money as its gift to the hands-on staff.

7. A family survival handbook can be developed (see next section).

An active family council with a strong and united voice could be seen by administration as a threat or as a subversive element. This would be an unfortunate situation for all involved. A family council can "hold one's feet to the fire," but if done with the spirit of partnership, the council can provide wisdom, experience, and helpful suggestions for change to the administration. Difficulties arise if a council sees its role as the final word on care situations or feels that it has the ability to change personnel or have them dismissed. In all situations, something can be learned from both the council and the administration. It is in listening to each other that care is improved, and the resident is the "winner." And that, of course, is what caregiving in a health care center is all about.

FACILITATING CHANGE: A FAMILY SURVIVAL HANDBOOK

At first, placement of a loved one in a nursing home can increase family members' stress, rather than decrease it. A family survival handbook can be similar to a family orientation program, except that the information is available immediately and can be reviewed again and again.

The Wealshire's Family Survival Handbook states:

> The Family Handbook has been developed by The Wealshire staff and the Family Council. It contains answers to questions that families have asked as they have moved their loved ones into The Wealshire and experienced the first year to 18 months of living there. The Handbook is not intended to be a policy manual or a treatise on caring for Alzheimer's residents. It is intended to provide commonly requested information and to point you to the proper source for additional information. As you use the Handbook, we ask that you pass along suggestions and additional questions whose answers will help make life easier for future residents and their families.

The table of contents of The Wealshire's Family Survival Handbook* includes the following topics:

The Wealshire Mission
The Disease
Living at The Wealshire
    Hours of Operation
    Clothing and Personal Items
    Daily Routine/Schedule
    Visiting and Taking Residents Out
    Religious Services
    Employee Gifts
Communication/Information
Resident Care
    Care Conferences
    Physicians' Services
    Personal Hygiene
    Housekeeping/Laundry
    Assessment of Resident's Condition
    The Advocacy Function
Billing
Support Groups
Appendix
    101 Things To Do When Visiting
    Doctors, Specialties, Schedules
    Ancillary Charges
    Wealshire Organization Chart, Phone Numbers
    Wealshire Floor Plan
    Glossary of Commonly Used Terms and Abbreviations
    Bibliography

INVOLVEMENT: "COULDS" VERSUS "SHOULDS"

Families can be invited to participate with their loved one in the nursing home as much as they wish, when they want to, and in ways in which they feel comfortable. Some families cling to caregiving and prefer to be at the nursing home all day. Others are anxious not to be involved and prefer infrequent visits, if at all. Because it is impossible to "know" all the information and history about a family, it is unfair to judge a family member's response to the resident.

> Sheila always had been a real "lady" and never used foul language. After her nursing home placement, Sheila's language ability continued to deteriorate and she no longer was able to control her words. She yelled loudly when her daughter came to visit and called her a "bitch." The daugh-

---

*With permission from The Wealshire Family Council, Lincolnshire, Illinois.

ter was aghast; this was so unlike her mother. She continued to visit daily, however, because she thought that she should be there and not let her mother down. In time, the swearing increased and the daughter became seriously depressed. She was able, with supportive help from the nursing home's social services, to realize that she could choose when she wanted to visit. Taking the emphasis away from feeling that she "should" visit to choosing or seeing that she "could" visit allowed her to take care of herself.

Some family members seem to need the staff to tell them not to visit so often; they think they "should." When they begin to understand that their decision to be involved or not is based on possibilities or "coulds" it can refocus their anxiety and allow for informed decision making. They are always invited to visit, but no expectations are expressed. Responding to "coulds" is by far more pleasant for most families.

VISITING: AN OPPORTUNITY FOR CONNECTEDNESS AND VOLUNTEERING

Nursing homes can take an active role in helping caregivers visit their loved ones. Planning ahead for the visit usually will lead to increased satisfaction. The nursing home can have simple activities available that the family can do with the resident or events that they both can enjoy, such as church services or sing-alongs. Often, special events or parties are a good way to involve families, not only for the valuable help that families contribute, but also because the visitors get to know other families and residents (see Appendix 13-4).

> Julie never really felt that she knew her dad. He always had been so busy with his factory while she was growing up. She found that as the dementia progressed he felt less pressured to "get to work" and more willing to sit with her. They enjoyed the nursing home activities together: singing, dancing, going to parties, and attending church. Although her dad had mid-stage Alzheimer's disease, Julie felt that the time they shared was deeply rewarding to both of them.

A nursing home with an active volunteer program can help families add quality to their visits. An involved family member, when appropriate, can include his or her loved one so that they can participate in their volunteer task together.

> Robert's wife has been on the Alzheimer's disease unit for more than 5 years. Robert has found that since he does not have family in the area, he wants to be with her constantly and has chosen to come in to the home to help at lunch and supper. Robert usually stays throughout the afternoon. Ruthie, his wife, appears to enjoy his company but is unable to have a conversation with her husband. Robert was invited to become a

volunteer, and he chose to do the facility's photocopying. Because Ruthie is in a wheelchair, he is able to bring her into the office as he runs the machine. She enjoys all the staff and volunteers coming in and out of the office and Robert feels useful and appreciated. Perhaps one of the greatest benefits of volunteering and visiting at the same time is that when Ruthie dies, Robert can choose to remain an active volunteer, if he wishes, and therefore continue to come to the home, where he will continue to receive staff and volunteer support.

SPECIAL OPPORTUNITIES: HOLIDAYS, FAMILY WEDDINGS, AND SPECIAL EVENTS*

Special family-related events should include the resident with dementia if at all possible (see Chapter 2). Detailed planning can make these occasions very special for all. For example, holiday traditions and past rituals will have to be modified to engage the loved one. Holidays are the time to start new traditions that enjoy the here and now. Perhaps Mother was the center of family "power" or the keeper of the family rituals or traditions. Mother was the one who set the table, decided what foods would be served, and was able to bring all the family members together by using her loving skills. Mother has no doubt changed if she has dementia. The holiday can hold within it past memories and emotions but this is now, and it is hoped that the family can let go of the past and celebrate the abilities and personal gifts of all present (see Appendix 13-5).

Family weddings also take special planning. The key to including someone with Alzheimer's disease in a family wedding or other special event is good planning, realistic expectations, adaptability, and flexibility. Even then, plans may need to be canceled at the last minute.

> Josephine attended her granddaughter's wedding, enjoying the ceremony with her husband, Vern. She had been brought by the coordinator of her nursing home's Alzheimer's disease unit. Vern lived in his daughter's home. He had been ill and could not continue caring for his wife. Josephine's daughter had wanted her mother to attend but thought she needed to give her full attention to the bride. It was a lovely, joyous event for all.

> Bertha's son, Scott, and soon-to-be-wife deeply desired to have Mother come to their wedding. Scott planned his wedding around his mother's needs. Bertha was an extremely active, pacing resident in a nursing home 1½ hours from the synagogue. Two staffpersons offered to take Bertha to the wedding and reception. A dressmaker arrived to measure

---

*With permission from C Hellen. Special opportunities: holidays, family weddings, and special events. Rush Alzheimer's Disease News 1992;spring:3.

Alzheimer's Disease: Activity-Focused Care

Bertha and obtain shoes and jewelry because Bertha could not tolerate a shopping trip. Scott arranged for a "stand-up" reception, held in the same building, that would feature food and refreshments being passed because his mother could only pace, stand, or lie down—she had not "sat" down for more than a year. He knew that she loved to dance and he hired a band that played her favorite music. A limousine was hired to drive his mother and the staff to the wedding and to wait outside in case she needed to return to the home quickly. Bertha loved the whole event, she waved poignantly at the guests because she recognized them, she stood or paced but it was not inappropriate, and she enjoyed the food and the dancing. Best of all, she was able to dance with her sons, including the groom and a son from out of town. She ate three petals from her gardenia wrist corsage, but otherwise she was great.

A year after Scott's wedding, Bertha's dementia limited her word-finding abilities and slowed her step. She still does not sit down, even to eat her meals. She looked at Peter's wedding pictures—her son that lived out of state had just gotten married. Bertha quietly said, almost to herself, "I should have been there."

Suggestions for a successful family event, for example a wedding, are as follows:

1. Ask, what does the family really want? Discuss the event with everyone involved, including the family, the bride, and bridegroom.
2. Do not become overwhelmed by "shoulds" such as, "Grandfather should attend because the groom is his only grandson."
3. Set realistic expectations. Look at the number of people attending, the time of day, the environment, the length of time to get there, noise, confusing surroundings, transportation requirements, and so forth.
4. Think about what is best for your loved one. Look at typical behaviors, best or worse times of the day, level of discomfort in strange situations or being around a lot of people—all of the possible pluses and minuses of participation. If the wedding is out of town, this assessment is extremely important because of the complete change of routine. The assessment and final decision should be flexible enough to change right up to the start of the event.
5. If the regular caregiver is a family member who will be busy with responsibilities during the wedding, find a substitute who is comfortable with your loved one and vice versa. The safest approach is to have two people giving care during the event.
6. Decide how long the person with dementia should be away from home. Attending just the wedding and not the reception might be wise.
7. Plan ahead! Allow enough time for hair styling, bathing, and dressing. Do not let the resident feel hurried. Talk quietly and simplify hygiene, grooming, and dressing as much as possible.
8. Dress the person in comfortable, familiar clothing in the style and color he or she has worn in the past. Be sure the clothing allows easy toileting. Make sure the shoes are not brand new and are comfortable.

9. Have an escape planned (e.g., a quiet spot to retreat to or cookies and snacks that can be used for distractions). A knotted handkerchief to "fiddle" with can be used to reduce anxiety. Have a car easily available so both the caregiver and the resident can leave early if necessary or immediately if the resident starts to become upset.

10. The final decision should be flexible enough to be changed right up to the start of the event. Do not be afraid to change your mind if your gut feeling is "no go."

PARTNERSHIP IN ACTION: PLAN-OF-CARE CONFERENCE

Family involvement in the care planning for their loved ones gives them an opportunity to share the caregiving. They can use the care planning conference with staff to voice concerns and express suggestions. As the staff share their goals and approaches to care, the family increases understanding about the cognitive, physical, spiritual, emotional, and psychosocial aspects of care.

The most effective care conferences are those that the family takes time to prepare for and attends. Families can think out their concerns and ideas before the conference using a family care conference form (see Appendix 13-6). This form reinforces the nursing home's commitment to be a partner with the family. If the family is not able to attend the conference, the form can be sent in to the care conference coordinator. After the conference, the coordinator can call the family and discuss the plan-of-care outcomes for their loved one.

As the dementia progresses, the family's participation in the care planning will allow them to express feelings about end-stage care and choices for interventions.

FAMILY SUPPORT: ONE TO ONE OR GROUPS

Family caregivers may experience various concerns and need support from the nursing home and other family members. A support group can be a safe arena for expressing feelings and concerns, a place to obtain practical information, and an opportunity to provide and receive support from others. A nursing home may have its own support group specifically for families of residents with dementia or a group for all families. Social services may recommend that a family member attend an Alzheimer's Association support group. At times, if appropriate, social services may recommend that a family member seek a professional counselor.

Informal support for family members is the responsibility of all staffpersons in a nursing home. At times, if the family is unreasonable or upset, this task can be very trying and difficult. A staff that is able to understand the grief and loss associated with a chronic disease, such as Alzheimer's disease, is best able to cope with stressed family members. Staffpersons are called to extend their caregiving to include the family members with the same respect and support given to residents. Families who sense that the staff truly care are often able to return the support to the staff, other residents, and other family members.

As part of the family-staff caregiving partnership and support, it is of great benefit when a staff member is invited by the family to speak about dementia to their community of friends, such as members of their church or service organization. The friends thus become more comfortable with knowing "how to visit" and what to expect, and this often allows the resident's friends to continue their previous relationship with the resident in the nursing home.

FAMILY SUPPORT: WHEN BOTH PARENTS HAVE DEMENTIA

When nursing home care involves spouses with dementia, the family members can be overwhelmed and in need of support. Caregiving can also be, at times, seemingly overwhelming to the staff as they try to support the husband and wife and respond to wishes and demands of their adult children (see Chapter 2).

Considerations include the couple's marriage history, their individual life stories, current needs and abilities, and their plan of care. The mother and father are first individuals and second a couple, usually. There are situations when the "couple" relationship outweighs considerations for focusing on one of them as an individual. Adult children can bring their own point of view into the situation, sometimes for the best and sometimes colored by past family history and perhaps not so beneficial for their parents. The adult children's fear of developing dementia as they age themselves because of their genetic history, while maybe not openly expressed, is a viable concern for the family.

Family members can be encouraged to consider the time they spend in a health care facility and use it wisely. Perhaps at times it is best to visit Mother and Dad together or perhaps there should be opportunities to have a quality visit with each one individually. The same can hold true when considering trips outside of the facility. Relationships, wellness, challenges, overall likes and dislikes, emotional responses, and cognitive abilities are all elements for decision making. It is hoped that the parents, together and separately, plus the family members can find dignity within this difficult situation.

Caregivers should recognize the often agonizing sadness family members encounter when both parents have dementia. Relationships can become strained between the adult children and the parents as they watch helplessly as the relationship between their parents changes. Attending a care conference where the staff and the family first discuss Mother and then, taking up another chart, discuss Dad, can also be overwhelming to staff. Counseling is advised for family members and should also be available for staff.

Each situation that involves a husband and wife is totally unique. The decisions about room placement, care emphasis, and how to support the personhood of each requires a tremendous commitment to caring for each person involved as well as offering and providing respect for them as husband and wife and for their family members.

PARTNERSHIP: EDUCATIONAL OPPORTUNITIES
AND FAMILIES AS TEACHERS

Families appreciate opportunities to learn more about dementia and its effects on their loved ones. A nursing home that has an educational forum several times a year enables both staff and family members to come together to increase understanding. Inviting family members to participate in staff training helps both groups. Staff become more sensitive as they hear the family's story about their loved one before placement in the home. Family members obtain increased awareness into the staff's responsibilities and how caregiving is implemented within the facility on a day-to-day basis.

Topics most requested from families are: how to visit, dealing with difficult behaviors, ways to communicate more effectively, appropriate meaningful activities, and what's new about Alzheimer's disease and current research.

Resources for speakers and videotapes can be obtained from the Alzheimer's Association, hospitals, and agencies working with the aging population. Attending physicians, consultants, and experienced staff can also be considered for presentations. Another source for family education is having a resource center of books and tapes to borrow.

Family members can be actively involved in the facility's training program. "Family Story" is an opportunity for family members to relate their stories of caregiving to the staff. Elements of the story should include how the family member first began to recognize the signs that "something is not right," a description of the emotional experiences during the beginning of the disease process, how it affected the loved one, what caregiving was like in the early stages and how the resident responded, what were the experiences of placement in a care facility, what change has occurred in the family member's life because of the placement, and how he or she thinks the loved one is doing. Staff listening to a family member are almost always amazed and impressed with the family's journey of caregiving beside their loved one.

Another opportunity for family members to join in with staff training is when the staffperson has selected their loved one for a resident case study (see Chapter 2, Appendix 2-5). Having the family member help with background information is helpful in preparing for the case study. When the family member attends the presentation of the case study, it is a wonderful opportunity for him or her to hear the thought, interest, and caring that goes into the study. For example:

> Caroline, an activity therapist, selected George for her case study. As Caroline gathered information about George from various disciplines and different shifts, she also worked closely with Anita, George's daughter. Finding out about George before admission and the details of his life history enabled Caroline to put together an intimate and detailed study about George. Anita was invited to attend the presentation of the study. She was clearly overwhelmed with the thought and content of the study as well as the warm feelings Caroline had for her father. At the close of the discussion, Anita went over to Caroline, gave her a big hug, and with tears and gratitude said, "Thank you for loving my dad so much."

Family members may offer excellent insight into Alzheimer's caregiving and their loved one's experience of dementia. Asking family members to be a copresenter, with a staffperson, at conferences can provide an outstanding opportunity to learn, teach, share, and enrich and strengthen the caregiving partnership.

Alzheimer's Disease: Activity-Focused Care

PARTNERSHIP: RESEARCH OPPORTUNITIES

Nursing homes are encouraged to observe and learn as they provide care to persons with dementia. At times, homes are involved in formal or informal research. Staff and families can learn a lot from each other. Families often enjoy the research activity and want to be included. Many think that their participation helps the tragedy of their loved one's illness have meaning. This thinking also encourages families to consent to a brain autopsy on the resident's death.

Research requests that involve the residents, the staff, or family members require careful consideration from the facility's ethics committee. Resident dignity, staff tolerance, and the efficacy of the research should be carefully weighed and discussed. The balance between demands on staff attention and their perception of their jobs and the amount of time they have available to spend on observations and charting should be looked at carefully. Possible outcomes and the significance of the information for others should be well discussed before entering a research project. Using family members as research participants will usually involve a great deal of staff time to set up and carry through. The question to ask, again, is how will participation in research affect resident care, the use of staff time, and involvement and the interest of family members, including their willingness to commit to active participation?

FAMILY AND THE DYING RESIDENT

Death always seems to be a surprise, even after years of a progressive illness or wishing that "it will soon be over." The last few weeks of caregiving can affect family members in various ways. The family involved in the decision making for the end stage of their loved one's care often will be better able to accept death (see Chapter 12).

A nursing home may allow the family to stay with the resident around the clock, providing a cot or a place to rest. At times, just having a staffperson hold their hands or inquire about their needs helps the family. Families are touched deeply when staffpersons whom they have close relations with, such as the Alzheimer's care director, are with them at the bedside. It is equally meaningful when staff attend the resident's wake or funeral. Family members of other residents often reach out to each other during this period and are loving and caring in their support.

A family member wrote the following note when her father, Bernie Boyle, died.*

> Dear Wealshire Family,
>
> My Dad died at 12:30 this morning—peacefully in my arms.
>   He was having a little difficulty with his breathing at the end, and could not seem to let go. I looked him straight in the eyes and sang, "Show Me the Way to Go Home," told him that I loved him, thanked him for all that he had done for me, and he took a deep breath and relaxed.
>   Life is good.
>
> THANK YOU

---

*Special thanks to Kathie Benson.

HEALTH CARE PROVIDER AND STAFF ISSUES

Staff, trained to be caring listeners, understanding, and supportive, can offer family members a strong hand to hold throughout their loved ones' journeys into Alzheimer's disease. At times, the commitment to co-partner the care is extremely difficult. Families arrive with multiple experiences and facets of their relationship with the residents. No staffperson has ever walked in their shoes. Staff judgmental attitudes are not helpful or acceptable. A support group for staff may be helpful in providing a safe arena in which to discuss feelings. Role expectations, for all involved with the resident, should be spelled out and understood.

At times, it is very difficult for staff when family members constantly complain about what are seemingly "small" issues. It is helpful for staff to recognize, name, and deal with "triggers" that seem to really aggravate each family. Perhaps it is Mom's fingernails, Dad's whiskers, or the wife who always wears the same dress. If these triggers are taken care of daily, perhaps the family can be more relaxed. It is especially difficult when staff think that a family member is on a "snoop patrol" just trying to find something wrong. When families think that care is not provided or is inappropriate, they should know where to go with their concern for help and immediate attention to the situation.

Family members are also clients and users of services in a care facility. Health care providers realizing and responding with positive support for family members of their residents can provide comfort for families. Connectedness can be maintained throughout the resident's stay in the facility and, it is hoped, can continue after the resident's death. In return, the facility will reap great rewards in support from the families as they encourage and appreciate staff, assist with outings and activities, and generally add to the overall well-being of everyone in the health care center.

SUMMARY

Families usually seek to be involved as continuing caregivers. They need ongoing reassurance and support outside of the nursing home as well as within. Because there are no "perfect homes" and no "right ways" to provide care, families are challenged as they cope to the best of their abilities.

Honest and open communications are the cornerstones of the caregiving partnership. Staff and family cannot help but be involved with each other. It follows that those who really care and support each other are apt to experience greater loss and sadness when they risk being vulnerable. They also are able to give and receive the greatest love and admiration.

SUGGESTED READING

Bell V. Tapping an Unlimited Resource: Building Volunteer Programs for Patients and Their Families. In NL Mace (ed), Dementia Care: Patient, Family and Community. Baltimore: Johns Hopkins University Press, 1990.

Bell V, Troxel D. The Best Friends Approach to Alzheimer's Care. Baltimore: Health Professions Press, 1997;321–336.

Cohen D, Eisdorfer C. The Loss of Self: A Family Resource for the Care of Alzheimer's Disease and Related Disorders. New York: W.W. Norton, 1986.

Coons D, Mace N, Whyte T. Quality of Life in Long-Term Care. New York: Ballantine Books, 1996.

Davis R. My Journey into Alzheimer's Disease. Wheaton, IL: Tyndale House, 1989.

Doka KJ (ed). Living with Grief: When Illness Is Prolonged. Washington, DC: Hospice Foundation of America, and Bristol, PA: Taylor and Francis, 1997.

Mace NL (ed). Dementia Care: Patient, Family and Community. Baltimore: Johns Hopkins University Press, 1990.

Mace NL, Rabins PV. The 36-Hour Day: A Family Guide for Caring for Persons with Alzheimer's Disease, Related Dementing Illnesses, and Memory Loss in Later Life (rev ed). Baltimore: Johns Hopkins University Press, 1991.

Wilken C, Farran C, Hellen C, Boggess J. Partners in care: a program for family caregivers and nursing home staff. Am J Alzheimer's Care Rel Dis Res 1992;7:8–22.

Books for Children

Fox M. Wilfrid Gordon McDonald Partridge. Brooklyn, NY: Kane Miller Publishers, 1985.

Guthrie D. Grandpa Doesn't Know Me Anymore. New York: Human Sciences Press, 1986.

Prillaman P. Papa, Are You There? Bloomington, IL: Alzheimer's Association, Corn Belt Chapter, 1982.

Books for Adolescents

Frank J. The Silent Epidemic. Minneapolis: Lerner Publications Company, 1985.

Young A. What's Wrong with Daddy? Worthington, OH: Willowisp Press, 1986.

A13-1
*Twelve Steps for Caregivers**

1. Although I cannot control the disease process, I need to remember I can control many aspects of how it affects me and my relative.
2. I need to take care of myself so that I can continue doing the things that are most important.
3. I need to simplify my lifestyle so that my time and energy are available for things that are really important.
4. I need to cultivate the gift of allowing others to help me, because caring for my relative is too big a job to be done by one person.
5. I need to take one day at a time rather than worry about what may or may not happen in the future.
6. I need to structure my day because a consistent schedule makes life easier for me and my relative.
7. I need to have a sense of humor because laughter helps to put things in a more positive perspective.
8. I need to remember that my relative is not being "difficult" on purpose; rather that his/her behavior and emotions are distorted by the illness.
9. I need to focus on and enjoy what my relative can still do rather than constantly lament over what is gone.
10. I need to increasingly depend upon other relationships for love and support.
11. I need to frequently remind myself that I am doing the best that I can at this moment.
12. I need to draw upon the Higher Power which I believe is available to me.

---

*Reprinted with permission from CJ Farran, E Keane-Hagerty. Twelve steps for caregivers. Am J Alzheimer's Care Rel Dis Res 1989;4:38–41.

A13-2

Care for Caregivers: Grappling with Guilt *

Guilt: The gift that keeps on giving.

—Erma Bombeck

Caring for persons with dementia can bring out the best and worst in the human personality. Compassion, concern, and loyalty are just a few of the characteristics of those who have accepted the labor of love. At the same time, caregivers often experience great frustration, anger, depression, and guilt in response to the stress of caring for those with a chronic illness. Guilt or self-reproach seems to stand out as the feeling experienced most frequently.

Although countless situations can induce guilt, a few examples can illustrate common dilemmas:

- The daughter of a person with Alzheimer's disease works a full-time job in addition to caring for her spouse and three children. She spends Saturdays helping her parents. On leaving for her home, she is distraught as both parents plead for her to spend more time with them.
- The son of a person with dementia begins to argue with his mother who is acting irrationally and ends up slapping her. He quickly realizes that his mother has a brain disorder and cannot control her behavior.
- The husband arranges for his wife with Alzheimer's disease to attend adult day care a few times per week. In her absence, he is unable to relax or participate in enjoyable activities.
- The wife of a person with dementia had promised her husband and herself that she would never place him in a nursing home. After several exhausting years of home care, she places him in a facility.

In some cases, guilt may serve a useful function; but persistent guilt can become a crippling problem for caregivers. Such guilt usually stems from unrealistic expec-

---

*Reprinted with permission from D Kuhn. Care for caregivers: grappling with guilt. Rush Alzheimer's Center Disease News 1991;summer:2.

tations put on oneself. Despite unbearable conditions, some caregivers expect that they can handle any problem that comes their way. Instead of freely choosing such challenges, they become caught in a trap of thinking they "should" or "ought to" be able to meet all needs at all times. When guilt becomes a dominant motive in the caregiving role, help is clearly indicated.

It is possible to move beyond feeling guilty. Some recommended "guilt-busters":

1. Acknowledge that you are in a no-win situation; the disease will worsen despite your best efforts.
2. Set realistic goals; take pride in focusing attention on offering care and comfort instead of a cure.
3. Accept your shortcomings; perfectionists are destined to be disappointed.
4. Find your sense of humor and hang on to it; laughter is good medicine without bad side effects.
5. Get some physical exercise; it is a proven way to reduce stress.
6. Share your thoughts and feelings with a compassionate listener.
7. Take a break and enlist someone to assist you on a routine basis.

Guilt may be impossible to dismiss altogether but at least it can be put in proper perspective. Talking with a confidant or others who care for persons with dementia may help normalize and minimize this painful feeling. If informal sources of support are ineffective, professional intervention with a counselor should be explored. After all, an emotionally healthy caregiver is one of the chief needs of a person with dementia.

A13-3
Preadmission Information Form

Resident: _____ Age: _____

Prefers to be called: _____

Number of years with dementia: _____ Right-handed: _____ Left-handed: _____

Please answer the following:
1. Describe the person and specific techniques you use in caregiving, including methods of clueing and breaking down a task. _____
   _____

2. List the resident's abilities. _____
   _____

3. List situations or things to avoid. _____
   _____

Awareness (attention span, ability to follow directions, orientation to self, you, environment): _____
_____

Communication (verbal and nonverbal abilities, language spoken, hearing and vision abilities and inabilities, useful words to obtain a response): _____
_____

Bathing: Prefers showers: _____ Prefers tub: _____
Describe process: _____
_____

Dressing and grooming (shaving, oral care, hair, etc.): _____
_____

Toileting (include bowel movement pattern, use of incontinence products, nighttime needs, ways of reminding resident to use the toilet): _____
_____

Eating and mealtime (food and beverage preferences, favorite meal, feeding ability, food consistency, help needed): _____
_____

Mobility (walking, getting in and out of chairs, bed, etc.): _____

Safety concerns (Does the resident eat unsafe things, go out of the house, need supervision, etc.?): _____

Daytime activities (Are they helpful? Past and current interests, daytime routine): _____

Sleep habits and nighttime activity (usual morning waking time): _____

Behaviors and responses (Is the resident cooperative, friendly, moody, trusting, suspicious, depressed, lethargic, wandering, pacing, rummaging, or combative? Does the resident experience a late afternoon or early evening increase in anxiety or fearfulness? List behavioral triggers or risk situations that elicit difficult behaviors that need refocusing. What refocusing techniques have been successful? List, discuss.): _____

Other important information and situations or things to avoid (e.g., noise, crowds, touch): _____

Caregiver: _____

Relationship to resident: _____ Date: _____

A13-4
Activity-Focused Nursing Home Visits

"Hi, Mom, how are you?" . . . and then what do you say? Visiting loved ones and friends in a nursing home can be fun and enjoyable or it can be a time of frustration and feelings of guilt.

There are many factors involved in a nursing home visit. Here are a few items to be considered:

1. *The resident*: cognitive, physical, and emotional well-being; past and current relationships; what is happening on the day of your visit
2. *You*: your cognitive, physical, and emotional mood; views of aging, including those for yourself; expectations
3. *The nursing home*: time of day; caregiving schedule such as bath time or medicine distribution; environment of the visit such as a busy, noisy family room or activity going on at the time of the visit

Planning ahead for your visit usually will lead to a successful, reciprocal enjoyment for all involved. Part of the preparation for such a visit invites you to see the event as an activity for both of you. Having something to do enables communication and will enrich the relationship.

OBJECTIVES AND CRITERIA FOR AN ACTIVITY

- Use an activity that will focus on the resident's ability or wellness and will help to promote a sense of belonging and a purposeful use of time.
- Select an activity that can be broken down into simple steps, modified, or adapted to ensure success.
- The activity must be safe for the resident and for others.
- Choose an activity that can be done on a one-to-one basis, or, if appropriate, in a small group for others to be included.
- Select activities that meet the resident's cognitive, physical, and psychosocial needs.

Cognitive-Focused Activities: Examples

- Word games (e.g., fill-in-the-blank, opposites, Trivial Pursuit Jr. (Horn Abbot Ltd., Ontario, Canada), categories, identifying pictures)
- Reminiscing (e.g., old pictures, scrapbook, fabric pieces, stories or objects from the past to encourage memories)
- Games with numbers or letters (e.g., spelling, Scrabble [Milton Bradley Company, Springfield, MA], flashcards)
- Use your imagination (e.g., pretend to go on a trip. Where would you go? What would you pack?)
- Adapt table games such as Scrabble, Yahtzee (Milton Bradley Company, Springfield, MA), checkers, cards, bingo, and dominos
- Sorting activities such as poker chips by color, buttons, lids and bottoms of containers, socks to be matched, straightening up drawers, organizing a box of costume jewelry
- Poetry (e.g., read favorite poems, make a game out of rhyming)
- Simple crafts (remember that crafts take many steps)
- Sensory games (use various smells, textures, or sounds from a tape)
- Music (e.g., singing, rhythm band, clapping—use old favorites)

Physical-Focused Activities: Examples

- Use balls, balloons (e.g., tossing them to each other, into a laundry basket or box, kicking)
- Tossing items (e.g., sponge flying disks, plastic horseshoes, beanbags)
- Exercises (make it fun, use a dowel for the resident's hands to hold)

Psychosocial-Focused Activities: Examples

- Parties—make a party out of anything (e.g., because it's Monday, or the first day of spring, the first day of the baseball season)
- Make things for others such as a scrapbook of old cards for a children's hospital
- Grooming (e.g., polish nails, groom hair, polish shoes, apply makeup)

NORMALIZATION ACTIVITIES

Normalization activities are activities that the residents would be doing if they were home and able to care for themselves. These activities give a real boost to residents' self-esteem and help them to cope with all of the changes they are experiencing. Sometimes the activity should be simplified, depending on the resident's cognitive abilities.

Normalization Activities: Examples

- Folding washcloths

- Simple cooking that does not require a stove, such as making sandwiches or fancy toppings for crackers
- Rolling coins
- Shining silverware or other objects
- Washing windows
- Washing hand laundry
- Sorting envelopes
- Planting a flower pot for a room
- Polishing shoes
- Sorting and looking through costume jewelry

A13-5
Coping with the Holidays* and Gift Suggestions

'Tis the season to be jolly. . . . A lot of time and effort goes into making the nursing home a special place for the holiday. Often, however, there is an underlying sadness and feelings of loss, change, and separation as residents, families, and staff try to focus on the season's joys.

Residents should be included in holiday festivities but not overloaded with activities or unreasonable expectations to participate. They may have an adverse reaction to the change in the everyday routine, the increased sensory stimulation from decorations and noise, and perhaps visitors who do not understand how to interact with someone with Alzheimer's disease. They enjoy doing simple decorating, singing, and subdued parties. Traditional music and worship services give them a sense of grounding and peace. Families are often disappointed when they realize that their loved ones can no longer respond to the beloved rituals of the holidays such as opening gifts or enjoying traditional foods.

Taking the resident home for the holidays, even if just for a few hours, has to be a personal decision, best made by the family with input from the staff. The nursing home usually becomes "home," a place of comfort and routine, and residents generally want to return after being away 2–3 hours. Going away from the care units can make residents with dementia feel anxious and insecure.

The best gift for the nursing home resident is a scrapbook with pictures of family, friends, places visited, favorite foods, poetry, places once lived . . . the joys of the past, all labeled, perhaps with comments. This can be a tool for reminiscing during visits with family and staff. Other gift suggestions are attractive bedspreads, a decorative pillow, a stuffed teddy bear, a night-light, knee-high stockings, leg warmers, costume jewelry, a cardigan sweater, fragrant lotions, and body powder.

Families are an important part of the holidays and often desire to feel supported and included. Staff members need love and support during the holidays because they also become deeply involved with residents and their families. Staff members should recognize their own feelings and develop ways to cope during this busy season, thereby setting the mood of love and caring for all.

The following is an example of a letter that a nursing facility sent to families of its residents:

---

*Reprinted with permission from C Hellen. Coping with the holidays. Rush Alzheimer's Disease Center News 1989;fall.

To Our Family Members At Holiday Time

We hope that you will be joining us for the holiday plans we have made for you and your loved ones. This is the time of year for creating new celebrations focused on shared moments together.

We have attached articles and gift suggestion ideas that may be helpful to you. Please know that we are looking forward to sharing our first holiday season here at The Wealshire with you.

Activity Ideas for Sharing Time Together: Families, Residents, and Staff

Drive about and see the lights
Visit a church or synagogue
Visit a Christmas tree lot
Watch children climb up on Santa's knee in a mall
Bake cookies, share them with the fire and police departments
Take pictures of the residents, frame pictures and assist the residents to make cards for their families, insert picture
Celebrate Christmas around the world by watching videotapes, looking at books, and preparing a special food from the selected country
Decorate a tree with residents' names and their family members
Gather a strolling group of carolers and visit everyone in the facility
Wrap gifts for family members
Make tree decorations using old cards, paper chains, strings of cranberries, etc.
Create a wall decoration by taking used cards, cutting off the backs, and starting with one card for the top of a card tree, tape it to the wall, three cards under that one, and so forth until the tree has the traditional shape—all size cards can be used
Practice carols so the residents can always sing back to visiting groups
Bake cookies for sharing with visitors
Make a mural of a holiday or a winter scene
Write a group letter to Santa that includes everyone's wishes
Make scrapbooks for children in the hospital during the holidays
Make wrapping paper using potato printing or by placing string in poster paints and then moving it about on a large sheet of paper
Make wrapping paper by spattering paint over cut out snowflakes using screening and a toothbrush and poster paint on large pieces of paper
Color pictures from a coloring book that has had the pictures enlarged and photo-copied (e.g., "The Night Before Christmas" or the Hanukkah story) then punch holes in the paper and place in a scrapbook so it is ready to read to visiting children

Gift Suggestions

LifeStory Book: see Family Services for information
Photo albums: pictures labeled
Scrapbooks: empty to be filled
Identification bracelet (Safe Return, Alzheimer's Association)
Exercise items (e.g., soft sponge ball, colorful scarves, plastic tubes for golf clubs, cassette tapes or videotapes that can be used by the group)
Tapes of familiar music, tape player

Alzheimer's Disease: Activity-Focused Care

Night-light

Bulletin board for the resident's room

Visitors' log and comment book so you can know who has been in to see your loved one (comments could tell about what worked well during the visit)

Goodies for visiting (e.g., makeup, fun jewelry, shoe-shine kit, cards, baseball cards, maps)

Cosmetics (e.g., after shave, powder, perfume, lip moisturizers, makeup bag)

Tissues in an attractive holder

Colorful mobiles

Stuffed animals and pillows for decorating the bed

The resident's old bedspread, re-cut if necessary, afghans

Beauty appointments

Family videotape

Tote bags or fanny packs for carrying "stuff"

Newspaper or magazine subscription

Activities:

    simple puzzles

    easy woodworking projects

    yarns to wind

    fabrics to fold and sort

    adult coloring books, nontoxic markers or crayons

Clothing

    one size too large is easier to put on

    cotton clothes are easiest to care for

    slippers with firm and nonslip bottoms

    lap cover or blanket

    jogging suits

    leg warmers

    washable cardigans

    mittens, scarves, ear muffs

    underwear

Please Remember Safety

We are all concerned that this be a safe holiday for all. Gifts should contain no small parts, sharp instruments, or toxic items. We also ask that you consider silk or artificial poinsettia plants, because ingestion of the plant's red leaves can cause the mouth tissue to be inflamed and could be toxic.

    Please check with staff for specific suggestions.

A13-6
Family Care Conference Form

Pre-Care Conference Questionnaire

The staff is reviewing the present status of, care being given to, and goals for the future of _____
on _____. We really care about your resident and hope that you will read the following questions carefully and respond with your ideas and thoughts. If you are unable to attend the conference, please complete this form and return to:

_____

_____

_____

_____

1. Are your resident's abilities and strengths being recognized and promoted? Any suggestions? _____

   _____

2. Do you think that your resident could be doing more for himself or herself? Explain. _____

   _____

3. Are there any changes or additions to your resident's daily care and routine that you think would benefit him or her? _____

   _____

4. What caregiving goal(s), techniques, and approaches do you think should be continued on behalf of your resident? Are there aspects of care that you want to see stopped? What do you want the staff to focus on during the next 3 months? Please be specific. _____

   _____

5. Are there any daily care activities or recreational activities that you or your family members would like to be doing for your resident? Examples: simple crafts, grooming, nails, etc. How can we help you? _____

   _____

6. Our staff welcomes information about our residents. Please describe any insights or information you have that would be helpful in our caregiving.

_____

7. Are there any specific family needs or concerns or resident needs at this time that we could be helping with? _____

_____

Thank you for your cooperation and input. If you have any further concerns or questions please feel free to contact _____.
Please bring this questionnaire with you to the conference, if attending. If not, please mail. You are welcome to review the plan of care when you visit.

Ability-Centered Plan of Care Glossary of Terms for Residents with Dementia

Care plans for persons with dementia should reflect the resident's abilities and personal difficulties and include dementia-specific approaches and interventions. Care plans are then able to reflect the caregivers' understanding of holistic care of persons with Alzheimer's disease and related disorders. For example, in facilities with a special care unit, the question, "Why is Mr. Jones being cared for on this unit rather than in the rest of the nursing home?" can be answered by looking at Mr. Jones's personalized dementia plan of care. The following are common terms used on care plans for persons with dementia and their definitions:

Ability-centered based interventions: care delivered by focusing on and using the resident's remaining strengths and abilities

Activity: all the daily "stuff" of life, the "whatever" that is, occurs, and happens affecting one's cognitive, physical, psychosocial, and spiritual personhood and well-being

Adapt task or activity: simulate resident's former occupation or involvement, assuring successful participation by using simplification and task breakdown

Agnosia: inability to recognize, understand, or interpret information coming in through the senses (e.g., turning toward a voice, recognizing a face or reading but unable to comprehend)

Anomia: inability to name objects

Aphasia: difficulty understanding or expressing language or both

Apraxia: inability to motor plan or be aware of body's relationship to space; inability to carry out a purposeful movement even when the muscle power and general coordination is adequate (e.g., moving a fork from the potatoes to his or her mouth)

Attention span and cooperation increase: this can be achieved by using bilaterally handheld objects, simplifying

Bridging: a sensory connection with the resident by having the resident hold in his or her hand the same item the caregiver is using, leading the resident to feel as though he or she is doing the task for himself or herself

Chaining: caregiver holds the resident's hand, arm, or leg to start the desired movement or activity, then the caregiver removes his or her hand to allow the resident to take over

Clueing systems: specific approaches for enabling the resident through the use of verbal, visual, or physical cues

Crossing the midline: moving arms or legs and eyes across the midline of the resident's body to the other side

Delusion: a false belief or wrong judgment

Distraction techniques: specific techniques for refocusing the resident when needed (e.g., food, singing, objects to be held, family names)

End chaining: same as chaining, except that the ending of the task or activity is started first, encouraging the resident to repeat the task or activity (e.g., the caregiver places the spoon of mashed potatoes in the resident's mouth and then removes his or her hand, leaving the spoon in the resident's mouth, and the resident then reaches up to the spoon and begins to self-feed)

Environmental competency: resident-needed environmental support for promotion of abilities or reduction of inabilities or both; can include color, noise, crowding, etc.

Excess disability: when a resident is affected by a condition (internally or externally caused) that makes the dementia and its symptoms more disabling than would be expected

Festination: acceleration of gait (e.g., the resident picks up speed when walking and cannot stop); sometimes happens when the resident is parkinsonian or has Parkinson's disease

Figure ground: differentiation between foreground and background form and objects

Gegenhalten response: resistance that is involuntary in arms or legs in response to being moved passively; usually, arms pull into the chest, making dressing and other activities of daily living difficult

Hallucination: misinterpretation of an object or event when none is present; hallucinations may be visual, auditory, olfactory, tactile, or gustatory

Hand-over-hand: caregiver places his or her hand over the resident's, and the two proceed together with the task or activity

Hyperorality: everything possible, including inappropriate items, are put into mouth

Labeled items, area, activities: labeling items in the environment to increase the resident's competency and cognitive abilities

Low stimulus threshold: resident requires an environment that is calm in content, color, noise level, and movement

Mirroring: caregiver does the same activity or procedure he or she wants the resident to do while facing the resident, encouraging the resident to copy the movement

Monitoring: caregiver watches the resident to assure safety and success

Alzheimer's Disease: Activity-Focused Care

Monitoring of nonverbal communication: caregiver watches the resident's nonverbal responses to assure the therapeutic value of continuing a specific activity or task

Multisensory clueing: the simultaneous use of verbal, visual, auditory, olfactory, or tactile cues, or all, when appropriate to help enable the resident's participation

Myoclonus: a twitching or spasm of a muscle or group of muscles; for example, a jerking movement of the arm or kicking response of a leg

Normalization task: specific task that reflects the resident's daily life work, a familiar task calling forth past experiences

One-step directions: providing instruction for the resident's active participation by giving one step at a time and waiting until that step has been completed before describing another step

Patrol: a one-to-one behavioral intervention when staff take half-hour periods with a verbally or physically acting out resident requiring constant attention or refocusing to calm the resident while relieving other staff and residents in the area

Perseveration: repetition of a word, phrase, or action; although often meaningless, the tone or the sound can be useful to interpret mood or need or both

Personhood: the "I" within each resident, his or her sense of self

Plantar proprioception: resident needs more sensory stimulation coming in through the bottom of the feet; therefore, he or she may need to walk with shoes off and just socks or barefooted for successful ambulation

Proprioception: interpretation of stimuli originating in muscles, joints, and other internal tissue that alerts and provides information about the position of one body part in relationship to another (e.g., feedback coming in through the visual, vestibular, and proprioceptive systems is required for balance competency)

Props: resident needs cueing for increasing awareness and comprehension, so props reflective of the topic, task, activity, or information being sought can enable resident's response

Refocusing: an approach to behaviors that helps difficult responses to be adapted to be more acceptable

Rescuing: a strategy used when a caregiver needs assistance with a resident who is becoming upset with him or her, whereby another caregiver approaches the situation and sends the first caregiver "away," allowing the resident to feel "rescued"

Restraint: two basic types (1) chemical: drugs prescribed to control mood, mental status, or behavior; (2) physical: any method, device, material, or equipment that cannot be removed by the resident that restricts freedom of movement or normal access to his or her body

Rhythmic sounds, words, movements: using rhythm to enable the resident to initiate task or activity involvement

Sensory bridging: when a task is being attempted, the resident holds a similar object to that of the caregiver, thereby sensing that he or she is actually doing the task as he or she bridges from himself or herself, to the caregiver, and back to himself or herself through the held item

Sequencing: placing information, concepts, tasks, and actions in order

Structured activity: resident is most successful when the activity or task presented for involvement is well defined, is broken down in understandable components, and follows a familiar routine

Task or activity breakdown: dividing the task or activity into many small steps that help to assure the resident's success

Task or activity simplification: simplifying the task or activity from one of complexity to one that is easier for the resident to follow

Task timing: yielding to the resident regarding the time a task takes and not superimposing a caregiver's time schedule, thereby assuring the resident's success

Therapeutic fib: "bent facts," supportive words or information in place of reality and facts that may demean the resident because he or she cannot remember, therefore allowing the resident's dignity and reducing or eliminating confrontations

Touch response: specific responses to being touched; where, when, and how to use as a therapeutic intervention

Wayfinding: assistance given with verbal or visual cueing so the resident can locate needed areas (e.g., room, toilet)

Index

Note: Page numbers followed by *f* indicate figures.

Aberration(s), as behavioral response, 221–223
Ability(ies)
  behaviors as expressions of, 196–197
  focusing on, effects on daily life care activities, 91
Ability-based interventions, defined, 419
Ability centering, 3
Ability-centered plan of care, 7, 15–17
Accusation(s), as behavioral response, 223
Active games, therapeutic benefits of, 307
Activity, defined, 419
Activities. *See also under specific type of activity*
  activity therapists' role in, 251–252
  age-appropriate, defined, 285–286
  analysis of, 247–249
    components of, 247
    example of, 247–249, 277–279
  aroma therapists' role in, 253
  art therapists' role in, 252
  assessment of, 250–251
  for behavioral refocusing and effective intervention, 269–270
  cognitive activities, 255–258
  cognitive qualities of, 246
  community partnership in, 263–264
  criteria for, 245
  daily life "stuff," 243–310
  dance and movement therapists' role in, 252
  for depression, 274–275
  drama therapists' role in, 252
  effective activities, grouping residents for, 250–251
  horticultural therapists' role in, 252

initiation of, inability in, as behavioral response, 225
intergenerational activities, 264–265
involving residents in, 253
for late-stage dementia care, 268–269
for loneliness, 274–275
male-oriented activities, 265–266
massage therapists' role in, 253
movement activities, 258–259
music therapists' role in, 252
normalization activities, 262–263
objectives of, 244–245
one-to-one activities, 267–268
personalized activities, 267–268
pet therapists' role in, 252–253
physical qualities of, 246
psychosocial activities, 259–260
psychosocial qualities of, 246–247
qualities of, 245–247
for refocusing "searching and discovering," 274
reminiscing kits for, 281–283
requirements for, 253–255
for residents with short attention spans, 266–267
for residents who pace and wander, 273–274
for sadness, 274–275
service for others' activities, 263–264
"shoestring" activities, 266–267
spiritual activities, 261
structured, defined, 421
success in, 244
supervisory personnel for, 251–253
terminal care–related, 363–364
therapeutic benefits of, 307–310
therapeutic value of, 249

Activities—*continued*
  for therapeutically reducing preva-
      lence, onset, or intensity of
      aggressive or combative
      behaviors, 270–273
  thinking activities, 255–258. *See
      also* Cognitive activities
  "wearable" activities, 266–267
Activities of daily living (ADLs), 87–126
  bathing, 93–97
  bridging, 93
  caregivers support policy and proce-
      dures for, 125–126
  chaining, 92
  clueing, 91
  consistency in, 90–91
  cultural issues in, 91
  disrobing, 97–100, 121–123
  distraction, 91
  dressing, 97–100, 121–123
  end chaining, 92–93
  factors affecting
      cognitive, 87–88, 107–108
      dementia, 87–89
      emotional, 88–89
      environment-related, 89
      physical, 88, 108
      psychosocial, 88–89, 108–109
  focusing on abilities in, 91
  guidelines for, 90–92
  hand-over-hand strategy, 92
  hands-on care strategies, 92–93
  health care provider issues in, 25,
      103–104
  hygiene, 93–97
  incontinence, 100–103
  mirroring, 92
  monitoring in, 90
  nonverbal input in, 91
  oral care, 93–97
  report form for, 115–118
  rescue strategy in, 92
  resident basic care information form
      for, 119–120
  sensory profile in, 89–90, 111–113
  staff issues in, 25, 103–104
  task breakdown in, 91
  timing in, 90
  toilet use, 100–103
Activities of service, pride in, 290–291
Activity therapists
  daily life activities supervised by,
      251–252
  job description of, 303–304
Activity therapy care conference
      report form, 305, 307–310
Activity-focused care, 1–17
  ability-centered, 7, 15–17
  defined, 1–2
Adapt task or activity, defined, 419
Administrator(s), "walk in shoes" of
      assistants by, 49–50
Affection, giving and receiving of,
      311–337. *See also* Intimacy,
      expressions of
Affirmation, life, LifeStory Book for,
      55–66. *See also* LifeStory
      Book
Aggression
  as behavioral response, 218
  physical, safety issues related to,
      211–216
Aggressive behaviors, activities for
      reducing, 270–273
Agitation, as behavioral response,
      216–217
Agnosia, defined, 419
Alzheimer's behaviors, 195–241. *See
      also* Behavior(s)
Alzheimer's care center, and local con-
      gregation, uniting of,
      343–345
Alzheimer's disease. *See also* Dementia
  activity-focused care for, 1–17
      ability-centered, 7, 15–17
      defined, 1–2
  Bill of Rights for patients with, 22–23
  care of patients with
      health care provider and staff
          issues related to, 9–11
      ten commandments of, 8–9
  challenges of, 13–14
  symptoms of, 13–14
Alzheimer's patient hospital transfer
      information, 373
  explanation and worksheet, 375–377

Ambulation, independent, promoting of, 162–165
Anomia, defined, 419
Anxiety
  as behavioral response, 216–217
  money-related, decreasing of, 29–30, 29f
Apathy, as behavioral response, 225
Aphasia, defined, 419
Apraxia, 419
Aroma therapists, daily life activities supervised by, 253
Art therapists, daily life activities supervised by, 252
Assisted movement, terminal care–related, 365–367
Attention span
  and cooperation increase, defined, 420
  short, activities for residents with, 266–267
Autopsy, 371

Baking, therapeutic benefits of, 307
Balance, in physical well-being, 183–185
Basic care information form, activities of daily living-related, 119–120
Bathing, in daily life care activities, 93–97
Beauty shop, therapeutic benefits of, 307
Behavior(s), 195–241. See also Behavioral responses
  aggressive
    activities for reducing, 270–273
    safety issues related to, 211–216
  analysis form for, 205–206, 231–234
  analysis of, examples of, 207–211
  assistance for, 204
  causes of, 201–203
  cognitive focus of, 202
  combative
    activities for reducing, 270–273
    safety issues related to, 211–216
  as communication, 71
  defined, 195, 201
  environmental focus of, 203

as expressions of abilities and inabilities, 196–197
  focusing of, guidelines for, 198–200
  health care provider and staff issues related to, 225–226
  location of, 204
  manifestations of, risk factors precipitating, 198
  pacing, examples of, 207–209
  patrol, 213
    defined, 421
  patterns of, tracking of, 205, 229–230
  persons involved in, 203
  physical aggression, safety issues related to, 211–216
  physical focus of, 202
  profile of, implementation of, 200–204
  psychosocial focus of, 202–203
  reasons for, 195–196
  "redistribution of stuff," examples of, 209–211
  refocusing of, activities of, 269–270
  resident security and, 206–207, 235–238
  rescue, 213
    defined, 421
  rummaging, examples of, 209–211
  safety issues related to, 211–216
  terminal care–related, 367
  timing of, 204
  understanding of, guidelines for, 198–200
  violent, safety issues related to, 211–216
  wandering, examples of, 207–209
Behavior analysis form, 205–206, 231–234
Behavior observation form, 229–230
Behavior profile form, 227–228
Behavioral responses, 216–225. See also Behavior(s)
  aberrations, 221–223
  accusations, 223
  aggression, 218
  agitation, 216–217
  anxiety, 216–217
  apathy, 225
  calling, 224–225

Behavioral responses—*continued*
  catastrophic reactions, 217
  combativeness, 218
  delusions, 221–223
  demanding, 223
  hallucinations, 221–223
  hyperorality, 220
  inability to initiate activities, 225
  inappropriate sexual responses, 220
  nocturnal wandering, 221
  pacing, 220
  patrol, 213
    defined, 421
  picking, 220
  redistribution of "stuff," 221
  repetitious movements, 220
  repetitious questioning, 224–225
  rescue, 213
    defined, 421
  rummaging, 221
  screaming, 224–225
  sleep disturbances, 221
  sundowning, 218–219
  wandering, 220
  withdrawal, 225
  yelling, 224–225
Bill of Rights, of Alzheimer's disease
        patients, 22–23
Bingo, therapeutic benefits of, 307
Breakfast, finger food ideas for, 153
Bridging
  in daily life care activities, 93
  defined, 420
  in eating process, 130
  sensory, defined, 421

Calling, as behavioral response, 224–225
Caregivers, family, 379–418. *See also*
        Family caregivers
Caregiving, as purposeful activity, 7–8
Catastrophic reactions
  analysis of, 239–241
  as behavioral response, 217
Chaining
  in daily life care activities, 92, 130
  defined, 420
Clergy
  in spirituality, 340

as support for persons with dementia
        and their families, 340–341
Clueing
  defined, 420
  effects on daily life care activities, 91
  multisensory
    defined, 421
    in eating process, 129
Cognitive abilities, 3–6
  centering of, in dementia impairment
    mild, 4
    moderate, 5
    severe, 6
Cognitive activities, 255–258
  dementia challenges affecting, 256
  examples of, 256–258
  qualities of, 246
Cognitive factors
  effects on daily life care activities,
        87–88, 107–108
  mobility affected by, 160–161
  physical restraint use affected by, 172
Cognitive participation, in activities
        of daily life, 255–258
Combative behaviors, reducing of,
        activities in, 270–273
Combativeness
  as behavioral response, 218
  safety issues related to, 211–216
Communication, 67–85
  behaviors as, 71
  choice of words in, 67–68
  connecting in, guidelines for, 68–71
  emotional needs behind words in, 69
  environmental effects on, assess-
        ment form for, 81–82
  environmental distractions in, 70
  eye contact in, 69
  facial expression in, 69
  health care provider issues in, 79
  implied, 76–77
  in late-stage dementia, assessment
        of, 78, 83–85
    profile form for, 83–85
  listening in, 68
  missing words in, 70
  multisensory cues in, 70
  nonverbal, 69, 76–77

effects on daily life care activities, 91
  monitoring of, defined, 421
posture in, 69
promotion of, environmental effects
        on, 78–79
respect in, 68–69
sensitivity in, 71
spoken, 71–76
staff issues in, 79
terminal care–related, 362–363
therapeutic fibs in, 70
touch in, 69, 78
verbal, 71–76
verbalization as basis for, 23
vocal, 71–76
voice, tone of, in, 69
well-being through, 71
word selection in, 69
Community, safety in, 206–207,
        235–238
Community and civic professionals
        training outline, 235–236
Compassionate connectedness, 261,
        339–354
  religious, spiritual, and sacred center
        assessment of, 353–354
  terminal care–related, 369
Compassionate relationships, 327–328
Competence, upholding and maintain-
        ing of, 3
Competency, environmental, defined,
        420
Congregation
  and Alzheimer's care center, uniting
        of, 343–345
  shared communion of love and sup-
        port in, 340, 341–342
Connectedness
  compassionate, 261, 339–354
    religious, spiritual, and sacred
        center assessment of,
        353–354
    terminal care–related, 369
  family, 393–394
  respected, 30–31
Consistency, effects on daily life care
        activities, 90–91
Cooking, therapeutic benefits of, 307

Coping, as focus of psychosocial sup-
        port group for residents with
        moderate impairment, 37
Couples with dementia, finding a bal-
        ance for, 31–35
  care goals for, 32
  current abilities and needs and, 32
  decision time in, 32
  family support in, 32–33, 397
  LifeStory in, 32
  living as roommates, 32
  marriage history in, 32
  staff support in, 33
Crafts, therapeutic benefits of, 307
Creative arts, therapeutic benefits
        of, 307
Crossing the midline, defined, 420
Cueing, multisensory
  in communication, 70
  in eating process, 129
Cultural issues, effects on daily life
        care activities, 91

Daily life, activities of, 243–310. See
        also Activities of daily living
        (ADLs)
Dance and movement, therapeutic
        benefits of, 308
Dance and movement therapists,
        daily life activities super-
        vised by, 252
Death
  creation of "cherished sentinel,"
        369–370
  impending, medical issues related
        to, 359–361
Delusion(s)
  as behavioral response, 221–223
  defined, 420
Demanding, as behavioral response, 223
Dementia
  both parents with, family support
        for, 397
  couples with, finding a balance for,
        31–35. See also Couples with
        dementia, finding a balance
        for
  discounting of patients with, 21–22

Dementia—*continued*
  effects on daily life care activities,
      87–126. *See also* Activities
      of daily living (ADLs)
  late-stage
    communication of, assessment of,
        78, 83–85
    sensory stimulation and activities
        for, 268–269
  mild impairment with
    cognitive and physical ability cen-
        tering and challenges in, 4
    personal challenges for persons
        experiencing, 13–14
    psychosocial ability centering and
        challenges facing, 20
  moderate impairment with
    cognitive and physical ability
        centering and challenges
        in, 5–6
    personal challenges for persons
        experiencing, 14
    psychosocial ability centering and
        challenges facing, 20–21
    psychosocial support group for,
        development of, 35–39. *See
        also* Psychosocial support
        group, for residents with
        moderate impairment
  nutrition for residents with, 151–152
  personhood in, indicators of, 19–20
  severe impairment with
    cognitive and physical ability cen-
        tering and challenges in, 6
    personal challenges for persons
        experiencing, 14
    psychosocial ability centering and
        challenges facing, 21
  well-being in, indicators of, 19–20
Depression, 25–26
  activities for, 274–275
Desserts, finger food ideas for, 154
Dietary department, role in food modi-
      fications and mealtime sup-
      port, 141–142
Dignity, terminal care–related,
      enabling of, 363–364
Dinner, finger food ideas for, 154

Disability(ies), excess, defined, 420
Discounting of dementia patients, 21–22
Disrobing, in daily life care activities,
      97–100, 121–123
Distraction
  defined, 420
  effects on daily life care activities, 91
Drama therapists, daily life activities
      supervised by, 252
Dressing, in daily life care activities,
      97–100, 121–123
Drum circle, therapeutic benefits
      of, 309

Eating
  as activity, 127–157
    assistance with, 143–145
    bridging in, 130
    chaining in, 130
    dietary department's role in,
        141–142
    dining environment and equip-
        ment support in, 142–143
    end chaining in, 130
    "feeder" in, humiliation associ-
        ated with, 136–138
    hand over hand in, 130
    health care provider and staff
        issues related to, 148–149
    implement behavior intervention
        tools in, 129
    increasing food consumed, 138–141
    interventions and facilitation
        in, 129–131
    mirroring in, 129
    mouth opening and swallowing
        facilitation in, 130–131
    multisensory cueing in, 129
    nutritional considerations, 138–139
      food approaches and adapta-
          tions, 140–141
      food setup, 139–140
      staff approaches to and interven-
          tions, 138–139
    sensory profile in, 128–129
    success with, 128–129
    task simplification and sequencing
        in, 129

behaviors associated with, 131–132
  problems due to, 131–132
    causes of
      cognitive challenges, 132
      environmental challenges, 136
      physical challenges, 133
      psychosocial challenges,
        134–136
  cognitive, physical, and psychosocial
    abilities related to, 128
  resident's history of, obtaining of, 128
  terminal care–related, 364–365
Educational activity, therapeutic bene-
    fits of, 308
Educational opportunities, for family
    caregivers, 397–398
Emotional factors, effects on daily life
    care activities, 88–89
Emotional needs, in communication, 69
Emotional support, terminal
    care–related, 361–362
End chaining
  in daily life care activities, 92–93
  defined, 420
  in eating process, 130
Entertainment, therapeutic benefits
    of, 308
Environment
  in communication, 70, 78–79
    assessment form for, 81–82
  effects on daily life care activities, 89
  physical restraint use affected by, 173
  problems due to, assessment of, 147
  safety of, in independent ambula-
    tion, 165
Environmental competency, defined,
    420
Environmental distractions, in com-
    munication, 70
Excess disability, defined, 420
Exercise, 159–193. *See also* Mobility;
    Physical wellness
  defined, 183
  for fitness trail, 187–188
  in physical well-being, 183–185
  therapeutic benefits of, 308
Expression, facial, in communication, 69
Eye contact, in communication, 69

Facial expression, in communication, 69
Falls, assessing for, 167–169
  form for, 191–193
Family(ies)
  clerical support for persons with
      dementia and their families,
      340–341
  grief, 356–357
  mealtime involvement of, 145–146
  problems due to, assessment of, 148
  support of, for couples with demen-
      tia, 32–33
  visits, therapeutic benefits of, 308
  weddings, 394–396
Family care conference form, 417–418
Family caregivers, 379–418
  activity-focused nursing home visits
      by, 409–411
  in admission to nursing home,
      admission day, 384–387
  care for, 405–406
  connectedness of, 393–394
  coping with holidays, 413–415
  "coulds" versus "shoulds," 392–393
  and dying resident, 399
  educational opportunities for, 397–398
  family care conference form, 417–418
  family council, 390–391
  family mentor program, 389
  family support for, 396–397
  family-related events for, 394–396
  gift suggestions for, 413–415
  grief experienced by, 380
  guilt of, 405–406
  health care provider issues related
      to, 400
  loss experienced by, 380
  new family orientation program, 389
  nursing home placement decisions
      made by, 380–382
    nursing home's response to, 382–384
    preadmission support factors for,
      383–384
  and partnership with staff, 387–389
  in plan-of-care conference, 396
  preadmission information form
      for, 407–408
  research opportunities for, 399

Family caregivers—*continued*
staff issues related to, 400
survival handbook for, 391–392
12 steps for, 403
visiting times, 393–394
volunteering by, 393–394
Family council, 390–391
Family mentor program, at nursing
home, 389
Family Survival Handbook, 391–392
Feeling(s), as focus of psychosocial
support group for residents
with moderate impair-
ment, 36
Festination, defined, 420
Figure ground, defined, 420
Finger food suggestions, 153–154
Fitness, therapeutic benefits of, 308
Fitness trail, 187–188
Food(s), problems due to, assessment
of, 147
Friend visit, therapeutic benefits of, 308

Games, support group, 45–46
Gardening, therapeutic benefits
of, 308
Gegenhalten response, defined, 420
Gift suggestions, 413–415
Grief, family, 356–357
as caregivers, 380
Guilt, of family caregivers, 405–406

Hallucination(s)
as behavioral response, 221–223
defined, 420
Hand-over-hand strategy
in daily life care activities, 92
defined, 420
in eating process, 130
Health care providers
activities of daily life issues related
to, 25, 103–104
Alzheimer's disease care issues
related to, 9–11
behavior issues related to, 225–226
communication issues related to, 79
eating and mealtime issues related
to, 148–149

family caregivers' issues related
to, 400
intimacy issues related to, 322–324
LifeStory Book issues related to, 60–61
physical well-being issues related
to, 179–180
psychosocial support group issues
related to, 41
spirituality issues related to, 350–351
support policy and procedures for
activities of daily living
issues related to, 125–126
terminal care issues related to,
371–372
Hobbies, therapeutic benefits of, 307
Holidays
coping with, by family caregivers,
413–415
family-related, 394–396
Homemaking, activities of, pride
in, 292–293
Horticultural therapists, daily life
activities supervised
by, 252
Hospice care, 358
Hospitality, activities of, pride in,
291–292
Hydration, problems due to, assessment of, 147
Hygiene, in daily life care activities,
93–97
Hyperorality
as behavioral response, 220
defined, 420
Hypersexuality, 316–320
as behavioral response, 220

Immobile residents, caregiving for,
166–167
Implied communication, 76–77
Inability(ies), behaviors as expressions
of, 197
Incontinence, in daily life care activities, 100–103
Intellectual activity, therapeutic benefits of, 308
Intergenerational activities, 264–265
therapeutic benefits of, 308

Intimacy
  benefits of, 313
  changing face of, 325–326
  essence of, 313
  expressions of, 311–337
    activity analysis of, 333–336
    in care facilities, 320–323
      guidelines for persons with
        dementia, 329–331
    health care provider issues in,
        322–324
    inclusiveness of, 312–313
    profile of, 314–315, 337
    responses to, 313–314
    self-directed, 315–316
    staff issues in, 322–324

Labeled items, area, activities, defined,
    420
Ladies' group, therapeutic benefits
    of, 308
Language of posture, in communica-
    tion, 69
Language of touch, 78
Life
  "activity" of, 2–3
  components of, 1
  meaning of,
    promotion of, 19–20
    search for, 2–3
LifeAffirmation, LifeStory Book for,
    55–66. See also LifeStory Book
LifeStory Book, 55–66
  content recommendations for, 58
  contraindications to use of, 56–57
  defined, 55
  family suggestions for, 58–59
  format suggestions for, 57–58
  health care provider issues related
    to, 60–61
  indicators for, 55–56
  letter to families, 63–66
  quality involvement in, 58–59
  staff use of
    guidelines for, 59–60
    issues related to, 60–61
Life work activities
  defined, 287–288

examples of, 289–294
  normalization, 262–263
  pride in, 293–294
Lincolnshire Police Department Resi-
    dent Checklist for the Weal-
    shire, 237–238
Listening, in communication, 68
Loneliness, activities for, 274–275
Loss, of family caregivers, 380
Low stimulus threshold, defined, 420
Lunch, finger food ideas for, 153–154

Male-oriented activities, 265–266
Massage, therapeutic benefits of, 308
Massage therapists, daily life activities
    supervised by, 253
Masturbation, responses to, 315–316
Meal(s), problems due to, assessment
    of, 147
Mealtimes. See Eating
Medical issues, terminal care–related,
    359–361
Men's group, therapeutic benefits
    of, 308
Ministry, creative, 343–345
Mirroring
  in daily life care activities, 92
  defined, 420
  in eating process, 129
Mobility, 159–193. See also Exercise;
    Physical wellness
  assisting, 165–166
  environmental safety for, 165
  factors affecting
    cognitive, 160–161
    dementia, 160–162
    physical, 161–162
    psychosocial, 162
  maintaining of, 164
  promoting of, 162–165
  task example of getting into a car,
    goals for, 189–190
  terminal care–related, 365–367
Monitoring
  defined, 421
  effects on daily life care activities, 90
Monitoring of nonverbal communica-
    tion, defined, 421

Mouth opening, in eating process, 130–131
Movement activities, 258–259
Movies, therapeutic benefits of, 308
Multisensory clueing, defined, 421
Multisensory cues
  in communication, 70
  in eating process, 129
Music program, therapeutic benefits of, 308
Music therapists, daily life activities supervised by, 252

Need(s), spiritual, appraising of, 339–340
Need to know, 30–31
Need to participate, 30–31
New family orientation program, at nursing home, 389
News and views, therapeutic benefits of, 309
Nocturnal wandering, as behavioral response, 221
Nonverbal communication, 69, 76–77
  effects on daily life care activities, 91
  monitoring of, defined, 421
Nonverbal responses, objectives of, 67
Normalization
  activities, 262–263
    defined, 287–288
  task, defined, 421
  therapeutic benefits of, 309
Nursing home(s)
  admission day at, 384–387
  residents of, meaningful activity opportunities for, creation of, 295–298
Nutrient-dense recipes, 155–157
Nutrition
  assessment of, in late or terminal care, 146–148
  in meal preparations, 138–141
  optimal, for dementia patients, 151–152
  terminal care–related, 364–365

One-step directions, defined, 421
One-to-one activities, 267–268
  therapeutic benefits of, 309

Oral care, in daily life care activities, 93–97
Outdoor walking group, therapeutic benefits of, 309

Pacing
  activities for residents who engage in, 273–274
  as behavioral response, 220
  examples of, 207–209
Pain
  recognition of, 357
  responding to, 357
Paranoia, as behavioral response, 223
Passive movement, terminal care–related, 365–367
Patrol, 213
  defined, 421
Percussion circle, therapeutic benefits of, 309
Perseveration, defined, 421
Personalized activities, 267–268
Personhood
  maintaining of, 19–53
    being valued, not "discounted," 21–22
    being included, 30–31
    compromised self-image and, 24–25
    couples with dementia and, 31–35
    depression and, 25–26
    development of a psychosocial support group and, 35–39
    integrated self-image and, 23
    interventions and support of psychosocial needs and, 26–30
    patient's bill of rights and, 22–23
    promoting life's meaning and, 19–20
    psychosocial ability centering and, 20–21
    staff and, 41
  preservation of, terminal care–related, 361–362
  reduced, physical restraints and, 173
  of staff, 40, 47–50
Pet care and therapy, therapeutic benefits of, 309
Pet therapists, daily life activities supervised by, 252–253

Physical abilities, 3–6
  centering of, in demenia impairment
    mild, 4
    moderate, 5–6
    severe, 6
Physical activities, 258–259
  dementia challenges affecting, 258
  examples of, 258–259
  qualities of, 246
Physical aggression, safety issues
    related to, 211–216
Physical factors
  mobility affected by, 161–162
  physical restraint use affected by, 172
Physical restraints, 171–172
  alternatives to, 174–176
    cognitive distraction techniques, 175
    environmental adaptations, 176
    physically based, 174–175
    psychosocial distraction tech-
      niques, 175
  cognitive effects of, 173
  defined, 171
  efficacy of, 171
  factors affecting use of
    cognitive, 172
    dementia, 172–173
    environmental, 173
    physical, 172
    psychosocial, 173
  issues related to use of, 171–172
  love and belonging needs for, 177, 178
  negative effects of, 173
  physical effects of, 174
  physiologic needs for, 177–178
  psychosocial effects of, 173
  safety and security needs for, 177, 178
  self-actualization needs for, 177,
    178–179
  self-esteem needs for, 177, 178–179
  social needs for, 177, 178
  types of, 171
  use considerations for, 176–179
Physical wellness, 159–193. *See also*
    Exercise; Mobility
  balance in, 183–185
  defined, 159
  exercise in, 183–185

fitness trail in, 187–188
functional maintenance and rehabili-
    tation programs for, 169–171
health care provider and staff issues
    related to, 179–180
strengthening in, 183–185
Picking, as behavioral response, 220
Plan-of-care conference
  family caregivers in, 396
  nursing assistants' activities of daily
    living report form in, 115
Plantar proprioception, defined, 421
Police department resident checklist,
    237–238
Posture, language of, in communica-
    tion, 69
Praise, thanksgiving, and worship cen-
    ter, creation of, 345–346
Preadmission information form,
    407–408
Problem solving, 205–206, 231–234
Proprioception, defined, 421
  plantar, 421
Props, defined, 421
Psychosocial activities, 259–260
  dementia challenges affecting, 259
  examples of, 259–260
  qualities of, 246–247
Psychosocial factors
  effects on daily life care activities,
    88–89, 108–109
  mobility affected by, 162
  physical restraint use affected by, 173
  terminal care–related, 361–362
Psychosocial needs, interventions for
    and support of, 26–30, 29f
Psychosocial support group, for resi-
    dents with moderate
    impairment
  development of, 35–39
  focus areas of, 36–37
  games in, 45–46
  health care provider issues related
    to, 41
  implementation of, 37–38, 43–44
  member selection criteria for, 36
  objectives of, 35–36
  observations in, 38–39

Psychosocial support group, for residents with moderate impairment—*continued*
  staff issues related to, 41
  theme facilitation plan for, 38, 45–46

Quality of life, enhancement of, community partnership and collaborating forces for, 299–301

Reading, therapeutic benefits of, 309
Recipes, nutrient-dense, 155–157
"Redistribution of stuff"
  as behavioral response, 221
  examples of, 209–211
Refocusing, defined, 421
Rehabilitation programs, for physical wellness, 169–171
Relationships, as focus of psychosocial support group for residents with moderate impairment, 37
Relaxation, therapeutic benefits of, 308
Religion. *See* Spirituality
Religious activity, therapeutic benefits of, 309
Reminiscence, therapeutic benefits of, 309
Reminiscing kits, for activities of daily living, 281–283
Repetitious movements, as behavioral response, 220
Repetitious questioning, as behavioral response, 224–225
Rescue strategy, in daily life care activities, 92
Rescuing, defined, 421
Research opportunities, for family caregivers, 399
Resident case study form, 51–53
Resident security, behaviors and, 206–207, 235–238
Resident volunteer, therapeutic benefits of, 309
Respect
  in communication, 68–69
  staff statement of, 40

Response(s), objectives of
  nonverbal, 67
  verbal, 67
Restraints, physical. *See* Physical restraints
Rhythmic sounds, defined, 421
Rummaging
  as behavioral response, 221
  examples of, 209–211

Sadness
  activities for, 274–275
  overwhelming, 25–26
Safety, in the community, 206–207
Safety issues, behavior-related, 211–216
Screaming, as behavioral response, 224–225
"Searching and discovering," activities for refocusing, 274
Security, of residents, behaviors and, 206–207, 235–238
Self
  acceptance, self-esteem and, 21
  actualization, physical restraint use for, 177, 178–179
  confidence, words affecting, 68
  eating, enabling of, 152
  esteem
    physical restraint use for, 177, 178–179
    self-acceptance and, 21
    validation of, 26
  identification of, facilitation plan for, 43–44
  image
    compromised, 24–25
    integrated, 23
  initiated activity, therapeutic benefits of, 309
Sensitivity, in communication, 71
Sensory bridging, defined, 421
Sensory processing, 89–90, 111–113
Sensory profile, in eating process, 128–129
Sensory stimulation
  for late-stage dementia care, 268–269

therapeutic benefits of, 309
Sequencing, defined, 421
Service
　activities of, pride in, 290–291
　for others' activities, 263–264
Sexual responses, inappropriate, as
　　　behavioral response, 220
Sexuality, overt, 316–320
Shaving, in daily life care activities, 96
Skill(s), sharing of, activities for, pride
　　　in, 289–290
Sleep disturbances, as behavioral
　　　response, 221
Snacks, finger food ideas for, 153–154
Sound(s), rhythmic, defined, 421
Special events, therapeutic benefits
　　　of, 308
Spirituality, 339–354
　clerical support for persons with
　　　dementia and their fami-
　　　lies, 340–341
　confused worshippers and, 340, 343
　congregation's shared communion
　　　of love and support and,
　　　340, 341–342
　creation of praise, thanksgiving, and
　　　worship center, 345–346
　health care provider issues related
　　　to, 350–351
　staff issues related to, 350–351
　terminal care–related, 369
　uniting of Alzheimer's care center and
　　　local congregation, 343–345
Staff
　activities of daily life issues related
　　　to, 25
　activities of daily living in dementia
　　　patients issues related to,
　　　103–104
　behavior issues related to, 225–226
　communication issues related
　　　to, 79
　eating and mealtime issues related
　　　to, 148–149
　family caregivers' issues related
　　　to, 400
　intimacy issues related to, 322–324
　LifeStory Book issues related to, 60–61

physical well-being issues related
　　　to, 179–180
　psychosocial support group issues
　　　related to, 41
　spirituality issues related to, 350–351
　support policy and procedures for
　　　activities of daily living
　　　issues related to, 125–126
　terminal care issues related
　　　to, 371–372
Staff empowerment considerations,
　　　47–48
"Staff Statement of Respect," 40
Storytelling, therapeutic benefits
　　　of, 309
Strengthening, in physical well-being,
　　　183–185
Stripping, as behavioral response, 220
Structured activity, defined, 421
Success, in activities of daily living,
　　　defined, 244
Sundowning, as behavioral response,
　　　218–219
Support, psychosocial aspects of,
　　　19–53. See also Psychosocial
　　　support group
Support group games, 45–46
Support group theme facilitation plan,
　　　example of, 43–44
Swallowing, facilitation with, in eat-
　　　ing process, 130–131
Swingin' singers, therapeutic benefits
　　　of, 309

Table games, therapeutic benefits of, 310
"Talking" touch, 362–363
Task(s)
　breakdown of, effects on daily life
　　　care activities, 91
　simplification, in eating process, 129
　timing, defined, 422
Task or activity
　breakdown, defined, 421
　simplification, defined, 422
Tea and talk, therapeutic benefits of, 310
Terminal care, 355–377
　activities in, simplicity of, 368–369
　activities of daily care in, 363–364

Terminal care—*continued*
autopsy following, 371
behavior in, 367
communication in, 362–363
compassionate connectedness
in, 369
considerations related to, 358–359
and death, 369–370
dignity in, enabling of, 363–364
eating in, 364–365
emotional support in, 361–362
health care provider issues related
to, 371–372
hospice care, 358
medical issues related to, 359–361
mobility in, 365–367
nutrition in, 364–365
nutritional assessment in, 146–148
personhood preservation in,
361–362
psychosocial issues related to,
361–362
spiritual support in, 369
staff issues related to, 371–372
Terminal stage, defined, 355–356
Therapeutic fib, 27–28, 72
in communication, 70
defined, 422
Timing, effects on daily life care activities, 90
Toilet use, in daily life care activities,
100–103
Tone of voice, in communication, 69
Touch
in communication, 69
language of, 78
"talking," 362–363
Touch response, defined, 422

Understanding, communication in,
67–85. *See also* Communication

Verbal communication, 71–76
Verbal responses, objectives of, 67
Verbalization, as basis for communica-
tion, 23

Violence, safety issues related to,
211–216
Voice tone, in communication, 69
Volunteering, by family caregivers,
393–394
Vulnerability, 21

Walking group, outdoor, therapeutic
benefits of, 309
Wander, activities for residents who,
273–274
Wandering
as behavioral response, 220
nocturnal, 221
examples of, 207–209
Wayfinding, defined, 422
Weddings, family, 394–396
Weight, maintenance of, 127
Weight loss, causes of, 127
Well-being
compassionate connectedness and,
339–354
compromised functional, physical
restraints and, 174
indicators of, 19–20
spiritual, appraising of, 339–340
through communication, 71
Wellness, physical. *See* Physical wellness
Wisdom, sharing of, activities for,
pride in, 289–290
Withdrawal, as behavioral response, 225
Word(s)
choice of, 67–68
missing, in communication, 70
Work, life, activities associated with.
See Life work activities
Worship services
activity-focused
examples of, 347–349, 349f
guidelines for, 346–347
of remembrance, 349–350
Worshippers, confused, 340, 343
Writing, therapeutic benefits of, 309

Yelling, as behavioral response,
224–225